The Human Brain and Its Universe, Vol. 1:
The World of Natural Sciences and Its Phenomenology

Hartwig Kuhlenbeck

The Human Brain and Its Universe

Second, revised and enlarged edition of "Brain and Consciousness"

Edited by Joachim Gerlach, Würzburg

S. Karger · Basel · München · Paris · London · New York · Tokyo · Sydney

Vol. 1

The World of Natural Sciences and Its Phenomenology

40 figures comprising 54 illustrations, 1982

S. Karger · Basel · München · Paris · London · New York · Tokyo · Sydney

National Library of Medicine, Cataloging in Publication

Kuhlenbeck, Hartwig, 1897–
    The human brain and its universe / edited by Joachim Gerlach. – Basel; New York: Karger,
    1982   v. 1
    2nd rev. and enl. ed. of: Brain and consciousness.
    ISBN 3-8055-1817-X (v. 1).
    Contents: v. 1. The world of natural sciences and its phenomenology.
    1. Brain   2. Consciousness   3. Psychophysiology   I. Gerlach, Joachim   II. Kuhlenbeck,
    Hartwig, 1897–   Brain and consciousness   III. Title   IV. Title: The world of natural
    sciences and its phenomenology
    WL 102 K95h

© Copyright 1982 by S. Karger AG, P.O. Box, CH-4009 Basel (Switzerland)
Typeset in Hong Kong by Asco Trade Typesetting Limited
Printed in Switzerland
ISBN 3-8055-1817-X

'Πῶς οὖν εἰκὸς βραχὺν οὕτως ὄντα τὸν
ἀνθρώπινον νοῦν μήνιγγι ἢ καρδίᾳ,
βραχέσιν ὄγκοις, ἐγκατειλημένον
μέγεθος οὐρανοῦ καὶ κόσμου χωρῆσαι
τοσοῦτον;'

'How then, is it natural that the mind
of Man, being so small as contained
in such narrow spaces as a brain
or a heart, should have room for
all the vastness of sky and universe?'
(*Philo Judaeus* 208, 90)

'Our entire experienced world of consciousness is, as *Schopenhauer* justly stated, a brain phenomenon, but the brain itself is a brain phenomenon.'
(*H. Kuhlenbeck* in *The Brain Paradox*)

Preface to First Edition (1957)

The relationship of brain and consciousness can be considered from the epistemological as well as from the neurological aspect. In this disquisition, I shall attempt to discuss both points of view, and to integrate these aspects into a unified presentation.

The purely neurologic subject matter constitutes the greater part, approximately two thirds of this presentation, and its validity or purpose retains, for practical intents, an intrinsic independence of any epistemologic interpretation.

Nevertheless, I believe that such an epistemologic interpretation, frequently avoided by the neurologist, is of substantial theoretical importance. Many authors evade the question by slurring over the crux at issue with a few generalities concealing the gist of the problem. However, some writers, conversant with the topic, have clearly recognized the elementary and essential fact that the experienced private perceptual space is not identical with the inferred public physical space. This recognition, of course, should imply the distinction of the two different space-time systems including their dimensions.

It has also been stated – not without justification – that the relation of brain and consciousness is to some extent a semantic problem. In this respect, the inherent deceptiveness of abstractions and of apparent verbal precision must be kept in mind: *fraus latet in generalibus*. While in theoretical systems of logic based upon digital rules, the principle of excluded middle can be considered valid, this principle is certainly not valid in many aspects of applied scientific and practical everyday thinking which operates rather according to analogue rules: Truth value is here not digital or binary, corresponding exclusively to one of the two values zero or one, but encompasses, within these two limiting values, innumerable intermediates between truth, that is significant conformity, and error, fallacy or falsity.

The costs for the publication of this monograph, which follows my *Summary on the Human Diencephalon*, have again been defrayed by the Woman's Medical College of Pennsylvania, this time from a special Psychiatry-Neurology Fund of the College. As before, I wish to express my appreciation to the College and to our Dean, Dr. *Marion Fay*, for the appropriation of this liberal subsidy.

H. K.

Preface to Second Edition

The monographs *Brain and Consciousness; Some Prolegomena to an Approach of the Problem* (1957) and *Mind and Matter; An Appraisal of Their Significance for Neurologic Theory* (1961) were originally conceived as companion volumes providing a philosophical background to the author's planned neurobiological series *The Central Nervous System of Vertebrates* (1967–1978) which was subsequently completed.

In elaborating said philosophical background, the concept of neurological epistemology was introduced, based on *Schopenhauer's* recognition that our world of consciousness represents a brain phenomenon. The empirical substantiated fact that consciousness is a result of brain function involves, however, the brain-paradox, which, in turn, provides the proof that the problem of brain-consciousness relationship is intrinsically insolvable. As regards consciousness, a valid descriptive definition could be formulated, stating that consciousness is a private perceptual space-time manifold or system, represented by its contents, which are sensory and extrasensory percepts. Upon this basis a 'mental geography' in *Hume's* sense could be given, that is to say, a 'delineation of the distinct powers of the mind'. These 'powers' have very definite limitations, but one can agree with *Hume's* opinion that 'it is at least a satisfaction to go so far; and the more obvious this science may appear (and it is by no means obvious) the more contemptible still must the ignorance of it be esteemed, in all pretenders to learning and philosophy' (*Enquiry Concerning Human Understanding*; 1750).

While, in accordance with *Berkeley's* 'esse est percipi' and *Hume's* additional elaborations, both perceptual matter and the extrasensory percepts of thought (reason) and emotion (affectivity) are 'mental', there obtains a self-evident 'dualism' between the domain of consciousness and the domain of unconscious 'existence', which remains incomprehensible, since devoid of space-time relationships, these latter being restricted to consciousness. This unavoidable 'dualism' was expressed by the author in terms of a transcendental neutralism implying an 'orderliness x' corresponding to the valid aspects of *Kant's* 'Ding an sich'.

Since, however, the natural sciences must, for practical purposes, discount non-observable other consciousness and consider the world as if existing in a public space-time independent of consciousness, a justifiable pragmatic fictionalism in *Vaihinger's* sense was adopted. Other relevant results included the anâtman (or non-self) concept introduced by Buddhism, rediscovered by *Hume*, and justly upheld by *Mach*, moreover the recognition that logical thought processes (reason) are based on the mechanics of 'material' circuit events involving 'switches', in accordance with *Boolean algebra*, as elaborated by *Shannon* and applied to the nervous system by *McCulloch* and *Pitts*. Finally, in accordance with *Hume*, the considerable difference between reason (logic) and affectivity (emotions) was emphasized. The former involves truth or falsity, respectively provability. Affectivity, although likewise based on neural circuit processes, involves axiologic evaluations, for which the laws of logic with respect to truth or falsehood do not hold.

In preparing a second edition of *Brain and Consciousness*, which has been out of print for several years, the attempt has been made, on the basis of the diverse above-mentioned results, to enlarge that treatise into an outline of philosophy in terms of natural sciences, neurological epistemology, brain mechanisms, and transcendental neutralism. This, besides necessitating numerous additions, such e.g. as a further elaboration of the principle of sufficient reason, also required a change of title, and a subdivision into three separate volumes. The two first ones follow the arrangement of the original edition. The third volume, entirely new, deals with the world of philosophy. It emphasizes an historical approach, stressing what could be called the evolutionary aspect of Human thought and this latter's intrinsic limitations, resulting in a 'scientific humanism' strongly influenced by the incomparable *David Hume*.

My esteemed old friend, colleague and former student Professor *J. Gerlach* who, in 1973, had already provided a German translation of the original edition, again has taken the trouble to help me by editing and proofreading the present work. In addition to many helpful discussions concerning the topics under consideration, he and Mrs. *Gerlach* have transcribed my longhand manuscript into the final form. It is a pleasure to express my thanks for their help. I am also obliged to my former secretary, Mrs. *Brennan*, who, after more than 20 years of efficient service, had to retire from her work, for still typing a substantial part of the manuscript of volume 1.

H. K.

Editor's Preface

By gladly undertaking the edition of the present volumes I am not only thanking my teacher in neurobiology and scientific method, under whose sponsorship I obtained my doctorate about 50 years ago, but also appreciate the opportunity to assist in the publication of his important work. On a neurobiological basis, he rigorously clarified the possibilities and limits of human scientific, philosophical and cultural activities, all of which are aspects of brain function. In particular, he thoroughly examined and supplemented the classical philosophical systems of *Locke, Berkeley, Hume, Kant, Schopenhauer,* and *Vaihinger.* Being their equal, he critically linked the valid aspects of their doctrines to modern science. This second, more comprehensive edition of *Brain and Consciousness* should contribute to the further understanding of the difficult and complex problems at issue, and the realization of the present work's high rank.

Joachim Gerlach

Table of Contents of the Present Volume

Volume 1: The World of Natural Sciences and Its Phenomenology

Table of Contents of the Complete Work

Volume 3: The World of Philosophy

I. Introductory Remarks

One of the most ancient references to the problem of the relationship between brain and consciousness is found in the *Hippocratic* writings. In the remarkable treatise Περὶ ἱερῆς νούσου (*On the Sacred Disease*) we read in section XX: 'Διό φημι τὸν ἐγκέφαλον εἶναι τὸν ἑρμηνεύοντα τὴν σύνεσιν' etc. – 'Therefore I assert that the brain is the herald of consciousness. The diaphragm ('αἱ δὲ φρένες') has a name due merely to custom, not to reality and nature, and I do not know what power the diaphragm has for thought and intelligence.' Additional significant statements are: 'Men ought to know that from the brain, and from the brain alone, arise our pleasures, joys, laughter and jests, as well as our sorrows, pains, griefs, and tears. Through it, in particular, we think, see, hear, and distinguish the ugly from the beautiful, the bad from the good, the pleasant from the unpleasant ...' (section XVII); 'In these ways I hold that the brain is the most powerful organ of the human body ...' (section XIX).

Historians of medicine assume that the views regarding the brain as the organ of consciousness can be traced back about 100 years earlier, namely to the physician *Alcmaeon of Croton* (ca. 500 BC) who associated with the *Pythagoreans*. He is reported to have stated: 'ἐν τῷ ἐγκεφάλῳ ἐστιν τὸ ἡγεμονικόν.' Although these views were rejected by the philosopher *Aristotle*, the early Greek physicians had thus already clearly recognized the relationship of brain and mind.

In the course of the centuries and especially within the last 100 years, a voluminous literature has arisen on this subject, since the questions involved are of particular import for three different groups of scientists: for the philosopher as a problem of epistemology, for the physicist and mathematician as a problem of concerning the relation of physics to perception, or the 'interpretation of physics in terms of what exists' [*Russell*, 1972],[1] and for the neurologist studying the organ of consciousness. Many treatises and papers have been published on 'Brain and Soul', 'Brain and Mind', and allied subjects [*Flechsig*, 1896; *Haeckel*, 1903; *Verworn*, 1919; *Mach*, 1922; *Lashley*, 1923; *Ziehen*, 1924; *Boring*, 1933; *Buscaino*, 1951; *Ebbecke*, 1959; *Ey*, 1963, 1968;

---

[1] He should, however, have added: 'of what exists independently of consciousness' or still better: 'what exists when there is no consciousness'.

Eccles, 1970; *Ornstein*, 1972; *Penfield*, 1975; *Popper and Eccles*, 1977; the diverse conferences and symposia with many participants: *Laslett*, 1950; *Abramson*, 1951, 1952, 1953, 1954, 1955; *Delafresnaye*, 1954; *Smythies*, 1965; *Karczmar and Eccles*, 1969; *Kenny* et al., 1972; and various others].

The problem, which for the present purpose I prefer to designate as that of the relationship between brain and consciousness, leads to many pitfalls resulting in considerable disagreement and confusion. Some of this confusion can be attributed to the ambiguous use of words with different connotations or even denotations, as well as to excessive and thereby confusing sophistication, which may be combined with marked deficiency *in secunda Petri*.[2] Despite its complexity, I believe that the gist of the problem can be formulated in fairly simple terms. In my old lectures on the central nervous system of vertebrates [*K.*, 1927] I have very briefly referred to the relation of consciousness to brain, merely indicating my fundamental viewpoint. Much later, in my summary on the human diencephalon [*K.*, 1954a], I have added some short comments. Regarding these latter remarks, a reviewer has stated that my discussion concerning cybernetics and consciousness 'suffers from the lack of sophistication in behavioral science which marks so much of the neurological literature of the past 50 years'. This was obviously meant as a criticism but I take it as a compliment, since it expresses exactly what I had intended, because behavioral science, as *Watson* [1925, 1929] justly stressed, must exclude or at least completely ignore the occurrence of consciousness. I shall also try to abstain from any unnecessary details of the alluded sophistication or rather sophistry entirely irrelevant to the topic here under consideration.

Consciousness is said to be undefinable insofar as it cannot be defined in terms referring to anything else than conscious experience or awareness: it stands for the sum total of all such experiences connected into an ordered manifold, which is the world system of a sentient being. In this respect, it constitutes the foundation of all definitions. Consciousness, although essentially undefinable, may be considered as synonymous with the terms 'soul' ('psyche') as well as 'mind' in the widest sense, but in view of its narrower connotations this latter term shall be avoided for the present. Consciousness must thus be regarded as the irreducible fundamental phenomenon, as 'Urphänomen' in the terminology of *Goethe* (1808) and *Schopenhauer* (1844).

Although a 'denotational definition' of consciousness, referring to one or more known other 'entities', thus becomes logically impossible, a structural or descriptive definition easily can be given: *consciousness is any private space-time manifold or system characterized by its contents, which are called 'percepts', 'perceptions', or 'sensations'*. Further details concerning these con-

---

[2] *Dialectica Petri Rami, pars secunda, quae est de 'judicio'.*

tents will be given further below, following the discussion of a variety of relevant data. Said definition of consciousness goes back to the author's old 'Vorlesungen' [*K.*, 1927] and was further expanded in the monograph *Mind and Matter* [*K.*, 1961] as well as in the first edition [*K.*, 1957] of the present treatise. Although not specifically elaborated in their writings, this concept of consciousness is, however, implied in the views of *George Berkeley, David Hume, Kant*, and *Schopenhauer*.

It should also be added that, with regard to the definition of consciousness, the problem concerning the definition of definition becomes relevant. Among the various authors who have discussed that topic, the following may here be mentioned: *Kant*, in his lectures on logic, *Schopenhauer*, in his comments to these lectures [*Schopenhauer*, Nachlass, vol. III, p. 34], *Poincaré* [1913a], *Tarski* [1946], *Ogden and Richards* [1946], *Russell* [1948], and myself (*K.*, 1961, 1968). It is evident that my definition of consciousness is a structural respectively descriptive definition, that is to say a proposition (*Urteil*) enumerating the significant known (i.e. 'experienced') components and relationships pertaining to consciousness. This definition presupposes the understanding of language and the occurrence of identical (i.e. 'common') experiences (contents) in an undefined number of separate (i.e. 'other') different Human consciousness-manifolds. *Mutatis mutandis* it can be extended to other sentient beings such as animals, possessors of a central nervous system (brain). Such extrapolation, however, based on inferences from observable behavior, becomes progressively more uncertain as the required degree of central nervous system differentiation decreases in the taxonomic or phylogenetic animal series.

II. The Materialistic Approach

1. The Physical World

Consciousness occurs in discontinuous periods. It seems to arise from nothingness and again to fade into nothingness. Yet, despite its discontinuity, continuous orderliness prevails. This orderliness is most conspicuous in the relationships of sensory spatial and temporal experiences referred to as material and leading to the concept of matter. Furthermore, consciousness is found to depend on, or to be the function of, a material complex, the brain.

It appears therefore possible to postulate the existence of a four-dimensional (space-time) material or physical world independent of consciousness; the assumption of such a world, also referred to as 'external world' independent of a perceiving conscious being, is indeed the basis of all natural science. 'Since, however, sense perception only gives information of this external world or of "physical reality" indirectly, we can only grasp the latter by speculative means. It follows from this fact that our notions of physical reality can never be final' [*Einstein*, 1934]. It should here be understood that 'perception' as well as 'sensation' (in connection with 'sense perception') imply consciousness, in contradistinction to mere 'sensory registration' which, although resulting in central nervous activities (e.g. reflexes), may remain entirely unconscious.

With respect to the so-called 'external world', *Planck* [1931] formulated two *'fundamental canons of natural philosophy'* as follows:

(1). There is a real outer world which exists independently of our act of knowing.

(2). The real outer world is not directly knowable.

Assuming, however, that this so-called 'outer world' or 'physical world' is indirectly knowable by inferences, the following argumentation and tentative description seems, *prima facie*, permissible.

In order to define the attributes of a physical world it would seem necessary to abstract all those qualities obviously inherent to consciousness and perception, that is all those related not only to brain activity but to the entire nervous system including the sense organs. The distinction between said qualities, known as secondary qualities, and the assumed inherent attributes of matter designated as primary qualities, has a long history. It goes back in principle to *Democritus* (ca. 400 BC) and was further elaborated by *Sextus*

Empiricus (ca. 200 AD) in his Outlines Pyrrhonism (II, 7 §70–75). Among the Scholastics, *Albertus Magnus* (*Albert von Bollstädt*, canonized as St. Albert), Bishop of Regensburg 1260–1262, famed as Doctor Universalis and teacher of *St. Thomas Aquinas*, was somewhat acquainted with this distinction, which was also used by *Galileo, Descartes*, and *Spinoza*. The best known definitions of primary and secondary qualities were given by *Robert Boyle*, and by *John Locke* (1689). This latter author stated that the secondary qualities are 'nothing in the objects themselves, but powers to produce various sensations in us by their primary qualities'. Secondary qualities appear in human consciousness in various forms, such as colors, sounds, tastes, smells, and are highly variable and inconstant. Primary qualities are constant, being inseparable from objects, and comprise solidity, extension, figure, motion, rest, number. It is evident that these so-called primary qualities represent (1) mass or inertia ('solidity'), (2) space ('figure', 'extension', 'rest'), and (3) time ('motion', 'number', i.e. succession), namely that, what in classical physics refers to the notation m, s, t (or m, l, t).

In *Newton's* view, the concept of mobile bodies is further stripped of the characteristics of extension, form, and orientation in space, leaving only the material point. According to *Newton's* system, as concisely summarized by *Einstein* [1934], physical reality is characterized by the concepts of absolute time (t, sec), absolute space (s, cm), material point, endowed with inertia (mass: m, g), and force (reciprocal action of material points; $m \cdot s \cdot t^{-2}$; $g \cdot cm \cdot sec^{-2}$; dyn). 'Force' thus refers to a change, namely acceleration, deceleration or pressure (resistance) in the motion or state of mass. It is a vectorial magnitude, which becomes closely related to 'energy' measurable by the magnitude of 'work' ($m \cdot s^2 \cdot t^{-2}$; $g \cdot cm^2 \cdot sec^{-2}$; erg) or of mass in the dimension of acceleration ($1/2\ mv^2$). Since the result of performed work depends on distance moved in relation to magnitude of force, that is, distance with respect to the direction of force (interaction), but irrespective of the path by which the distance has been traversed, work is expressible in terms of scalar magnitudes.[1]

Physical events are to be regarded as the motions, governed by fixed laws, of material points in space. The material point is our only mode of representing reality when dealing with changes taking place in it. This atomistic and mechanistic theoretical scheme postulates the material point as the solitary representative of the real, insofar as the real is capable of change. All happen-

---

[1] Some confusion in the formulations can result from the fact that the notation s is sometimes used for speed, as e.g. in the expression $1/2\ ms^2$ which is commonly given as $1/2\ mv^2$, where v stands for velocity. Instead of s for space, l (length, cm) is also used. As regards speed (s) versus velocity (v), cf. further below footnote 3.

ings are interpreted purely mechanistically as motions of material points according to *Newton's* laws of motion.[2]

The attempts to base all physics upon this scheme of classical mechanics subsequently failed, particularly under the impact of *Faraday's* and *Maxwell's* field theory which, in turn, led to an attempt to develop physics entirely upon the concept of fields, that is spatial states. In this connection, *Einstein*, by eliminating the concepts of absolute space, absolute time, and luminiferous ether, formulated the theory of relativity [1905], based on the speed[3] of light in vacuo as the fundamental constant c.

The special theory of relativity implies the four-dimensional space-time concept subsequently developed by *Minkowski* [1908] and states that the laws of nature are invariant with respect to *Lorentz* transformations or in other words that a law of nature does not change its form if one introduces into it a new inertial system with the help of a *Lorentz* transformation on s, y, z, t. It has shown the role which the universal constant c plays in the laws of nature and has demonstrated that there exists a close connection between the form in which time on the one hand and the spatial coordinates on the other hand enter into those laws. A further consequence of the special theory of relativity is the connection between mass and energy in the formula $E = Mc^2$. Mass is convertible into energy and energy is convertible into mass. The two conservation laws of mass and energy are thus combined into one, the conservation law of mass-energy. The general theory of relativity provides a further analysis of the four-dimensional space-time continuum. It extends the validity of the theory from inertial coordinate systems to gravitational fields and regards the equivalence of gravitational mass and inertial mass as an essential feature, introducing concepts of *non-Euclidean* geometry into the description of the physical world.

In other words, and roughly speaking, *Einstein* elaborated a geometrical construction of space, time, and mass relationships based on the assumption of c as an invariant. A different interpretation of the *Fitzgerald-Lorentz contraction* and of the *Lorentz transformation* is given, such that space, time, and mass become thereby variables. In the special theory, acceleration

---

[2] The three laws of motion are commonly expressed as follows. (1) Any body remains in its state of rest or of uniform motion in a straight line with constant speed unless acted upon by a force. (2) The change in motion is proportional to the acting force and takes place in the straight line which is the direction of the force. (3) Action and reaction are equal and opposite (German: *Prinzip der Wechselwirkung*).

[3] This speed equals roughly 300,000 km/sec. It should be added that physicists now generally use speed as a scalar, and velocity as a vectorial magnitude. In the present elementary discussion, this distinction does not become relevant. Speed and velocity are here less rigorously taken as synonyms.

is not included, and the space remains *Euclidean* (parabolic). The general theory includes acceleration, and the space becomes non-Euclidean (elliptic, *Riemannian*).

With regard to the special theory of relativity, *Einstein's* first derivation of the mass-energy relationship contained a serious mathematical error, which was not noticed until many years later [cf. *Brancazio*, 1975]. Nevertheless, *Einstein's* conclusion was still correct and became properly supported by his subsequent elaborations.

It was shown that, if the *Newtonian* definition of linear momentum (p) as product of mass (m) and velocity (v) is used ($p = mv$), this momentum is not conserved in all inertial reference frames and would have to be redefined in accordance with special relativity as

$$p = \frac{m_0 \cdot v}{\sqrt{1 - v^2/c^2}}$$

where m_0 represents the rest mass. From this equation of relativistic linear momentum the relativistic mass, varying with the body's speed, becomes

$$m = \frac{m_0}{\sqrt{1 - v^2/c^2}}$$

Newton's equation $F = ma$ (Force = mass × acceleration) can also be expressed

$$F = \frac{\Delta p}{\Delta t} = \frac{\Delta(mv)}{\Delta t}$$

In relativistic mechanics this equation becomes

$$F = \frac{\Delta p}{\Delta t} = \frac{\Delta(m_0 v/\sqrt{1 - v^2/c^2})}{\Delta t}$$

and $F = ma$ appears only as a low-velocity approximation.

Newtonian kinetic energy (KE), is defined by equation $KE = 1/2\, mv^2$. On the basis of the relativistic force equation, relativistic kinetic energy becomes then

$$KE(rel): 1/2\, m_0 c^2 \left(\frac{1}{\sqrt{1 - v^2/c^2}} - 1 \right)$$

which reduces to $KE = 1/2\, mv^2$ as a low velocity approximation [cf. *Brancazio*, 1975, for a detailed but elementary mathematical proof].

The relativistic mass can also be expressed as

$$KE(rel) = \frac{m_0 c^2}{\sqrt{1 - v^2/c^2}} - m_0 = mc^2 - m_0 c^2$$

which can be rearranged as

$$mc^2 = m_0 c^2 + KE$$

Since *Einstein* had shown that the mass of a body changes when electro-magnetic energy is emitted or absorbed in accordance with the equation

$$\Delta E = c^2 \Delta m$$

he concluded that mass is a form of energy. He then defined the rest energy E_0 of a stationary body by the now famous equation

$$E = m_0 c^2.$$

The total energy E is then

$$E = mc^2 = \frac{E_0}{\sqrt{1 - v^2/c^2}}$$

Energy and momentum can be related by the expression

$$E^2 = m_0{}^2 c^4 + p^2 c^2 = (m_0 c^2)^2 + (pc)^2$$

For a body at rest (p = O) this becomes again reduced to $E = mc^2$.

As regards general relativity, *Einstein's* field equation, pertaining to a family of ten equations, relates the distribution of matter in a region of space to the curvature of the four-dimensional geometry of the region. It includes (1) the tensors $R_{\mu\nu}$ (*Ricci curvature tensor*), $g_{\mu\nu}$ (metric tensor), and $T_{\mu\nu}$ (stress-energy tensor), each representing an array of ten independent quantities, moreover (2) the universal constant of gravitation G. The mathematical complexities are here extreme and even caused considerable difficulties for *Einstein*, who required coaching and help from a specialized mathematician. Further comments on tensors and their significance for biology are given on pages 36–37, volume 3/II of the present author's *Central Nervous System of Vertebrates*. A concise and useful elementary introduction to the relativity theories is included in *Brancazio's* text on the *Nature of Physics* [1975].

Einstein's field equation

$$R_{\mu\nu} - 1/2\, g_{\mu\nu}R = -\frac{8\pi G}{c^4} T_{\mu\nu}$$

represents the keystone of general relativity, in accordance with which matter determines the properties of space. The natural motion of a freely moving body is here along a geodesic in *Riemannian space-time*. In other words, space, depending on matter (i.e. mass and energy) must be considered a plenum, and space without matter, i.e. empty space, has no logical existence in this model. Thus, the paradox of a 'curved empty space' vanishes, quite apart from the inevitable postulate that space does not exist apart from time, and vice versa.

It should also be emphasized that *Einstein's* theories of relativity concern physical ('objective') events, in principle detectable by instruments, and thus measurable. In other words, the theories concern the behavior of 'physical clocks' and 'measuring rods'. *Russell* [1962] therefore justly remarked that the 'philosophical' consequences of relativity are neither so great nor so startling as is sometimes thought. The theories throw very little, in fact no light whatsoever on the time-honored controversies such as those between 'realism' (materialism) and idealism.

With regard to the constant c it also should be added that, in accordance with the elaborations by *De Broglie* and others on wave theory, phase velocity and group velocity must be distinguished. Phase velocity may far exceed c. However, no energy and no message (including that in the mass of material bodies) can travel faster than c. In other words, it is impossible to send a change faster than c [cf. e.g. *Rothman*, 1960].

The general theory of relativity, deduced from assumed basic principles, became supported by various subsequent actual observations confirming the theoretical predictions, but still remains open to some criticisms [cf. e.g. *Brancazio*, 1975].

Einstein proposed that gravitation is not a 'force' but a consequence of the *Non-Euclidean* geometry of space-time created by the presence of 'matter'. The curved paths of bodies respectively of energy quanta moving through gravitational fields represent the natural motions of these bodies along a geodesic which is not located in three-dimensional space but rather in four-dimensional space-time. It has been pointed out that by his geometrization *Einstein* did not 'explain' gravitation any more than *Newton* did, but merely re-interpreted it in terms of different unexplained concepts, that is to say by explaining *ignotum per ignotius*.

Another criticism is directed at *Einstein's* failure to 'explain' the concept of inertia. This latter was interpreted by *Mach* as a result of interaction between 'bodies' (*Mach's principle*). The inertia of a 'mass' is thereby due to the presence of other 'masses' in a system such as the universe. An attempt has been made to modify general relativity by incorporating in it additional terms accounting for *Mach's principle*.

Be that as it may, the fundamental concepts and the basic framework of general relativity seem nevertheless firmly established. *Einstein's* relativity has thus, at an advanced level, replaced the *Newtonian* concepts of classical physics. These latter, however, remain a convenient and sufficiently accurate operationally valid first approximation in dealing with many aspects of physical phenomena. At the ordinary macroscopic level, classical physics has not been 'falsified' nor replaced by relativistic physics.

While one of the failures of classical mechanics was connected with the finite speed of light, that is its avoidance of being ∞, other inconsistencies between deductions from mechanics and experimental facts were related to the finite magnitude, that is the avoidance of being zero, of *Planck's* constant h. For a theoretical explanation of this behavior it was necessary to postulate that the energy of a mechanical system can only assume certain discrete values whose mathematical expressions were always dependent upon *Planck's* constant h. This conception proved to be essential for *Bohr's* modification of *Rutherford's* model of the atom. Not only matter (mass) but also energy was assumed to have a granular structure. There are thus elementary quanta of mass as well as of energy. New difficulties arose in the interpretation of radiation. Certain phenomena are better explained by the wave concept and others by the particle concept. Physicists have undertaken to find mathematical formulations for suitable interpretations of the quantum character of systems and phenomena, resulting in the attempts of *de Broglie and Schrödinger, Heisenberg, Born,* and *Dirac.* Quantum physics establishes statistical laws applying to large numbers of events; probability distributions are given.

Heisenberg's uncertainty principle states that, as regards particles, simultaneous measurement of their position and momentum, respectively of the thereto relevant functions (called complementary variables) is subject to an inherent limitation related to the finite value of *Planck's constant h.* In simplified form, this can be expressed by the equation

$$\Delta x \cdot \Delta p \geqq h; \text{ more exactly: } \Delta x \cdot \Delta p \geqq \frac{h}{4\pi}$$

where x is the uncertainty in the position of a particle, and p the uncertainty in its momentum. It does not restrict the exactness of a position measurement alone or of a momentum measurement alone. However, if x could be made exact, p would become entirely uncertain and vice versa. Again, if the expression mv_x for momentum is adopted, then we have

$$\Delta x \cdot \Delta m v_x \geqq h \quad \text{or} \quad \Delta x \cdot \Delta v_x \geqq \frac{h}{m}.$$

This, of course, means that the smaller the mass m of the particle, the more significant becomes the uncertainty relation between position and momentum. It will obviously be very important for electrons and photons, but utterly negligible in the case of a thrown brick.

Said theoretical formulation requires, within the domain of its validity, the renunciation of the complete 'determinability'[4] of position and time for a

---

[4] 'Determinability' evidently means here ascertainability, indicability, measurability or predictability. The ambiguity of the word 'determine' should be stressed. It may, on one hand, mean (a) to ascertain, to indicate, or to predict, etc., but (b) on the other hand may mean to cause, to originate, to conduce, to decide, to conclude. If, according to this second sort of denotation, determinism subsumes causality, then it is evidently unjustified to equate uncertainty or unpredictability [(related to a) with indeterminism (related to b)]. Quantum physicists claiming that the uncertainty principle eliminates determinism (b) qua causality base their belief upon this faulty reasoning which is both a semantic and logical error related to a confusion of statistical events with ascertainable dynamic individual events.

particle whose momentum and energy are known, and the renunciation of the complete prediction of (small-scale) future events.

In *Schrödinger's* quantum mechanics which expand *De Broglie's* wave concept, the product

Extension in space of wave × Range of wave numbers

is approximately 1, or, in other words these two magnitudes are the reciprocals of each other. Thus, if the range of wave number is small, the extension in space is great. This can also be expressed as

$$\Delta x \cdot \Delta \frac{1}{\lambda} \geqq 1.$$

From this, by *De Broglie's* formula

$$\Delta \left(\frac{1}{\lambda} \right) = \frac{\Delta p}{h}$$

the expression

$$\Delta x \cdot \Delta p \geqq h$$

may be obtained, which is again *Heisenberg's* uncertainty relation. It can also be said that a particle whose momentum and energy are accurately determined by measurement and observation becomes diffused through an extended region of space, whereby the corpuscular aspect is entirely lost.[5] On the other hand, if the position of the particle is accurately determined at a given instant, the corpuscular aspect of the particle manifests itself, and the particle's momentum and energy cannot be stated. Similarly, an uncertainty relation obtains between the energy of a physical system and the time interval during which the system is known to possess approximately a given energy. This relation can be expressed by the formulation

$$\Delta t \cdot \Delta E \geqq h.$$

---

[5] In other words, we have here an event which, *in Whitehead's* words, 'is nothing at any instant. It requires its whole period in which to manifest itself.' *De Broglie* [1955] refers to *Zeno's* flying arrow, which would be at rest, if it occupied, at any instant of its flight, an exactly determined position. *De Broglie* remarks: 'That which is in a point cannot be in motion or evolve; what moves and evolves cannot be in any point.' More crudely speaking, it would be impossible to answer the question 'at what instant was the note of frequency sounded', since frequency already implies a series of repetitive events over a time interval. Quite evidently, a vibratory process of a certain frequency must, in order to manifest that frequency, occur during a period of time with magnitude > 0, that is, of greater magnitude than an instant, corresponding, in the dimension of time, to a mathematical point.

In communication and information theory, the physical limitations of a channel become of significance. If a channel with bandwidth Δv is used, then the shortest signals that can be transmitted have a duration

$$\Delta t \cdot \Delta v \cong 1.$$

We have here, as it were, an analogy with the uncertainty relation of quantum mechanics, that is to say, a pair of complementary respectively conjugate variables. A basic signal, of finite time and frequency bandwidth, is regarded as a unit of information, and designated as logon [*Gabor*, 1946]. It represents, for a given channel, the unit out of which any message, which the cannel is capable of transmitting, may be considered to be construed [*Cherry*, 1952].

Reverting to *Heisenberg's* uncertainty relation, some authors, including *Heisenberg* himself, have confused said mathematical and logical principle, which is purely theoretical, with an impossibility of the rigorous determination of small-scale events, because of the atomistic structure of any experimental apparatus. Thus, *Heisenberg* claims that, in order to measure the position of a particle with high velocity, it must be 'illuminated' by radiation of very short wavelength, but such high energy radiation would thereby change the velocity of the particle by a correspondingly large amount. Hence, its velocity cannot be measured accurately at the same time as its position. If the velocity is measured by 'illumination' of low energy, the position is relatively uncertain.

Quite evidently, such account is highly fanciful, since there is no practically possible experimental apparatus whose operation could be described as the 'illumination' of a particle (e.g. electron or photon) so that its position could be 'seen' and so measured. It is, moreover, not clear why the disturbance of the observed particle by the procedure of observation could not be allowed for and properly calculated. Again, the position of an electron in any except isolated points of its course can be determined only by inference from observed macroscopic events implying causality.[6]

While modern atomic theories, based on the concepts of positive and negative charge, mass, and energy, have tried to draw a picture of the material world in terms of as few elementary constituents as possible, the number of postulated negative, positive or neutral elementary particles has constantly increased. It appears likely that most of these particles are not elementary but compound systems. Yet, the present state of these theories remains in many respects unsatisfactory. Attempts at a unified theory of elementary particles

---

[6] The faulty reasoning by confusion of theoretical mathematically respectively logically resulting uncertainty with an uncertainty derived from fictitious experimental arrangements and considerations was clearly recognized by *Hesse* [1962] who discussed the relevant points at issue.

have been considered; it is also possible that the concept of 'particles' may have to be abandoned altogether and replaced by the abstract concept of 'events'.

Since, as *Einstein* emphasized, our notions of physical reality can never be final, new theories or logical systems, supplementing or replacing some of the present ideas of relativity and quantum mechanics, might perhaps be worked out.

It can thus be seen that the concept of the physical world as assumed by modern physics is far removed from the physical world of *Newton's* system; however, physicists are compelled to admit that there is no general theoretical basis for physics which can be regarded as its logical foundation [*Einstein*, 1950; *Dirac*, 1963]. The field theory has failed in certain spheres, and the translation of the field theory into the scheme of quantum statistics has not yet been accomplished in an altogether satisfactory manner. Up to his death, *Einstein* has continued in his attempts to formulate a unified field theory. *Heisenberg* likewise made inconclusive attempts at the elaboration of a mathematical so-called *World Formula*. Previously, and in accordance with the so-called minimal principles formulated by *Fermat* (1601–1665), *Maupertuis* (1698–1759), *Lagrange* (1736–1813), *Hamilton* (1805–1865) and others, a mathematical quasi-unification of physics including general relativity was attempted by *Hilbert* (1862–1943) who elaborated a mathematical expression which he called the *'World Function'*. All physical happenings are presumed to be predictable from the knowledge of that function whose integral, taken over space-time, becomes a minimum. The share contributed by gravitation to the world function is the curvature of space-time. Gravitation, as it were, represents a continual tendency of the universe to 'straighten itself out'. This, according to *Whittaker* [1948] is the gist of General Relativity in a single sentence. 'Forces' or 'interactions' become thereby eliminated from the mathematical model. As to the principle of least action, further comments can be found on pages 377–378 in volume 3/I of the present author's treatise on the *Central Nervous System of Vertebrates*.

Still more recently, an inconclusive and still unconvincing attempt has been made to obtain a unification of the laws of physics by introducing a so-called 'supergravity theory' [cf. *Freedman and Nieuwenhuizen*, 1978]. In this theory, of which several versions have been elaborated, the gravitational force arises from a symmetry of particles with vastly different properties whereby, as the ultimate result, and in the opinion of proponents of this approach, a unified theory of all four basic 'forces' in nature could perhaps be worked out. As is well known, these four 'forces' are gravity, quantum electrodynamics, weak force, and strong force (cf. further below p. 14). Recently, attempts were made to combine the weak force with electromagnetism. The strong force is described by a quantum field theory, while 'supergravity' is also described in terms of a quantum field theory which is presumed ultimately to unify all forces in nature.

Various, still not altogether convincing but seemingly promising unified field theories have been elaborated, which are meant to include electromagnetic, strong nuclear and weak forces. The status of such attempts at a single quantum field theory was briefly discussed in a comment by *Robinson* [1979].

As regards contemporary views concerning structure, configuration and events obtaining in the postulated physical world, all 'forces', that is to say interactions ('Naturkräfte'), are now generally subdivided into four kinds, namely (1) gravitational interaction, (2) electromagnetic interaction, (3) strong interaction between nuclear atomic particles such as for instance protons and neutrons (also called nucleons), and (4) weak interaction between certain other atomic particles.

(1) Gravitational interaction, of fundamental importance at the large-scale level, is far too weak for relevance at the small-scale, atomic level. It may be mediated by energy quanta called gravitons.

Because gravitational radiation is exceedingly weak if compared with other interactions, the detection of 'gravitational waves' by instruments poses substantial difficulties and has not been accomplished beyond doubt at the time of this writing, although some progress in methods for detection has been made. A recent paper by *Boughn* [1980] discusses the hitherto obtained results and the design of suitable instruments for recording of 'gravitational waves'.

(2) Electromagnetic interaction, mediated by energy quanta called photons, is a 'force' of significance both at the large-scale and small-scale level. It affects the motion of atoms and of 'matter' outside the atomic nucleus. It involves thus all ordinary physical phenomena except gravitation. Electromagnetic interactions are, moreover, found between all particles carrying electric charges or magnetic moment, but at the short distances at which strong interaction operates, they only amount to a few percent of the pertinent magnitudes.

(3) Strong interaction operates between protons, neutrons, and other particles, all of which can be subsumed under a set of particles called hadrons.

(4) Weak interaction essentially operates in the decay of unstable particles in which nuclei emit electrons and 'particles' called neutrinos. It thereby involves diverse sorts of particles.

At the time of this writing there is, moreover, the questionable possibility that still another, very poorly understood type of nuclear interaction might obtain.

The relative strength of the four fundamental forces is estimated as follows:

Gravitational	1		10^{-38}
Weak (certain decay interactions)	10^{25}	or	10^{-25}
Electromagnetic	10^{36}		10^{-36}
Strong (nuclear)	10^{38}		1

It should, however, be kept in mind that gravitation, despite its weakness, is an additive force, considerably increasing with mass. Thus, as far as large cosmic masses are concerned, and even on the much smaller scale of our solar system, gravitation far outweighs electromagnetism in strength.

It is, moreover, evident that the 'mechanics' of classical physics based on the Newtonian concepts of material points, endowed with inertia, and of force (cf. above p. 5), are complex multifactorial manifestations of matter and energy involving the four interactions of present-day physics. *Newtonian* 'mechanics', which still remain operational valid as sufficiently accurate first approximations, particularly but not exclusively at the macroscopic level, include dynamics and statics as well as acoustics and mechanical thermodynamics. The causal explanations of these 'mechanics' in the narrower sense, in addition to gravitational and inertial mass are based on 'collision', 'pressure' and 'pull' (German: *Stoss, Gegenstoss, Druck, Zug*). Yet, even in present-day atomic physics, the interpretation of cloud chamber respectively bubble chamber phenomena is, to a large extent purely 'mechanistic' in the old 'classical' sense (collision: '*Stoss*' and '*Gegenstoss*').

The concept of atoms, propounded more than 2000 years ago by *Leucippus* (about 440 BC) and *Democritus* (about 400 BC), although greatly modified and expanded, became firmly established by the 19th and 20th century developments of physics. It is, in fact, now possible to visualize (in the sense of making visible) atoms by at least two procedures, namely by means of *Bragg's* method using composite X-ray diffraction photographs, and by means of *E. W. Müller's* field ion microscope.

Atoms are indeed 'indivisible' insofar as a particular atom cannot be further divided without losing the chemical and physical characteristics of the element. This means that the atom cannot be divided, like a piece of homogeneous material, into two or more 'identical' parts. Atoms, however, consist of smaller constituents and differ in quantitative aspects, which, in turn, involves differences in behavior. Some atoms are stable, while others disintegrate or decay, emitting radiation. The radiation emitted by decaying elements such as radium was shown to consist of positively charged helium nuclei (α-rays), negative charged units (β-rays) consisting of electrons, and high-energy photons (γ-rays, representing high-frequency X-rays). The probability of disintegrating within a given time, that is to say the rate of disintegration, can be statistically ascertained and is constant for any particular radioactive atomic species. The term 'half-life' indicates the time required for half a population of radioactive nuclei or particles to disintegrate and corresponds to a reduction of measurable radioactivity by 50%). The orderliness characterizing 'half-life' is a statistical one based on the exponential law of decay as indicated by the expression e^{-at}.

The simplest atom seems to be the stable hydrogen atom. According to the *Rutherford-Bohr* model, further elaborated by *Sommerfeld* and others, it consists of a nucleus, of positive charge, the proton, which contains almost all of the atom's mass. Around that nucleus travels an electron in one of several permissible elliptic orbits which are quantized, that is to say related to integral multiples of *Planck's* constant h. The quantum number of the orbital radius (the principal quantum number) is designated as n.

For the innermost orbit, an approximate diameter of 10^{-8} cm has been calculated, which is designated as the Ångström unit. By absorption of energy, the electron 'jumps instantaneously' ('quantum jump') from an inner to an outer orbit of higher energy. Conversely, it may 'instantaneously' drop, with emission of energy, from an outer into an inner orbit. To these emissions of energy at various frequencies correspond specific spectral lines. As regards the orbital velocity of the electron, respectively the periodicity of the orbital events, the *Rydberg* constant of roughly 10^{15} cps is an appropriate example indicating time scales involved.

Do planets jump orbits? Like Mars...

The radius of the nucleus is estimated at about 10^{-12} cm. Compared to an atomic radius of 10^{-8}, this is one ten-thousandth (10^{-4}) of the atom's size. Thus, the distance between 'planetary' electron and central nucleus is roughly comparable to that between sun and outer planets. The mass relation of electron to nucleus (ca. $1:1,835$) is likewise comparable to that between sun and some planets. The size of nucleus and of electron, however, seems to be about the same in this model. Again, if the nucleus would be 1 cm in diameter, the hydrogen atom would have a diameter of about 100 m. The 'emptiness' of atomic physical space with respect to the distribution of 'mass' is evidenced by this model.

In order to account for spectral phenomena, it became necessary to assume further periodicities. A second quantum number (l, orbital quantum number) was provided by postulating a precession of the elliptic orbit. A third one (m_L, magnetic quantum number) was provided by assuming a rotation of the orbital plane, and a fourth one (m_s, spin quantum number) was introduced by assuming a rotation of the electron around an axis, with an angular momentum equal to $1/2 h/2\pi$ and with a corresponding magnetic effect.

About 1925 *Pauli* elaborated his exclusion principle, postulating that, in a system containing more than one electron, no two of the electrons can occupy the same quantum state, that is to say, can have the same set of quantum numbers n, l, m_L, m_s. This principle applies not only to electrons but to all particles with half integral spin. *Pauli's* principle provided the key to the electron structure of all atoms as arranged in the periodic table.

It was shown that, in atoms with higher nuclear charge than that of the hydrogen atom, the innermost allowed orbit can accommodate two electrons provided they have opposite spin.

Successive higher levels include a number of different orbits with different energy levels in terms of angular momentum, each again available for two electrons with opposite spin. When all of these states are occupied, the corresponding subshell is filled, and additional electrons must assume other states. The outer energy level electrons of atoms are also known as the volume electrons, since they are assumed to take part in chemical changes. In this respect there are inactive atoms, such as those of the noble gases, with closed outer shells or stable configurations, and active atoms with unstable configurations. Thus, in the carbon atom, two electrons occupy the inner shell, and four the outer shell which, in accordance with the theory, can 'accommodate' eight. Hence, in this atom, the second shell is only 'half full'. This characterizes the carbon atom as an almost 'unique' sort. In combining with other atoms by sharing electrons, carbon may form bonds with as many as four atoms at a time, thereby providing the possibilities for the exceedingly large amount of organic macromolecular compounds.

Pauli, moreover, postulated an intrinsic angular momentum, that is to say, a spin and intrinsic magnetism of the nucleus. The atom displays thus three angular momenta, namely, (1) the orbital angular momentum of the electrons, (2) the spin of the orbiting electrons, and (3) the spin of the nucleus.

After the neutron was discovered by *Chadwick* in 1932 the picture of atomic structure was further elaborated by considering the atomic nucleus as made up of Z protons and A minus Z neutrons, Z being the atomic or charge number, and A the mass number. Accordingly, the notation for the hydrogen atom became $_1H^1$, the charge number being the subscript at left, and the mass number the superscript at right. For deuterium, an isotope[7] of hydrogen, the notation is $_1H^2$, thereby indicating a nucleus consisting of a proton combined with a neutron ($_0n^1$). Discounting isotopes, helium becomes $_2He^4$, carbon $_6C^{12}$, and oxygen $_8O^{16}$. In accordance with *Pauli's* principle, several 'shells' of orbits become required as the number of 'planetary' electrons increases. This is of particular importance for the chemical reactivity of the atoms, whose valence by means of the covalent chemical bond depends upon electrons in the outermost or valence shell. The above-mentioned almost unique property of the carbon atom is the result of the distribution of electrons upon an inner shell with two, and an outer shell with four electrons.

The chemical properties of the elements were found to be periodic functions of their atomic weight as indicated by the mass number, upon which the periodic table of elements is based. On the other hand, the chemical reactivity,

---

[7] Isotopes are atoms with identical charge number but different mass number.

respectively the 'valence', depends on the behavior of the electrons manifested by electrostatic, by so-called covalent, or by 'metallic' bonds, as the case may be [cf. e.g. *Pauling*, 1960].

There are, up to isotopes of uranium such as $_{92}U^{238}$ and $_{92}U^{235}$ somewhat over 90 sorts of atoms with a variety of isotopes, representing 'natural' elements. Within this range, a few unstable 'artificial' elements, filling empty spaces in the periodic table, have been created by suitable nuclear reactions (e.g. technetium $_{43}Tc^{99}$). There are likewise additional artificially created isotopes as well as several 'transuranic' elements (e.g. the notorious plutonium $_{94}Pu^{239}$).

Since about hundred years ago it became evident that all the almost unlimited diversity of anorganic and organic matter resulted from the patterned arrangement, into 'molecules', of chemically bonded atoms pertaining to the limited number of different 'elements' consisting of 'atoms'.

The atomic notation based on mass and charge recently modified by superscribing the mass number to the left side remains valid, although, after 1925, the atomic model elaborated by *Bohr, Sommerfeld* and others became replaced by the quantum mechanics of *Heisenberg, Schrödinger, Born*, and *Dirac*. The *Bohr-Sommerfeld* model, nevertheless, represents a useful first approximation describing atomic properties with a modicum of 'visual representation' of the atom. The quantum theories, on the other hand, with complete abandon of classical postulates, provide entirely abstract mathematical formulations of atomic events. *Heisenberg's* approach is based on operations with matrices and is also known as matrix mechanics. Very shortly thereafter, *Schrödinger* elaborated his wave equation, involving a wave function ψ, and based on the concepts originated by *De Broglie*. *Schrödinger's* first wave equation is a generalization of *De Broglie's* equation for the motion of a free electron, and can be given as follows:

$$\left(\frac{ih}{2\pi c}\frac{\delta}{\delta t} + \frac{e^2}{cr}\right)^2 \psi = \left[m^2c^2 - \frac{h^2}{4\pi^2}\left(\frac{\delta^2}{\delta x^2} + \frac{\delta^2}{\delta y^2} + \frac{\delta^2}{\delta z^2}\right)\right]\psi$$

e represents here the charge of an electron, $i = \sqrt{-1}$, h is *Planck's* constant, r the distance from the nucleus, ψ is *Schrödinger's* wave function, and m is the electron's mass. This first equation did not fit experimental results because it did not take into account the spin of the electron, which was not known at the time.

Schrödinger's second wave equation (in which E represents energy), is an approximation to the original equation. It can be given as follows:

$$\left(E + \frac{e^2}{r}\right)\psi = \frac{h^2}{8\pi^2m}\left(\frac{\delta^2}{\delta x^2} + \frac{\delta^2}{\delta y^2} + \frac{\delta^2}{\delta z^2}\right)\psi$$

As regards weaknesses of the *Schrödinger* equation, the following five deficiencies have been pointed out : (1) the *Schrödinger* equation cannot be solved exactly for anything more complex than a one-electron atom; (2) it is not adaptable to a relativistic formulation; (3) it does not thereby account for the fine structure of the hydrogen spectrum; (4) it does not account for the electron spin; (5) the *Pauli* exclusion principle cannot be derived from *Schrödinger's* theory. Despite the apparent difference between *Heisenberg's* and *Schrödinger's* theories it became evident that matrix mechanics and wave mechanics were mathematically equivalent.

Although superior to the *Bohr-Sommerfeld* model, *Heisenberg's* and *Schrödinger's* theories still involved shortcomings which were partly avoided in the relativistic quantum mechanics elaborated by *Dirac* in 1928 and thereafter.

Such relativistic treatment appeared appropriate in view of the very high velocities obtaining in the collisions of high-energy particles. The orbiting electrons within the atomic 'shells', however, move at a relatively much slower speed, corresponding to roughly 1% of the speed of light (c) in the first hydrogen orbit. The velocity of electrons 'inside' heavier atoms is assumed to be somewhat greater, but still remaining within only a few percents of c. Although such velocities of a few thousand km/sec are considerable, the relativistic effect still remains negligible.

Again, *Einstein's* incorporation of *Minkowski's* space-time concept into the relativistic theory can be regarded as of particular significance. *Dirac's* elaboration thus unites, to some extent, relativity and quantum mechanics.

Dirac's equations led naturally to a quantum number corresponding to the spin but also implied the existence of states of negative energy, negative mass, and infinite charge density which appeared to contradict the prevailing concepts and led to the postulate of '*antimatter*'. Although *Einstein* had eliminated the notion of a luminiferous ether, *Dirac* introduced what could be called a 'new ether' by postulating a negative energy continuum. Thus, the 'vacuum' or 'empty' space is assumed to represent the condition in which all the negative mass and negative energy electron states are occupied. An anti-particle, namely the positron (anti-electron), becomes then a hole (the absence of a negative energy particle) in the sea of negative energy states, that is, 'a hole in the vacuum'. An electron with positive energy will fill this hole, whereby electron and positron disappear and two energy quanta (photons) are created. The total energy of the two photons is equivalent to the mass of the two disappearing particles. This is the process of annihilation which represents the complete conversion of mass into energy ($e = mc^2$).

The theoretical basis for antimatter arose from *Dirac's relativistic wave equation. For the energy of the free electron the relativistic formula*

$$E^2 = (m_0 c^2)^2 + (pc)^2$$

as shown above on page 8 holds. For an electron at rest, this equation reduces to

$$E^2 = (m_0 c^2)^2$$

To solve the equation, the square root of both sides is taken, which has two mathematical solutions, namely $E = m_0 c^2$ and $E = - m_0 c^2$. The first solution is the relativistic rest energy of the electron, but the second one gives a negative energy. This negative solution might be rejected as mathematically correct but physically meaningless. As regards the moving free electron, the equations become

$$E = +\sqrt{(m_0 c^2)^2 + (pc)^2}$$

and

$$E = -\sqrt{(m_0 c^2)^2 + (pc)^2}.$$

The positive solution has, at the non-relativistic limit of small velocities, the approximate value pointed out above on page 8. The negative solution becomes

$$E = -m_0 c^2 - 1/2 \, m_0 v^2.$$

Instead of rejecting the negative solution, *Dirac* pointed out that there was no theoretical reason why a negative energy solution should be rejected. He showed, moreover, that the negative solution was required to maintain the logical and mathematical consistency of the relativistic wave theory and to make certain predictions of the theory agree with observations. *Dirac* thus proposed a theory of the electron in which the negative energy solutions are given a 'real', 'physical' status. Discounting the strange features of these negative formulations, it must be admitted that they correspond to some still incomprehensible respectively unknown aspects of the obtaining physical orderliness, since deductions resulting from said mathematical model were found to agree with actual observations.

In 1932 the positron was accidentally discovered, in 1955 the antiproton, and in 1956 the antineutron were detected, thereby confirming valid aspects inherent in *Dirac's* bizarre theoretical formulations predicting the now well-substantiated existence of antiparticles and of antimatter.

It is of interest that positron tracks in cloud chambers were observed as early as 1927 but erroneously interpreted as backward directed electron tracks, since a positron moving in one direction displays, in a magnetic field, the same deflection of its track as an electron moving in the opposite direction. In 1932, however, *Anderson*, who was unaware of *Dirac's* theory, unequivocally determined the direction in which a secondary cosmic ray particle was moving and thereby concluded that this particle, equal in mass to the electron, had a positive charge [for further details cf. *Brancazio*, 1975].

Despite the spectacular success of quantum theories two main difficulties remain. The first one is the apparent impossibility to formulate a consistent 'explanation' or 'description' of the orderliness 'behind the rules for present quantum theory' [*Dirac*, 1963]. Since, however, statistically accurate results which agree both with mathematical equations and with the outcome of experiments are obtained, the physicist may remain unconcerned with that difficulty. This latter concerns, however, the philosopher who would like to have a coherent and satisfying description of nature.

The second sort of difficulties arises from the fact that the present laws of quantum theory are not always adequate to give any results. If one pushes the laws to extreme conditions, to phenomena involving very high energy or very small distances, one sometimes gets results that are highly ambiguous or not really sensible at all. Equations that look satisfactory do not have any solutions, since certain quantities that ought to be finite become actually infinite and have to be manipulated by arbitrary methods in order to yield definite results. But it seems quite impossible to put such so-called '*renormalization*' procedure on a mathematically sound basis.

After practically all the major questions concerning atomic structure had been more or less satisfactorily answered, physicists began with an intensive study of the atomic nucleus.

This involved the 'bombardment' of the nucleus with charged particles and subsequently also with neutrons. These latter, however, because of their uncharged nature, are not only more difficult to detect but also more difficult to control. Already about 1919 *Rutherford* had succeeded in changing a few atoms of nitrogen into atoms of oxygen by placing a source of α-particles in nitrogen gas (cf. fig. 1, p. 25). The nuclear transformation involved may be indicated by the sequence

$$^4\text{He} + {}^{14}\text{N} \rightarrow {}^{17}\text{O} + {}^1\text{H}$$

Later on, numerous experiments of this type were performed, leading to the fission of uranium ($^{235}_{92}\text{U}$) by neutrons. *Hahn* and his collaborators showed, in 1939, that the impact of a neutron causes the uranium nucleus to split, with further emission of neutrons, into smaller fragments (including an isotope of barium) and with concomitant release of enormous quantities of energy. This energy corresponds to the reduction of the resulting mass with corresponding partial conversion into energy by 'exoergic' reaction. Said nuclear fission if propagated by a sufficient number of thereby emitted neutrons, becomes a 'chain reaction', either uncontrolled and explosive as in the atomic fission bomb, or controlled as in nuclear reactors.

Apart from some fluctuations in the light nuclei, the nuclear binding energy per particle tends to increase rapidly to a maximum around 60 (e.g. nickel, $^{58.7}_{28}$Ni with isotopes) and then to decrease gradually. Any nuclear reaction where the particles in the resultant nuclei are more strongly bound than the particles in the initial nuclei will release energy. Thus, in general, free energy may be gained by combining light nuclei to form heavier ones, or by breaking very heavy ones into two or three smaller fragments. The former procedure is 'fusion', and the latter is 'fission'. As regards nuclear fusion, *Bethe* had, about 1938, elaborated a theory explaining the long-lasting heat of the sun by a cycle of nuclear transformations involving carbon, hydrogen, nitrogen and oxygen, eventually leading to the formation of helium. This self-perpetuating pattern of chemical (nuclear) reactions, gradually transforming mass into energy, was assumed to proceed in the following sequence:

(1) $^{12}_{6}C + ^{1}_{1}H \rightarrow ^{13}_{7}N$

(2) $^{13}_{7}N \rightarrow ^{13}_{6}C + ^{0}_{1}e$

(3) $^{13}_{6}C + ^{1}_{1}H \rightarrow ^{14}_{7}N$

(4) $^{14}_{7}N + ^{1}_{1}H \rightarrow ^{15}_{8}O$

(5) $^{15}_{8}O \rightarrow ^{15}_{7}N + ^{0}_{1}e$

(6) $^{15}_{7}N + ^{1}_{1}H \rightarrow ^{12}_{6}C + ^{4}_{2}He$

whereby the carbon-hydrogen reaction (1) starts again.

The net effect is the transformation of hydrogen into helium and positrons (here designated as $^{0}_{1}e$), and the release of about 30,000,000 eV energy.

Another cycle, also outlined by *Bethe*, involves a chain of hydrogen and helium reactions of the following type:

(1) $^{1}_{1}H + ^{1}_{1}H \rightarrow ^{2}_{1}D + ^{0}_{1}e$

(2) $^{2}_{1}D + ^{1}_{1}H \rightarrow ^{3}_{2}He$

(3) $^{3}_{2}He + ^{3}_{2}He \rightarrow ^{4}_{2}He + 2^{1}_{1}H$

with a corresponding release of energy. It is now believed that the proton-proton chain is mainly responsible for the conversion of hydrogen to helium inside stars of comparatively small mass like the Sun, while the carbon-nitrogen cycle is assumed to be of most importance inside main-sequence stars of larger mass.

Additional details of nuclear transformation cycles involving beryllium or beryllium and lithium have been elaborated. Various questions concerning these events in the interior of stars still remain incompletely elucidated, but the general principles of the obtaining mass-energy transformation can be evaluated as satisfactorily understood.

In dealing with atomic particles, it became convenient to use a unit of energy called electron volt (eV). This is the energy gained by an electron or a single charge particle accelerated through a potential difference of 1 v. The work done on any particle of charge e accelerated through a potential difference of V volts is V_e. If the particle starts from rest and no energy is lost in collisions with other particles, V_e will be the kinetic energy gained:

$$1/2\ ms^2 = V_e$$

This energy will be eV if the unit of e is the charge of one electron. It is a very small unit and for energy released in, or required for nuclear reactions, the relevant magnitudes are denoted by 10^6 (MeV) or 10^9 (GeV) electron volts. As mentioned above, nuclear reactions releasing energy are called exoergic. The total mass of the reactants is here greater than the total mass of the products. On the other hand, if the total mass of the reactants is less than the total mass of the products, the reaction is endoergic. In such reaction, energy must be supplied, either kinetic at sufficiently high speed, or by high-energy photons. Energy is here 'absorbed' to create mass, while in exoergic reactions, mass is converted into energy. The amount of energy absorbed or emitted in a nuclear reaction is designated as the Q value:

$$Q = c^2\ \text{(total mass of reactants)} - \text{(total mass of products)}.$$

If Q is positive, mass has been converted into energy (exoergic reaction), and if Q is negative, energy has been converted into mass (endoergic reaction).

Subsequently to the early experiments, a systematic study of atomic nuclear structure was undertaken by numerous investigators. Nuclear particles are much more firmly bound to each other than electrons to nuclei or atoms to each other in molecules. To break up a most strongly bound molecule, such as e.g. CO, about 11 eV of energy are required. Per contra, to break up the deuteron, one of the least firmly bound nuclei, an energy of somewhat more than 2 MeV becomes necessary. This high energy requirement, however, does not apply when the bombarding missiles are neutrons, which, being uncharged, can more easily penetrate the nucleus. Thus, in some instances, slow (or 'thermal-velocity') neutrons are more efficient for nuclear fission than fast ones.

Slow neutrons cause fission in one uranium isotope (^{235}U) but not in another (^{238}U), and fast neutrons have a lower probability of causing fission in ^{235}U than thermal neutrons. Fast neutrons can be slowed down by so-called 'moderators' such as heavy water or graphite. In general, the steady production of atomic power requires a slow-neutron-induced fission chain reaction occurring in a mixture or lattice of uranium and moderator, while a fission bomb[8] requires a fast-neutron-induced chain reaction in ^{235}U or

---

[8] A detailed historical account concerning the first atomic fission bombs is given by *Smyth* [1945].

^{239}Pu, although both slow- and fast-neutron fission may contribute in each case.

The agents commonly used to initiate nuclear reactions are neutrons, deuterons, protons, alpha particles, occasionally also heavier particles, and gamma rays. As regards the uncharged neutron, which is more difficult to handle than charged particles and gamma rays, there are artificial sources, such as bombarding for instance beryllium or boron by alpha particles, and a natural source is provided by the secondary particles of cosmic rays.

For the production of charged particles with very high energies a diversity of accelerators has been devised, such as the straight-line linear accelerator, the cyclotron, and the synchrotron. The largest synchrotrons can generate particle energies up to 400 GeV, and still much more powerful ones are being planned. Fast charged particles can be detected by light flashes which are emitted by the particles' impact upon, e.g. zinc sulfide screens (scintillation counter). Scintillation counters can also be used to detect gamma rays. Of particular importance are additional devices which depend on the particles' ionization effect. Thus, the *Geiger counter* indicates the arrival of a particle, while the *Wilson cloud chambers* and the various bubble chambers provide images of particle tracks. Such tracks can also be obtained by using photographic emulsions. Thus, from the tracks it becomes possible to determine mass, speed, charge, spin and to some extent lifetime of a particle.

Neutral particles, such as the neutron, leave no tracks, but their path can be inferred[9] from other tracks formed by charged particles pertaining to a related chain of collisions and respectively decays (fig. 1–3).

Generally speaking it can be assumed that the particles found in the atomic nucleus occupy distinct, quantized levels within the nucleus. Such levels, representing a 'nuclear shell structure', are roughly comparable to the distinct energy levels of electrons in the *Bohr-Sommerfeld* atomic model. Nuclei were likewise found to exhibit absorption and emission line spectra, differing from the atomic ones by a much higher energy.

Before briefly discussing the diverse types of particles discovered in atomic physics, reference to a general classification scheme seems perhaps appropriate. All particles can be divided into two groups according to their

---

[9] Discounting decay, such chains of events are thus interpreted in terms of rather elementary mechanical causality. Thus, the track of a neutron is identified by its effects, such as recoil of protons or other nuclei when struck by said neutron. Even atomic physicists denying causality on the basis of their interpretation of quantum mechanics thereby apply causal thinking to 'atomic events'. *Von Neumann* [1932], who emphatically denies causality, justly remarked that no experiment proves causality. He did not, however, seem to realize that experiments are designed to produce effects whose interpretation consciously or unconsciously implies causal thinking. In other words experiments do not prove causality but already imply causality [cf. *K.*, 1961, pp. 209–210].

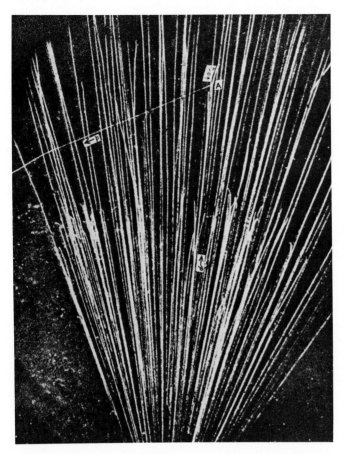

Fig. 1. Cloud chamber photograph of tracks of alpha particles in nitrogen [after *Blackett* from *Massey*, 1960]. At the point A an alpha particle has collided with a nitrogen nucleus, producing a proton (p) and an ^{17}O nucleus whose tracks are visible.

intrinsic spin. Those with half integer spin (s = 1/2, 3/2, 5/2, ...) follow the *Pauli exclusion principles*, and those with integer spin (s = 0, 1, 2, 3, ...) do not.[10] The former are called *fermions*, and the latter *bosons*. Two different sorts of statistics thereby obtain, namely the *Fermi-Dirac statistics* for fermions, and the *Bose-Einstein statistics* for bosons.

Paraphrasing a simile used by *Whittaker* [1948], let us assume an empty railroad train boarded by a (significantly less than capacity) crowd of passen-

---

[10] Otherwise formulated, fermions have a spin of odd multiples of $h/2\pi$, and bosons are particles with a spin of even multiple of $h/2\pi$.

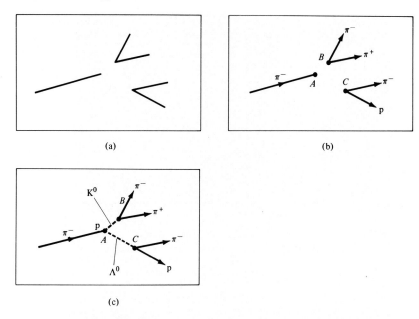

Fig 2. Diagram illustrating analysis of particle tracks in a photographic emulsion exposed to cosmic rays from *Brancazio,* 1975]. Examination of the tracks (a) indicates that a high – energy negatively charged pion colliding with a proton at rest in the emulsion created two neutral particles, a kaon and a lambda baryon, the former decayed at B into a positive and negative pion. The lambda particle decayed into a negative pion and a proton. K^0: neutral kaon; Λ^0: lambda baryon; p: proton; π^+, π^-: positive and negative pion.

gers. If every passenger selects his compartment and seat at random, without regard to the presence of other passengers, a distribution in accordance with the *Maxwellian statistics* would result. If passengers prefer compartments to themselves or at least corner seats, the distribution would be comparable to *Fermi-Dirac statistics.* If, on the other hand, the passengers are gregarious, do not wish to be alone, and select compartments with company, some compartments would be empty, and others quite full. This distribution could be considered analogous to the *Bose-Einstein statistics.* In other words, depending on particular parameters, altogether different sorts of statistics can result. Roughly speaking, in *Maxwellian statistics,* the dice are 'honest', the results of their throw being 'equiprobable'. In the two other statistics, the dice are 'loaded', e.g. in favor of the 1 in *Fermi-Dirac,* and in favor of the 6 in *Bose-Einstein* statistics. Again, the 'equiprobable' *Maxwellian* statistics, without significant constraining parameter, represents here, as it were, a sort of

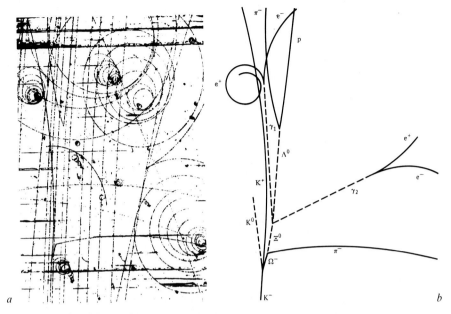

Fig. 3. Bubble chamber photograph (a) and its interpretation (b), showing the discovery of the omega minus particle [Brookhaven National Laboratory, from *Brancazio*, 1975]. A negative kaon, entering at lower left bottom, struck a stationary proton, producing uncharged kaon, positive kaon, and omega minus. This latter decayed into uncharged sigma baryon and negative pion. The further decay of the sigma particle involved an uncharged pion (not shown) that immediately decayed into two protons (γ_1 and γ_2). Each photon then converted to an electron pair. The dashed lines in the diagram represent the paths of neutral particles which leave no tracks in a bubble chamber. The other tracks in the photograph were made by charged particles not involved in the analyzed reaction.

limiting case between the two other statistics, comparable to the parabola as the limiting case between ellipse and hyperbola.

Dirac's concept of antimatter with mutual annihilation applies only to fermions. Identical bosons with opposite charge do not annihilate each other and do not represent antimatter in the same sense as fermions.

If the known particles are arranged in order of decreasing mass, four groups or 'families' can be distinguished [cf. e.g. *Brancazio*, 1975].

(1) The *baryon* family comprises the two 'nucleons' proton and neutron, moreover so-called hyperons (lambda, sigma and xi particles) which are heavier than the nucleons. All are fermions. The lightest member of the group is the proton which is the only stable baryon. All others decay in one or more steps to the proton. Thus, a free neutron decays with a half-life of about 12 min. Each baryon, including the uncharged ones, has a distinct antibaryon with which it annihilates. The difference between uncharged baryons and

antibaryons (e.g. neutron and antineutron) involves the direction of their magnetic fields.

(2) The *meson* family is a group of bosons with masses between the baryons and the leptons discussed further below. Baryons and mesons have also been classified as hadrons (cf. above p. 14). There are so-called pions and kaons, uncharged or with negative or positive charge. All mesons are unstable. All the known baryons and mesons seem to be composite structures, and, with the single exception of the proton, are unstable.

(3) The *lepton* family includes the well-known electron of rest mass 1, the much heavier muon of rest mass 207, which could roughly be described as a kind of heavy electron, and their associated neutrinos (muon neutrino, electron neutrino). All are fermions with corresponding antiparticles and are stable, except the muon. The nature of this group and the relationships between its members are poorly understood, particularly with respect to the large mass of the muon and the apparent existence of two neutrinos.

(4) The *massless*[11] *bosons* are represented by the photon which is the quantum transmitting the electromagnetic interaction, and the still hypothetical graviton, presumed to be the quantum transmitting the gravitational interaction. As regards the photon, it should be understood that there obtains an undefined, very large number of diverse photons differing from each other by their energy (related to frequency and wavelength, respectively). Under certain conditions high-energy photons (> 1.02 MeV) can disintegrate into an electron-positron pair (particle and antiparticle pair) displaying similar curved tracks diverging in opposite direction. This phenomenon illustrates a transformation of energy into mass.

The conservation laws obtaining for nuclear reactions state that, in these reactions, certain physical quantities must be conserved: mass-energy, linear momentum, angular momentum, spin, and charge. Another conserved quantity is the nucleon number. On the basis of these conservation laws, fairly valid predictions as to the outcome of proposed nuclear reactions can be made. Such predictions as well as further specifications have been particularly elaborated as regards the baryon and meson families of particles.

Some very short-lived baryons and mesons are designated as 'resonances', which might be a temporary association of particles.

Again, family members tend to be clustered in charge groups or multiplets of one, two or three particles of the same mass (singlets, doublets, triplets). This charge-grouping effect is defined by a quantum number called isospin suggested by *Heisenberg* in 1932 as isotopic spin [cf. e.g. *Robson*, 1973].

---

[11] Photon and graviton, with rest mass zero and charge zero, were occasionally also called leptons, together with neutrino and antineutrino, which likewise have zero charge and zero mass.

Several short-lived particles, including charged k-mesons, three sigma particles, and two xi particles with peculiar properties are called *strange particles*, and a quantum number '*strangeness*' (S) was introduced. The electric charge can be directly measured. But even if one could not measure it, one might, by noticing which particle reactions can occur and which cannot, discover its rule. In exactly this way, the number 'strangeness' which, in the strong interactions at least, never changes, may be said to have been discovered. One can assign to each hadron a number S (S = 0 for protons, neutrons, and pions; S = -1 for sigmas; S = $+1$ for positive kaons, etc.), so that the total strangeness does not change in a strong interaction.

The *baryon number* (B) formulates a principle of baryon conservation such that the total baryon number remains constant in all reactions.

S and B can be combined into a new quantum number Y, called hypercharge because it is equal to twice the average charge of all the members of a given multiplex. Hypercharge and strangeness are conserved in electromagnetic and strong interactions, but not in weak interactions.

Baryons and mesons can be classified according to their isospin and hypercharge. One can thus recognize five subfamilies of baryons and four meson subfamilies of baryons and four meson subfamilies instead of more than 80 different particles. On the basis of mathematical group theory, *Gell-Mann* and *Ne'eman* have originated theories defining the relationships between the (I, Y,) values of diverse hadron subfamilies designated as 'special unitary groups' (SU). Of importance are here also the conservation principles concerning the quantum numbers I, Q, S, B, and Y referred to above (for Q cf. p. 23).

The group of eight mathematical relationships describing various absolute and partial conservation principles is called SV(3). It predicts that among the hadrons there should occur multiplets of eight kinds of particles with a predicted relation among their quantum numbers and their masses. *Gell-Mann* named this group of relationships the 'eightfold way'.[12] These relationships severely limit the possible combinations of I and Y that a particle can display but predicted the occurrence of a meson (μ^0) that had not yet been observed. It was then subsequently discovered with exactly the predicted properties.

The mathematical relationships of the 'eightfold way' led to another group of I-Y combinations for a decuplet of ten particles. A missing, but predicted member of this decuplet, the omega-minus, was then subsequently

---

[12] This name was borrowed from the 'noble eightfold way' or 'path' of *Hînayâna Buddhism* leading to enlightenment: right knowledge, right aims, right speech, right conduct, right way of earning a livelihood, right effort, right concentration, right meditation.

discovered, after more than 50,000 bubble chamber photographs were analyzed (cf. fig. 3).

Further developments in particle theory led to the assumption that all hadrons are composite structures consisting of various combinations of three distinct fundamental subparticles, which *Gell-Mann* called '*quarks*',[13] characterized by fractional charges. All quarks have spin 1/2. The u-quark has charge number $+2/3$, and the d and s quarks each have charge numbers of $-1/3$. To each quark corresponds an antiquark. Finally, a fourth quark c of charge $+2/3$, characterized by a property called '*charm*' has been postulated. '*Charm*', like 'strangeness' does not correspond to any physically observable property, but both represent arbitrary designations for quantum numbers whose existence is implied by the results of certain experiments [cf. e.g. *Metz*, 1975; *Robinson*, 1976]. *Feynman* [1974] moreover suggested quanta called '*gluons*', supposed to hold the quarks together. Still another inferred quark quantum number, called '*color*' has been postulated [cf. e.g. *Schwitters*, 1977].

At the time of finally reviewing the present text, evidence for the existence of a 'fifth quark' was reported on the basis of the discovery of the so-called *ypsilon particle*, which represents the heaviest hyperon [*Lederman*, 1978], and of further experiments at the '*Deutsches Elektronen Synchrotron*' (DESY) near Hamburg [*Robinson*, 1978].

It is not unlikely that, by the time the present text should appear in print, further concepts in the rapidly expanding domain of the 'new physics' of particles might be elaborated, either substantiating or contradicting respectively invalidating the previous models. Again, as regards the terminology of diverse particles, e.g. of hyperons, various changes of the nomenclature which I have adopted from *Brancazio* [1975] were introduced.

The charm theory predicts that there are many more particles to be found. One such particle, which could not be formed by any 'allowed' combination of the original three quarks, was discovered in 1974 by two independent groups of investigators who called it I respectively psi. It is a hadron of three times the mass of the proton, being thus one of the heaviest particles known, with a longer lifetime than comparable hadrons and seems to represent a charmed particle. Yet, many dubious questions still remain, and so far, nobody was able to extract a quark from a hadron, and at the time of this writing, not all particle physicists seem to be entirely convinced that quarks exist.

---

[13] The term 'quark' is said to have been taken from one of the meaningless sentences in *James Joyce's Finnegan's Wake*': 'Three quarks for Muster Mark.' *Joyce's* writings illustrate *Shakespeare's* saying: 'such stuff as madmen tongue, and brain not' (*Cymbeline*, V, 4). In German the work '*Quark*' stands for a kind of soft 'cottage cheese' and, in the vernacular is used with the connotation of 'nonsense', comparable to the terms 'bilge' or 'boloney' ('bologna') in vernacular American English. Thus, *Mephisto*, in the Prologue to *Goethe's* Faust, exclaims: 'In jeden Quark begräbt er seine Nase.'

The invariance of mechanical 'laws' under a transformation of uniform velocity is known as the invariance under *Galilean* transformation, which is a characteristic symmetry principle of *Newtonian* mechanics. Another aspect of symmetry laws involves conservation of momentum under space displacement and rotation (angular momentum). Thus, the symmetry principles became firmly established in physics. The relationship of symmetry and conservation laws assumed particular importance following the elaboration of the relativity and quantum theories.

Besides the apparently well-substantiated mass-energy conservation principle a so-called principle of symmetry is expressed by the once widely accepted CPT theorem, which involves a number of dubious questions. C-invariance assumes the exchange of positive and negative charge such that to each charged particle there corresponds an antiparticle combined with the interchange of right and left, symbolized by P (parity). This means that the mirror image of a 'real' process should also be a 'real' process, or in other words, that if a physical description is replaced by its mirror image, no detectable difference should be noticed. P-invariance thus concerns the symmetry of 'handedness'. The principle of time reversal invariance states that all elementary processes can proceed equally well in both directions. Mathematically, this means that the equations of motion are invariant to a change of sign of the variable representing the time.[14] Four-dimensional symmetry, introduced by the special theory of relativity [*Einstein*, 1905] but elaborated in an appropriate mathematical formulation by *Minkowski* [1908] is not quite perfect. The lack of complete symmetry lies in the fact that the contribution from the time direction (c^2dt^2) does not have the same sign as the contributions from the three spatial directions $(-dx^2, -dy^2$ and $-dz^2)$ as, e.g. shown in the equation

$$ds^2 = c^2dt^2 - dx^2 - dy^2 - dz^2.$$

---

[14] 'Time reversal' is postulated by some atomic physicists for certain events involving the behavior of particles in relativistic physical space-time, as e.g. represented in the *Feynman diagrams* [cf. *Hoffmann*, 1959]. Accordingly, in terms of causality (which, however, is denied by various quantum physicists), certain effects could precede their causes. Be that as it may concerning the thereby obtaining mathematical formulations, it seems evident that the perceptual time of consciousness, which is the only experienced and 'actual' time, has an inevitable vectorial property, with an irreversible sequence from past through present to future and thus does not display reversal. It is also quite evident that time, which represents a dimension of the space-time coordinate system, as already implied in *Schopenhauer's* views and rigorously demonstrated by *Minkowski*, significantly differs from the dimensions of space by its directional property 'flow' characterized by irreversible (asymmetric) 'succession'. In relativistic physics the difference between space dimensions and time dimension is shown by the fact that this latter (w), in the coordinate system xyzw assumed to be ct, where c is the velocity of light, requires the use of the operator i (that is $\sqrt{-1}$) in relation to the time dimensions.

This equation is the expression for the invariant distance in four-dimensional space-time. The symbol s is the invariant distance; t is time; x, y and z are the three spatial dimensions; the d's are differentials.

Time symmetry or asymmetry appears related to reversible or irreversible processes in the physical world, manifested, *inter alia*, in thermodynamics as well as in biologic events. It also involves the diverse still controversial problems of isolated closed systems *versus* open systems, of micro-states *versus* macro-states, of so-called branch systems, of randomness, and of predictability.

Time reversal can, of course, easily be visualized by running a motion picture film backwards. Thus, by means of time-lapse cinematography, one could see a just hatched chick grow back into a blastoderm or into an undifferentiated ovum. A pendulum at rest would begin to swing with gradually increasing amplitudes of oscillation. Both events in reverse sequence would be time-asymmetric. Effect precedes here cause. Although this cannot only be imagined but actually demonstrated, this reverse sequence does not occur in the actual world of sensory experience and represents here qua 'material events' an 'impossibility', and qua abstract formulation, logically a contradictio in adjecto. On the other hand, the mirror image of a swinging pendulum in normal time sequence would display P-invariance.

Since the reports by *Yang* [1958] and *Lee* [1958] it has been shown that nonconservation of parity obtains in various weak interactions. Thus, both a neutrino and an antineutrino are apparently 'left-handed', that is to say, with counterclockwise spin. Thus left-handed and right-handed processes are not in all cases necessarily equivalent. Other instances of CP symmetry variations in weak interactions, as well as a violation of symmetry under reversal of time, have been indicated [cf. *Kabir*, 1968].

In view of all the mentioned difficulties and unresolved problems, it could be stated that the question concerning the 'ultimate nature' of postulated physical matter (i.e. mass and energy as well as 'interactions') is still far from being solved.

It seems evident that the questions 'what is mass', 'what is energy', 'what is electricity', 'what is magnetism' cannot be answered in a much more satisfactory manner than at the time of the early 19th century scientists, although much more, in great detail, and even in fairly rigorous mathematical formulation is now known about the behavior of 'matter', 'energy', 'electricity' etc., that is to say, of the observable and measurable relationships displayed by the phenomena subsumed under the above-mentioned terms.

Schopenhauer quotes *Kant's* definition of material bodies, namely that '*Körper krafterüllte Räume sind*', and remarks with regard to his own concept of 'matter': '*Ursach und Wirkung ist also das ganze Wesen der Materie: ihr Seyn ist ihr Wirken, in welchem ihr ganzes Daseyn besteht*'. This can be interpreted as being in full agreement with the concept of matter based on *Einstein's* elaborations. The thereby involved problem of causality shall be considered further below in the next section dealing with the controversial aspects of that postulate.

Schrödinger [1953] believes that with respect to the question 'what is matter'? the wave-particle dualism afflicting modern physics is best resolved in favor of 'waves'. He is, however, compelled to admit that there is no clear picture of matter on which physicists can agree.

At present, approximately 200 different atomic respectively nuclear particles have been identified, and even specialists encounter considerable difficulties in their attempts at dealing with this variety and establishing some sort of suitable classification. It seems that, in addition to a perhaps relatively small number of truly 'elementary' particles, an undefined number of different unstable fragments may result from high energy bombardment, whereby the large number of randomly resulting fragments is, nevertheless, subject to intrinsic constraints as regards the possible constitution of the thus obtained splinters.

Turning now from the small-scale aspect of the physical world to the macroscopic aspect as dealt with by the mechanics of classical physics, the fundamental concepts introduced by *Galileo*, *Descartes* and *Newton* remain valid and imply both causality and strict determinism. It cannot be said that *Newton's* model of mass, force, and energy concepts with their subsequently formulated g-cm-sec notation has been 'disproved' or 'falsified' by the new physics. It was merely shown that *Newton's* model represents a fully valid first approximation which, for many practical purposes, still remains more useful than the mathematical formulation of the new physics required for the description of small-scale and very large-scale levels, structures and events.

Proceeding next to the cosmic aspects of the very large-scale physical world, it is of interest to compare the 'emptiness' of atomic space (cf. above, p. 16) with the 'emptiness' of astronomic space. Since the extremely large figures thereby involved are difficult to conceive, *Newcomb*[15] made use of a helpful model in terms of mustard seeds, peas, and apples, which other authors imitated. *Wells* [1947] adopted it in the following manner. If we represent our Earth as a little ball of ca. 2.5 cm in diameter, the Sun would be a big globe almost 3 m across and nearly 300 m away, that is about 4 min walking time. The Moon would be a small pea ca. 75 cm from the Earth. Between Earth and Sun there would be the two inner planets, Mercury and Venus, at distances of about 115 and 215 m from the Sun. All around and

---

[15] Cf. *Schorr* [1929] and *Baker* [1932]. This model, however, dates back to the *Herschels* (father and son, 1738–1822; 1792–1891). Cf. also *L. Kuhlenbeck* [1904] vol. 3, pp. 208–209.

about these bodies would be emptiness until Mars, ca. 450 m beyond the Sun. All these planets are somewhat smaller than our Earth. Beyond Mars and an intervening belt of numerous very small planetoids, Jupiter, about 30 cm in diameter, would be nearly 1.6 km away from the sun. Saturn, a little smaller, 3.2 km off, Uranus 6.4 km off, and Neptune almost 10 km off. Still farther off, the small planet Pluto.

At this scale, Proxima Centauri, the nearest star in our galaxy would be about 80,000 km away.

It should, however, be understood that this 'emptiness' of astronomic space is only apparent and concerns the distance between large celestial bodies. Actually, said space is filled with gravitational interactions and electromagnetic radiation. In addition, it contains thinly scattered particles, atoms, and molecules, as well as 'dust' and 'dust clouds'.

Reverting now from the small-scale model to actual measurements, the average distance between Earth and Sun roughly 150,000,000 km, is designated as the astronomic unit (AU). Another unit of astronomic measurements is the light year, namely the distance traversed by light in 1 year. It corresponds to about 9.5×10^{12} km. Still another unit is the parsec, that is to say the distance at which the parallax[16] would be 1 sec of arc. It corresponds to about 3.26 light years, i.e. to somewhat more than 30×10^{12} km. No star is as close to us as this, Proxima Centauri being at a distance of about 4.3 light years. This compares with a distance of about 8 light minutes (corresponding to the AU) between Sun and Earth.

The stars are not distributed at random, but tend to cluster in large concentrations called galaxies. Our own galaxy, the Milky Way, seems fairly typical. Its general shape and size is shown in figure 4. It consists of a roughly spherical nucleus surrounded by a flattened disc-like region of spiral structure. The plane of this disc formed by the spiral branches is the equatorial plane of the galaxy. At the edges of this region, the density of stars falls off gradually, becoming effectively zero at a distance of 20,000 to 30,000 parsec from the center. Our Sun is located at a distance of about 10,000 parsec from the galactic center and a little less than 100 parsec from the equatorial plane.

In the neighborhood of the Sun, the mean distance between stars is about 1.3 parsec. Towards the galactic center the concentration increases to possibly as much as 10 times or more than near the Sun. In various regions of the galaxy, there are, moreover, rather dense aggregations of stars called open clusters and globular clusters. These latter are generally located in the galaxy's outskirts. Altogether there are perhaps between 10^{11} and 10^{12} stars in our Milky Way galaxy, whose central star clouds may correspond to 5×10^{10}

---

[16] The parallax of a star is measured from opposite points of the Earth's orbit, whose diamter (ca. 300,000,000 km) thus becomes the required baseline.

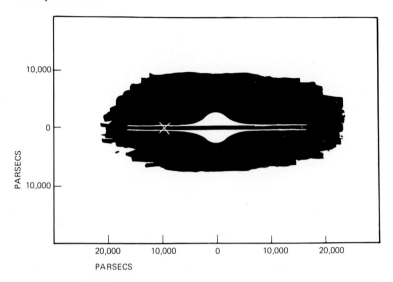

PARSECS

Fig. 4. Diagram illustrating the size and shape of our Milky Way Galaxy and the approximate position of the Sun (x). Note the dark obscuring cloud at the galaxy's equator [from Massey, 1960]. Distances indicated in parsecs. This sketch should be compared with figure 5 showing astronomic photographs of similar galaxies.

solar masses, while the mass of the entire galaxy is estimated to be a little more than 10×10^{10} solar masses. An average galaxy may include about 2×10^{11} or more stars.

This galaxy is presumed to rotate about an axis through its center, perpendicular to the equatorial plane. Not being a rigid body, the galaxy's speed of revolution varies with distance from the center, increasing to ca. 290 km/sec at about 9,000 parsec and then gradually decreasing. It may take about 200 million years to complete a rotation, and perhaps about 20 complete revolutions might have occurred since formation of the galaxy.

Out to a distance of ca. 3×10^9 parsec, which is approximately the limit of astronomic observability with the largest telescope (*Mt. Palomar* 500 cm reflector), there are about 10^9 or perhaps 10^{10} galaxies, apparently separated by average distances in the order of 10^6 parsec, although some degree of 'clustering' or 'grouping' may obtain. It has, moreover, been claimed that 'hierarchical clustering' of the galaxies represents 'a basic factor in cosmology' [*de Vaucouleurs*, 1970].

As regards the large numbers estimated for cosmic distances, numbers of galaxies and stars, as well as time scales in cosmic evolution, it should also be kept in mind that a substantial degree of uncertainty still obtains, allowing for

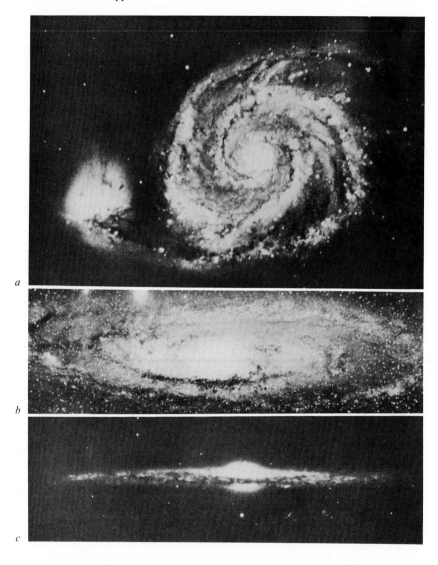

a

b

c

Fig. 5. Three spiral galaxies presumably comparable to our Milky Way Galaxy [from *Jeans*, 1931]. *a.* Galaxy in constellation Canes Venatici (Mt. Wilson Observatory), seen in polar view. *b.* Galaxy in constellation Andromeda (Yerkes Observatory), seen in slant view. *c.* Galaxy in constellation Berenice's Hair (Mt. Wilson Observatory), seen in equatorial view. Figure 5b: This galaxy, at a distance of ca. 450,000 parsec from our solar system, is said to contain about 10^{11} (hundred billion) stars.

considerable divergence in the extrapolated figures proposed by the different authors within the last decades. It is evident that these figures as here given in the text should be taken with a grain of salt and cannot represent more than reasonable approximations which may become subject to considerable corrections.

Thus, if the absolute distance of the great cloud of galaxies in the constellation Virgo could be determined, then their red shift, in combination with accurate age determinations from the relative abundance of nuclear isotopes, would help to obtain more reliable figures.

The red shift/distance relation (*Hubble's constant*), when directly extrapolated back to the point of zero expansion, yields an age for the universe ranging from 8×10^9 to 20×10^9 years, depending upon the distance chosen for the Virgo galaxies.

The difficulty lies in finding the distance to the galaxies, for the measurements have proven to be shifting and unreliable [*Gingerich*, 1977]. As the just cited author points out, *Sandage* gave the distance of the galaxy in Virgo as 22×10^6 light years in 1956. In the past decade, a distance twice as great has been commonly accepted, and *Sandage's* most recent determination is about 77×10^6 light years. At present, the relevant procedures, particularly concerning the more distant galaxies, still remain unreliable. *Hubble's* discovery of the red shift and the thereto related problems of cosmogony will be discussed further below on page 52. Many of these galaxies are similar in size and structure to our Milky Way. Thus, about two-thirds of known galaxies have a spiral structure (fig. 5). Others are elliptical in equatorial section, but without spiral arms. About 2% of all galaxies have irregular shapes. It seems possible although not certain, that the normal sequence of a galaxy's evolution is through the elliptical to a spiral structure with gradual opening out of the spiral (fig. 6).

The nearest galaxies, the two *Magellanic clouds*, are about 25,000 parsec away and of the irregular type, containing about one-tenth as many stars as the Milky Way. The well-known *Andromeda galaxy* (fig. 5b) is about 200,000 parsec away, being roughly comparable in structure, size, and star content to our own Milky Way galaxy.

Despite the apparent 'emptiness' of cosmic space, this latter, besides being traversed by the multitude of electromagnetic radiations, gravitational interactions, and particles (cosmic rays), contains dispersed amounts of intragalactic and extragalactic tenuous dust and gas, which condense to true diffuse '*nebulae*'. Some of these nebulae are dark, absorbing light, while others are faintly luminous, presumably by the effect of light from bright and large neighboring stars.

Generally speaking, it appears rather certain that the entire astronomically observable universe (or cosmos) consists of the same particles, atoms,

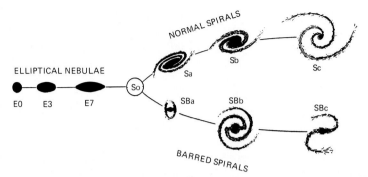

Fig. 6. Diagrammatic sketch showing the possible evolution of elliptical and spiral galaxies [from *Hubble*, 1936]. E_0, E_3, E_7: stages of elliptic nebulae; So: hypothetical transitional stage; S_a, S_b, S_c: stages of normal spirals; SB_a, SB_b, SB_c: stage of barred spirals. It should be emphasized that *Hubble's* classification of galaxies was originally meant to be purely empirical, without necessarily implying evolutionary connections between the different kinds. According to *Hoyle* [1975a, b] 'we still cannot say with any certainty whether or not such connections exist'.

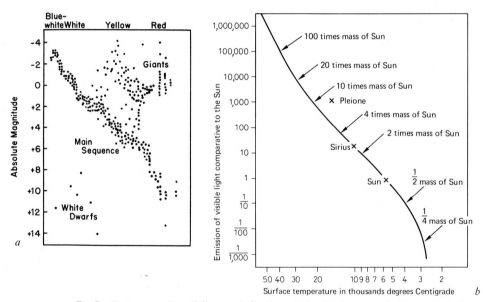

Fig. 7a. Hertzsprung-Russell diagram indicating relationship between absolute magnitude and color, respectively spectral class of stars [from *Dunning* and *Paxton*, 1941]. The units of absolute magnitude are here given by the 'classical' conventional ratio 2.5 of brightness differing by one so-called 'magnitude'. Thus a star of apparent first magnitude is 2.5 times brighter than one of second magnitude, As regards stars brighter than those of first magnitude, the units then become 0 and negative: 0, −1, −2, etc.

Fig. 7b. Hertzsprung-Russell diagram indicating details of the main sequence [from *Hoyle*, 1955].

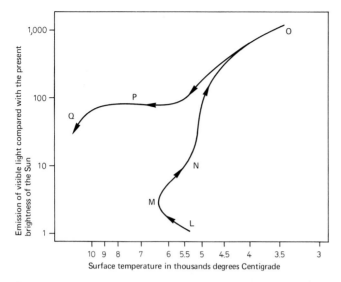

Fig. 8. Diagram indicating assumed evolution of a medium-sized star such as our Sun [from *Hoyle*, 1955]. L to Q is explained in the text. After evolving from the main sequence at M, the star is already in its death throes. Considerable fluctuations in size and luminosity may complicate the track from N to O and toward P. Evolving stars of considerable mass can develop pulsational instability with periodic oscillations. Such stars, that, as it were, zigzag back and forth in the giant zone of the luminosity-color diagram are the so-called 'Cepheid variables'.

and elements present in our solar system and planet.[17] Moreover, the same physical interactions and physicochemical orderliness ('laws of nature') seem to obtain.

With regard to the nature of stars, it became possible to plot, in the *Hertzsprung-Russell diagrams*, star populations on a grid of absolute luminosity (absolute magnitude) as ordinate, and spectral class (surface temperature) as abscissa (fig. 7a, b). This arrangement showed that most stars, including our Sun, lie near the diagonal from lower right to upper left, which represents the *main sequence* from '*red dwarfs*' to '*blue-white giants*'. Above the main sequence are to the right the 'red giants', and below, to the left, the 'white dwarfs'.

In addition to the differences in size, there are differences in type, related to the star's age, whereby type I (younger) and type II (older) stars are

---

[17] It is here of interest that the element helium was first discovered, by means of spectral analysis, in the Sun, and only subsequently was found to be also present in our Earth.

distinguished, our Sun being perhaps a late (i.e. relatively young) type I star. Some differences in structure and in distribution of atoms respectively atomic fuel also seem to obtain.

On the basis of the *Hertzsprung-Russell* diagram and of numerous additional data, it became possible to infer the evolution of a medium-sized star such as our Sun (fig. 8). Perhaps 4 or 5 × 10^9 years ago, such star was formed by gravitational collapse in a nebula, the nuclear reaction (cf. above, p. 22) ignited, and the star matured from infrared radiation to join the main sequence as a yellow star. Some billion (10^9) years later, with gradual consumption of nuclear fuel, it leaves the main sequence at M, becoming a red bloated giant (N-O) up to 100 times its main sequence size. It then shrinks again to a blue star of about original size (P), finally contracting (Q) to a white dwarf and presumably at the end burning out to a cinder. During the expansion process of our Sun to red giant, the Earth's oceans would boil off and all life on our planet, should end. The bloated Sun may engulf as well as melt the inner planets Mercury and Venus, perhaps also our Earth and Mars. Subsequently becoming a shrunk white dwarf possibly of a size comparable to that of Mars, the remaining core of the Sun then reaches a density so great that 1 cm^3 of its material would weigh about a ton.[18] It is not possible to determine with sufficient certainty the exact time of our Sun's expansion, but this latter event may not begin before some million or even 1 or 2 × 10^9 years. Thus, it has been estimated that only about one third of our Earth's life duration has elapsed.

With regard to these evolutionary processes, related to nuclear reactions, details of the size of a main sequence star becomes of significance [cf. *Chandrasekhar*, 1939]. Only stars below a certain mass which does not exceed about 1.4 times that of the Sun (*Chandrasekhar limit*)·can degenerate to a white dwarf.

Larger and more massive stars begin their final evolution as exploding stars known as *novae* and *supernovae*. A typical nova increases suddenly in brightness which exceeds from about 30 to 100,000 times that of the Sun. This

---

[18] The density of matter is evidently also much greater in the interior than at the surface of normal medium-sized stars. Upon collapse, of course, the atoms, which essentially consist of 'space' (cf. above p. 16) rather than of 'mass', can evidently become greatly 'compressed'. This results in states of 'matter' differing from the well-known gaseous, liquid, and solid states. Even in the core of a planet, such as our Earth, believed to consist of nickel-iron under considerable pressure at a temperature of perhaps 5,000–6,000 °C, and with a radius of ca. 3,450 km, the outer portion may be molten liquid, and the inner one in a peculiar 'solid' state. The pressure is here believed to be about 4,000 tons/cm^2 It will be recalled that the solid outer crust has a thickness of between 35 to 3 or 4 km, resting upon a mantle of roughly 2,900 km thickness surrounding the core, and consisting of hot rock in a plastic or semi-plastic state.

brightness is maintained for a week or two and then declines steeply. The end result of this process is a dense neutron star about 10 miles in diameter, whereby the gravitational force crushes the atoms. The density is such that 1 cm^3 would weigh 100 million tons or more.

Still larger and more massive stars of perhaps about and over 10 solar masses explode as extraordinary *supernovae*, which may radiate at 200 million times the rate of the Sun for about a fortnight. The end result of this evolutionary process is believed to be a so-called '*black hole*' with an extreme density far exceeding that of neutron stars and a concomitant gravity so strong that not even light can escape its boundaries, since the light quanta become trapped by the gravitational pull. Such black holes are presumed to grow by attracting gases and radiation.

It should, however, be mentioned that, while the concept of 'black holes' was elaborated and is upheld by competent astronomers or astrophysicists [cf. e.g. *Chandrasekhar*, 1977; *Wald*, 1977; *Thorne*, 1977], other likewise competent ones have remained sceptical up to the time of this writing [cf. *Metz*, 1978].

The occurrence of supernovae (suddenly visible temporary 'new stars') has been recorded several times, e.g. in 1572 (in the constellation *Cassiopeia*), in 1604 (in *Ophiuchus*), in 1901 (*Nova Persei*), in 1918 (*Nova Aquilae*), in 1920 (*Nova Cygni*), and in 1925 (*Nova Pictoris*). The Chinese recorded a supernova in AD 1054, which was apparently not noticed in the Dark Ages of the West. That supernova's exploded remnants, however, have been identified as the *Crab nebula*. Again, so-called planetary nebulae, which appear as luminous rings, surrounding a star at a late evolutionary stage, (e.g. the *Owl nebula* in *Ursa major* or the *Ring nebula* in *Lyra*), have been interpreted as shells of gas expelled by the star during an explosion in the process of decay.

As regards ordinary novae, numerous instances are recorded by astronomic observations. According to a recent theory [cf. e.g. *Hoyle*, 1975a, b], ordinary novae are supposed to result from binary systems of which one member is a white dwarf. This latter is said to receive material, especially hydrogen, from its companion star. The final outcome, following fusion processes of said hydrogen is an ejection of material from the white dwarf, a violent shedding of its skin of acquired material, that is similar, in principle, but not in degree, to the outburst of a supernova.

There are, moreover, variable stars with fluctuating brightness and pertaining to diverse categories. Thus, some red giants are long-period variables with regular cycles, and others with irregular fluctuations. The so-called *Cepheid* variables display fluctuations with great regularity, varying not only in brightness but in spectral class. By virtue of a relation clearly established between the period of the fluctuation and the absolute magnitude such Cepheids have become highly important distance indicators or 'cosmic yardsticks'. They appear in various parts of our Milky Way galaxy, in the globular clusters, and in other galaxies. Wherever a Cepheid is observed, the distance can be determined.

There are furthermore *binary stars*, that is to say double or even multiple stars revolving around each other. In eclipsing binaries, such as the *Algol binaries*, the fainter companion eclipses the brighter one as seen edgewise, thereby cutting off much of the system's light.

Subsequently to World War II, astronomy by optical observation became supplemented by *radio-* and *X-ray astronomony*. Although extraterrestrial radio sources were already noticed about 1932, this was not followed up in a systematic fashion until large parabolic aerials (radio telescopes) and multiple aerial arrays (long base line interferometers) were constructed. *Interferometers* are widely separated radiotelescopes that can measure the arc size of distant objects by recording the interference patterns. Radio emissions were recorded from the Sun, from regions within our galaxy, and from extra-galactic sources including so-called radiogalaxies. In addition to the quasi-stellar radio sources (*quasars* or '*quasi-stellar objects*') to be discussed further below, at least six distinct classes of radio stars were detected besides our Sun: *red dwarf flare stars*, *red supergiants*, *a blue dwarf companion* to a red super-giant, *exploding stars* (*novae*), pulsars, and *X-ray stars*.

Pulsars emit rapid, strong, and almost perfectly periodic bursts of radio waves. They are believed to be rapidly rotating neutron stars with an intense magnetic field.[19] This latter is assumed to constrain the emission of energy into a narrow beam that flashes like a lighthouse beacon as the neutron star rotates. A pulsar in the *Crab nebula* (remnant of a supernova explosion) pulses about 30 times a second.

X-ray astronomy, using X-ray detecting instruments carried by satellites, likewise detected X-ray pulsars in addition to other astronomical sources of said radiation. Although black holes are not assumed to emit radiation, it seems possible that such emission could result in the neighborhood of a black hole pulling in matter from a close companion star. Some randomly fluctua-ting X-ray sources thus have been interpreted as caused by the presence of a black hole.

Some of the above-mentioned radio emission sources designated as quasars were identified with very faint star-like optical objects emitting

---

[19] Magnetic fields such as surrounding the Earth and producing, inter alia, the *van Allen radiation* belts on both sides of the magnetic equator, moreover magnetic fields on Sun, stellar, interstellar, and galactic ones are doubtless of considerable importance, but in part still poorly understood. A variety of controversial views concerning this topic has been expressed and requires further clarification.

strongly in the ultraviolet as well as in the radio range of the spectrum, and fluctuating in brightness over short periods of time. Such quasars emit an enormous amount of energy, up to 100 times more energy than normal galaxies. In addition, many quasars display an extraordinary red shift of the spectrum. In accordance with *Hubble's* interpretation of the red shift as a *Doppler effect* indicating speed of recession and distance, to be discussed further below with respect to cosmology and cosmogony, such quasars would be located tens of billions of light years away, receding with incredible velocities. However, it has been questioned whether the red shift is entirely due to the *Doppler effect* of recession. In the case of the quasars, the large red shift might be either (1) gravitational, (2) due to collapse velocities of clouds of material falling back toward the center of compact galaxies, or (3) due to some as yet unknown factor.

Although quasars are still rather poorly understood and interpreted by a number of different as well as conflicting theories, it seems likely that at least some quasars are located in neighboring galaxies and in our own. Galaxies may begin with an enormous quasar explosion in their nucleus [*Unsöld*, 1975]. Such explosions in the center of galaxies could possibly be remnants of the primordial cosmic explosion discussed further below [cf. e.g. *Oort*, 1975].

Hoyle [1975b] points out that, although the radio method first led to quasars being discovered, it turned out that the property of radio emission is comparatively rare. The cited author therefore prefers the term 'quasi-stellar objects' (QSO) for compact objects radiating with a power output comparable to that of an entire galaxy.

There is little doubt that, at the present period of the universe, new stars originate and old ones decay. They appear to originate from the interstellar gas clouds by condensation and gravitational contraction. These protostars are relatively cool and predominately radiate in the infrared range. A star decays after many million or some billion years when its internal fuel of nuclear energy has been substantially used up. As end-stages of decay, and depending upon the star's mass, white dwarfs, neutron stars and black holes seem to result [cf. e.g. *Kippenhahn*, 1975].

Concerning the overall problems of cosmology and cosmogony, it is perhaps pertinent to recall some aspects of their historical development.

Although in the Old World (discounting thus the *Mayas* and their Calendar), astronomy may be said to have sprung from *Mesopotamia*, cosmology, as distinct from purely mythological concepts, dates only from Greece [cf. *Dreyer*, 1953].

The *Babylonians* and other *Mesopotamians* supposed the Earth to be a great hollow mountain, encircled by water, and the heaven a solid vault, whose foundation rested on the deep which also supported the Earth (fig. 9a). The *Egyptians* imagined the whole universe to be like a large box, the Earth

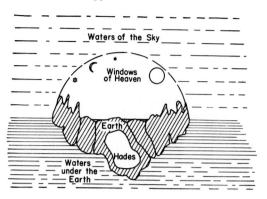

Fig. 9a. Ancient Babylonian conception of the universe [after *Whitehouse*, from *Dunning and Paxton*, 1941].

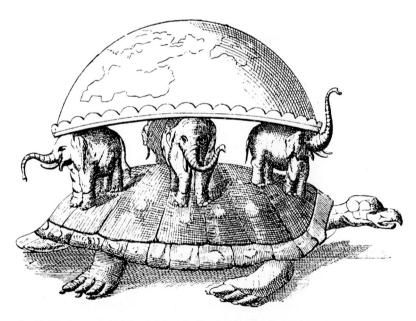

Fig. 9b. Hindu cosmology conceiving the Earth as supported by the four World elephants standing on the back of a tortoise [from *Sir Oliver Lodge*, 1893, 1960]. In the Ramâyâna these elephants are named *Bhadra* (N), *Saumanasa* (W), *Mahâpadma* (E), and *Virûpâksa* (S).

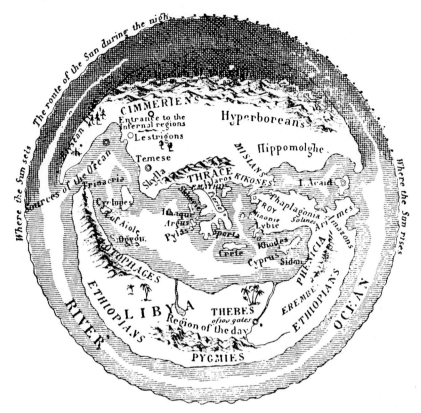

Fig. 9c. Ancient Greek (e.g. Homeric) concept of our Earth [from *Lodge*, 1893, 1960].

being its bottom, with *Egypt* as the center, and the sky being the ceiling, supported by columns or by mountains.

Hindu cosmology, somewhat later than the *Mesopotamian* and *Egyptian* concepts and perhaps dating back to about 1000 BC, assumed Earth to be a vaulted hemisphere, supported by four World Elephants resting on the back of a tortoise, whose support remains unexplained (fig. 9b). The famed *Hindu* epic poem *Râmayâna*, attributed to *Vâlmîki*, and presumably already extant before 500 BC, describes in two phantastic episodes (Book I 39, 40) how the *Sagarids* (the 60,000 sons of King *Sagara* of *Ayodya*) were digging through the Earth and, before being burnt to ashes by the fury of *Vishnu*, encountered and saluted the four World Elephants.

The earliest *Greek Ionian* philosophers (between 600 and 500 BC) presumably influenced by *Babylonian* concepts, considered the Earth to be a flat disc, presumably floating on water, and surrounded by the wide river *Oceanus* (fig. 9c). The *Pythagoreans* (about 500 BC), however, apparently first recognized the spherical form of the Earth, which was also recognized by their younger Eleatic contemporary *Parmenides*. The Earth was generally presumed to be at the center of the universe.[20] *Anaxagoras* (ca. 460 BC) believed that the celestial bodies moved around the Earth in the following order: the Moon, the Sun, and the five planets. *Plato* (ca. 380 BC) and *Aristotle* (ca. 350 BC) essentially adopted a similar view. *Eudoxus* (floruit ca. 340 BC) introduced the concept of concentric respectively homocentric spheres which *Aristotle* accepted. *Apollonius* (ca. 230 BC), *Hipparchus* (ca. 130 BC) who also discovered the precession of the equinoxes, and *Ptolemy* (ca. 140 AD) introduced and elaborated the concept of *epicycles* to account for the peculiar appearance of planetary motions. *Ptolemy's* geocentric system[21] with its concentric spheres and epicycles became then firmly established until the so-called *Copernican Revolution*.

There is, however, little doubt that *Aristarch of Samos* (floruit ca. 281 BC) elaborated a heliocentric system in which the Sun and the fixed stars are immovable, while the Earth, turning around its axis, is carried in a circle around the Sun. No original writing of *Aristarch* on this particular topic is extant, but his theory is unmistakably quoted by *Archimedes* and by *Plutarch*.[22]

---

[20] Already before *Ptolemy*, *Cicero* (about 50 BC) refers to the geocentric system, placing, in his *Somnium Scipionis*, the concentric 'spheres' in the following order: Moon, Mercury, Venus, Sun, Mars, Jupiter, Saturn.

[21] *Philolaus* (ca. 410 BC) gives an account of the *Pythagorean* system in which a so-called 'central fire' is assumed to exist. Around this 'fire' the Earth and all heavenly bodies, namely Moon, Sun, the five planets and the sphere of fixed stars are said to move in circular orbits. The 'central fire' is thus not the Sun, and cannot be seen from the part of the Earth in which Greece is located. Since the moving bodies are only nine, while ten is a *Pythagorean* perfect number, a tenth moving body, the '*Counter-Earth*' (*Antichthon*) was invented, supposed to be invisible because located between the Earth and the 'central fire' and always keeping pace with the Earth.

[22] The most detailed reference is that given by *Archimedes* (287–212 BC) in his treatise *The Sand Reckoner* (φαμμίτης) in which an attempt is made to calculate the number of sand grains that would fill the entire universe. *Archimedes* introduced here an exponential notation and obtained an interesting estimate corresponding to about 10^{63}. It will be recalled that the total number of elementary particles in the entire astronomical universe has been estimated at about 10^{78} to 10^{80} by present-day authors. *Plutarch's* (ca. 100 AD) mention of *Aristarch's heliocentric theory* in his treatise *On the Face of the Moon* is shorter, but likewise unequivocal. Still shorter is a reference by the sceptic *Sextus Empiricus* (ca. 200 AD) in the treatise '*Adversus mathematicos*'. Other very brief and perhaps garbled references to *Aristarch's* heliocentric concept are found in the compilations by the *Byzantine doxographic writers* (e.g. *Stabaeus, Galenus, Simplicius*, and others).

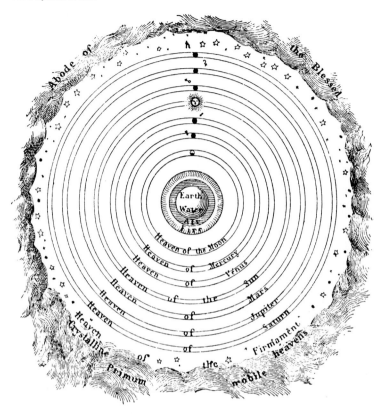

Fig. 10. Medieval concept of the Ptolemean geocentric system, simplified by omitting the required epicycles [from *Lodge*, 1893, 1960].

Herakleides (perhaps 350 BC), whose writings are lost, but are quoted by *Diogenes Laertius* (ca. 200 AD) and by the *Byzantine doxographers*, is also reported to have remarked that if the Earth moved in some way and the Sun stood still in some way, the 'irregularity' (ἀνωμαλία) observed relatively to the Sun could be accounted for. This rather vague statement has been interpreted to mean that *Herakleides* at least suggested the possibility of an heliocentric system.

Medieval cosmology, however, adopted the *Ptolemean geocentric system*, whose ultimate rotating sphere was that of the fixed stars (fig. 10). A well-known description of the various spheres is included in *Dante's Divina Commedia* (1331) and even after the treatise of *Copernicus* had appeared, in *Canto X* of *Os Lusiadas* by *Camões* (1572).

Copernicus, in 1543, re-introduced the heliocentric system, but, since he retained the concept of circular orbits, was thereby compelled to retain a number of complex epicycles and other artificial features of the *Ptolemean system*. *Copernicus*, moreover, did not contest the old concept of the sphere of fixed stars.

The great philosopher, cosmologist, and martyr *Giordano Bruno* (1548–1600) however, who following *Copernicus* had adopted the heliocentric system, expressed views that can be summarized as follows [cf. *L. Kuhlenbeck*, 1904].

(1). The Earth is only approximately spherical, being flattened at the poles.

(2). The Sun itself rotates around its axis.

(3). The precession of the equinoxes is due to the interaction between the heavenly bodies.

(4). The fixed stars are very distant suns.

(5). Around such stars rotate, but not in strictly circular orbits, planets which remain invisible because of their great distances from us.

(6). The comets are a special sort of planets. Since they appear only rarely it can also be assumed that the number of planets orbiting around our sun is not yet ascertained.

(7). The worlds and world systems are impermanent, subject to change and to decay, but their energy or substance remains, merely becoming recombined in different ways.

Kepler, who made use of the observations obtained by *Tycho Brahe* (1546–1601),[23] showed that the planetary orbits were elliptic, and formulated his well-known three laws. On the basis of *Kepler's* discovery, and on that of the laws of falling bodies, established by *Galileo*[24] at about 1638, *Newton* [1687, 1833, 1934] was then enabled to formulate in rigorous mathematical terms the law of gravitation, which had been anticipated by his contemporary *Robert Hooke* (1635–1702).

As regards dimensions (sizes and distances) in or of the universe, the Greek astronomers had a very fair idea of the size of the Earth as well as of distance and size of the Moon. Thus, *Aristarch* (ca. 130 BC) rather accurately determined the size of the Earth and *Hipparchus* (ca. 130 BC) calculated in

---

[23] *Tycho Brahe* was enabled to build the observatory of Uranienburg, on the island of Ven near *Elsinore*, with the most accurate instruments then available before the use of the telescope (invented by *Lippershey of Middleburg*) was introduced by *Galileo* about 1609. *Brahe* also elaborated a peculiar geocentric system differing from that of *Ptolemy*, and, as it were, incorporating some of the features of the *Copernican system*.

[24] *Galileo*, however, did not realize the principle of inertia and thus failed to formulate the three laws of motion. He still maintained, with *Aristotle*, the perfection of circular motion [cf. e.g. *Dreyer*, 1953, p. 414].

likewise rather accurate manner distance and size of the Moon. For a proper calculation of distance and size of the Sun and planets, however, the instrumental means at the disposal of astronomers were altogether insufficient until the invention of the telescope. The still more difficult problem of finding the distances to the stars by parallax was not solved before this was accomplished by *Bessel* and others at about 1838. This method, moreover, giving results in the order of magnitude of half a second of arc and less, proved to be applicable only to the nearest stars. For the greater distances it became subsequently necessary to use other yardsticks, such as spectroscopy and behavior of *Cepheid variables*.

Turning now from cosmology to cosmogony, it will be recalled that several ancient mythologies assumed some kind of unorganized 'Chaos' out of which subsequently Earth and Heaven, and respectively Gods originated, the latter taking part in the further development of the World. Thus, there is the Theogony of *Hesiod* (ca. 800 BC), who was perhaps a younger contemporary of *Homer* (if this latter actually was an historical personality). This was followed by a number of diverse myths elaborated by various Greek writers, as summarized in the treatise by *Moritz* [1791]. The original Chaos brings forth a personalized Earth, which, by itself, procreates light, *Pontus*, and *Uranus*, subsequently begetting with *Uranus* a generation of *Titans*, from which finally *Jupiter* (Zeus) originated, followed by the *Olympic pantheon*.

In ancient *Hindu Vedic cosmology*, the world originated independently of Gods. These latter then merely had regulating and ruling power.

Thus, the *Song of Creation* in the *Rigveda* (Mandala X, Hymn 129) states:

1.   Then was not non-existent nor existent; there
     was no realm of air nor sky beyond it.
     . . .

     . . .

4.   Thereafter rose Desire in the beginning. Desire,
     the primal seed and germ of Spirit.
     Sages who searched with their heart's Thought
     discovered the existent's kinship in the non-existent.
6.   Who verily knows and who can here declare
     it whence it was born and whence
     comes this Creation.
     The Gods are later than this World's production.
     Who knows then, whence it first came into Being?
7.   It, the First Origin of this Creation, whether It
     formed it all or did not form it.
     Whose eye controls this World in Highest Heaven,
     It verily knows it, or perhaps It knows not.
     . . .

7. (var.) Whence this Creation has its origin
           Whether created whether uncreated,
           He who looks down from heaven's highest seat,
           He only knows-or does He know not either?'

In later *Hindu* thought, the supreme *Brahman* was not a personal being, but an abstract absolute principle, whose 'emanations' are the individual 'souls', represented by the *'atman'* or *'self'*. The creation of the world is conceived as a 'disjunction' or 'disruption' of the Brahman's unity into innumerable individual 'forms' or 'manifestations', which represents a cosmic catastrophe, disaster or misfortune [*ein kosmisches Unglück*; cf. *Krause*, 1924], from which escape must be sought.

In ancient *Chinese cosmogony*, neither *Confucianism* nor *Taoism* conceive a personal creation, but only an evolution in accordance with 'cosmic law'. The *'Tao'* (*Path, Road*) as the 'first cause' brings forth from the original Chaos the two 'fundamental male and female creative principles' *Yang* and *Yin*.

The unattractive, weird, and in part nightmarish *Japanese cosmogony* compiled, from oral traditions, in two different versions (*Kojiki*, '*Records of Ancient Matters*', 712 AD; *Nihongi*, '*Chronicles of Nihon*', ca. 720 AD) gives approximately the following account.

In the beginning neither force nor form was manifest and the world was a shapeless mass that floated like a jellyfish upon water or the yolk in an egg. Then, in an unaccounted way, earth and heaven became separated; dim Gods appeared and disappeared. A male and a female Deity, *Izanagi* and *Izanami*, produced the islands of *Japan*. Generations of myriads of deities subsequently evolved. The Sun-Goddess *Ama-terasu-no-o-mikami* played an important role, the emperors of Japan being the divine descendants of this Deity [cf. e.g. *Hearn*, 1910].

Creation of the World by a personal God was not a very common notion and is essentially found in the following mythologies.

In later, and particularly in popular versions of the manifold and widely differing *Hindu* cosmologies and cosmogonies the abstract and impersonal *Brahman* became the highest God *Brahmâ*, the creator of the world, and Lord of Creation (*Prajâpati, Îshvara*).

Another personal God as world creator or 'maker' of all things is the *Jehovah* of *Judeo-Christian* mythology and its Moslem adaptation *Allah*. As proclaimed in *Genesis I, 1*, God, in the beginning, created Heaven and earth. This latter, at first, seems to represent the *Chaos* (Hebrew: *Tohuwabohu*), being without form, void and dark, while the spirit of God moved upon the face of the waters.[25]

In Greek philosophy, *Plato* (e.g. in the *Timaeus*), and *Aristotle* likewise postulated a personal God ($\theta\varepsilon\acute{o}\varsigma$) as the creator. This God, however, as in all mythologies except the Judaeo-Christian (and Moslem), did not create the

---

[25] This allusion to water, and other aspects of Old Testament mythology are evidently derived from the earlier *Babylonian cosmogonic notions*.

world out of nothing, but on the basis of a more or less undefined given 'something' or 'orderliness'. *Plato's* God is the δημιούργος, and *Aristotle's* God the 'Prime Mover' (ἀεχὴ τῆς κινήσως).

Only the Judaeo-Christian (and Moslem) mythology seems to assume the creation of the world out of nothing by a creator.

The *Greeks*, however, as *Dreyer* [1953] justly pointed out, eventually shook themselves free from mythological trammels. Philosophy, as distinct from religious speculations assuming the activity of capricious supernatural beings or similar mystical powers governing or influencing the phenomena, originated only in Greece, and does not date further back than the first half of the 6th century BC. These early thinkers endeavored to find the norms or 'laws' manifested by the phenomena of nature, postulating an impersonal general 'cosmic orderliness' correlating all these phenomena. Following the collapse of *Greco-Roman* civilization, and after a millenium of *Dark Ages*, this freedom of thought gradually arose again in Western civilization, leading to further advances in science and independent philosophic thought.

With regard to astronomic observations relevant to cosmology, *William Herschel* (1738–1773) who built improved telescopes, discovered, catalogued, and described a large number of nebulae. *Kant* [1724–1804] conjectured that they were very remote galaxies of stars, '*island universes*', while *Herschel* concluded that at least some of them were not composed of stars, but were composed of a 'luminous fluid'. *Kant* and subsequently with greater details *Laplace* (1749–1827) formulated a theory tracing the development of the Sun and its planetary system to the contraction and rotation of a gaseous nebula. Some of the spiral nebulae (observed with the large telescope of *Lord Rosse*) were accordingly interpreted as being solar systems at an early stage of development. Said telescope, however, and subsequent further improvements, revealed so-called nebulae as simply distant clusters of stars. This was also indicated by the spectral pattern of dark lines of such distant nebulae which could not be resolved into star aggregations. Yet, other nebulae, displaying spectra of bright lines, were definitely identified as gaseous.

Additional progress in astronomical observations included, among others, the discovery of the planet *Uranus* by *W. Herschel* in 1781. The planet *Neptune*, inferred by *Leverrier* and by *Adams* on the basis of deviations in the orbit of *Uranus*, was subsequently found in 1846 at the calculated location. Many asteroids, forming a belt between the orbits of *Mars* and *Jupiter*, were discovered after 1801, in the course of the 19th and 20th centuries. Discounting the comets, with their eccentric orbits, their tenuous composition of meteoric matter and gases, and their tails caused by a repelling effect of the Sun's radiation, the apparently outermost planetary member of the solar system was discovered in 1930 and named *Pluto*. The comets, on the other hand, are generally believed to be material left over from the primeval process in which the Sun and the planets were formed. In contradistinction to 'meteors', assumed to be remnants of comet matter, 'meteorites' are believed to be fragments of bodies from the swarm of 'planetoids' or 'asteroids', which orbit in a region of the solar system between *Mars* and *Jupiter*.

As regards the diverse satellites of various planets, the first ones discovered (besides our own Moon) were four of *Jupiter's* moons observed by *Galileo*; the two small satellites of *Mars*[26] were discovered by *Hall* in 1877.

A particular important development in cosmogony resulted from the discovery by *Hubble* [1936] that the spectral lines emanating from the distant galaxies are shifted toward the red end of the spectrum (cf. fig. 11). This red shift is interpreted in accordance with the *Doppler effect* to indicate a recession from the observer at a speed proportional to the shift. The inferred recessional velocity was found to be proportional to the galaxy's distance. The thus presumed uniform (linear) expansion of the universe occurs in all directions, such that the most distant galaxies are receding at extreme velocities, estimated at more than 16,000 km/sec for those much over 100 million light years away. This expansion, however, does not indicate that our local galaxy must be at the center of the universe: in a steadily expanding medium non-expanding clusters of matter are uniformly distributed, every cluster moves away from every other; an observer on any cluster would see the others all receding from him at a rate proportional to their distance. There could of course, somewhere be a center, but this problem, with respect to finite or infinite size of the universe, will be considered further below.

In contrast to the above-mentioned receding distant galaxies, nearby ones show not only a much less pronounced shift toward the red end of the spectrum but some such galaxies display even a shift toward the blue end. In other words, some of these are receding from us, and some (e.g. the *Andromeda galaxy*) are approaching us. This latter motion, however, seems mostly due to the fact that the Sun takes part in the galactic rotation. The velocity of

---

[26] It is of interest to note that several centuries ago, *Kepler*, in a letter to *Galileo*, had already expressed belief in their existence [cf. *Dunning and Paxton*, 1941]. This may perhaps explain the strange fact that *Jonathan Swift*, in *Gulliver's travels'* (1726) casually mentions the discovery of two satellites of *Mars* by the *Laputian astronomers*. Still more strange is here the coincidence that *Swift's* statements about their periods of revolution (10 and $21\frac{1}{2}$ h) correspond quite closely to their subsequently observed periods (7 h 31 min and 30 h 17 min). The erudite but highly eccentric psychoanalyst *Velikowsky*, whose weird theories of *World's in Collision* and *Ages in Chaos* can hardly be taken seriously despite the possibility of occasional true guesses concerning diverse generalities in accessory minor topics, believes that *Swift* obtained his information from an old manuscript based on actual observations of these moons at a time when *Mars* was close to the Earth. I am not inclined to accept this interpretation [cf. the comments on *Velikowsky* in *K.*, 1961, p. 517].

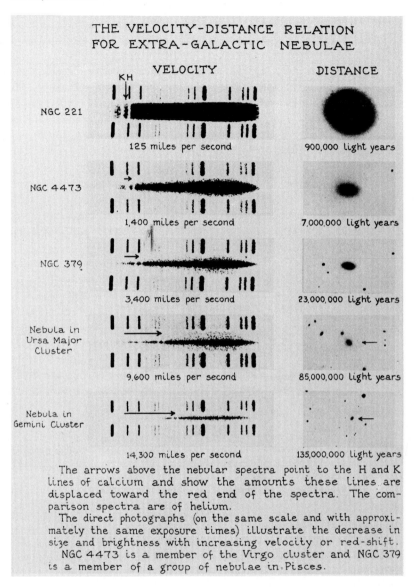

THE VELOCITY-DISTANCE RELATION
FOR EXTRA-GALACTIC NEBULAE

VELOCITY · DISTANCE

NGC 221

125 miles per second · 900,000 light years

NGC 4473

1,400 miles per second · 7,000,000 light years

NGC 379

3,400 miles per second · 23,000,000 light years

Nebula in
Ursa Major
Cluster

9,600 miles per second · 85,000,000 light years

Nebula in
Gemini Cluster

14,300 miles per second · 135,000,000 light years

The arrows above the nebular spectra point to the H and K lines of calcium and show the amounts these lines are displaced toward the red end of the spectra. The comparison spectra are of helium.

The direct photographs (on the same scale and with approximately the same exposure times) illustrate the decrease in size and brightness with increasing velocity or red-shift.

NGC 4473 is a member of the Virgo cluster and NGC 379 is a member of a group of nebulae in Pisces.

Fig. 11. Velocity-distance relation displayed by the red-shifts in the spectra of extra-galactic nebulae [from *Hubble*, 1936].

approach of the *Andromeda galaxy* to the center of our galaxy is apparently quite small. With regard to the overall significance of the red shift,[27] however, it would follow that, at a given time in the distant past, all extant and observed galaxies started out from a common location with exceedingly dense crowding. Depending on the value of the so-called *Hubble constant*, calculated from the red shift, the expanding universe may thus have started out about $10–15 \times 10^9$ years ago[28] from an exploding superdense concentration of subatomic matter, presumably more dense than that of the black holes. This theory of the primordial explosion,[29] propounded by *Lemaître* [1946], *Gamow* [1952] and others, does not seem unlikely. Within a given, relatively short time, the present types of atom were formed. The first atomic nuclei formed from elementary particles were presumably protons and neutrons, whereby initially only hydrogen and helium in the approximate proportion H : He $\cong$ 10 : 1 originated. In a hierarchy of condensations, galaxies and within these at least some planetary systems resulted.

A diffuse cosmic background thermal radiation at roughly 3°K has been detected and could be interpreted as the final dwindling remnant of the primeval fireball, whose temperature is estimated at 10^{12} degrees.

With regard to the 'history of matter', *Gamow* [1952] and others assumed that a variety of atoms became successively formed in a very short time following the primordial 'fireball' or 'explosion'. At present [cf. e.g. *Hoyle*, 1975a] it is widely believed that the material of galaxies was initially composed of hydrogen and perhaps helium only. The heavier elements are then presumed to have been produced by nuclear fusion processes inside stars. Sub-

---

[27] There are, however, several still dubious problems concerning the significance of the red shift. Although the *Doppler effect* most likely plays here a substantial role, other factors such as large gravitational fields (e.g. in the quasars) or other still poorly understood physical effects might be involved.

[28] The determination of the life span of the universe in terms of billion (10^9) years [now also called Eons or Aeons, AE, cf. *Unsöld*, 1975] based on galactic distances and velocities of recession is encumbered by so many hidden assumptions and pitfalls that all estimates remain subject to substantial revisions. There is, however, no reason to discard the exploding universe models on the evidence of inadequate time scale alone [cf. also *Singh*, 1961]. It should also be noted that a cosmologic Eon (10^9 years) is not to be confused with the geologic Cryptozoic Eon whose duration, although presumably in the order of magnitude of 10^9, remains nevertheless unspecified.

[29] The highly vulgar designations '*Big Bang*' and '*Urknall*' are now generally used by contemporary scientists to designate this presumed origin of the present universe. One is here reminded of *Don José Ortega y Gasset's* remark in '*La rebelión de las masas*': '*Lo característico del momento es que el alma vulgar, sabiéndose vulgar, tiene el denuedo de afirmar el derecho de la vulgaridad y lo impone dondequiera.*' Both the English and the German terms, moreover, are asinine, since the assumed event was outside the zonic range, quite apart from the fact that nobody could have been there to 'hear' or witness it.

sequently to their production inside stars, the elements were scattered into space by stellar explosions. Thus, the common materials providing the basis of life, such as carbon, oxygen etc., including metals, are believed to have been produced in stellar furnaces at temperatures up to a billion (10^9) degrees, being flung violently into space before the sun and planets of our system were formed. The parent stars, accordingly, 'are by now faint white dwarfs or superdense neutron stars which we have no means of identifying' [*Hoyle*, 1975a].

There are, moreover, with respect to the theory of the primeval fireball, certain difficulties concerning the existence of antimatter. Unless the universe is asymmetric in the sense that it consists exclusively of 'ordinary' matter ('koinomatter'), there should be equal quantities of 'koinomatter' and antimatter. But a homogeneous mixture of matter and antimatter at great density would result in immediate annihilation and the expanding universe should contain photons, electrons and positrons, as well as rapidly decaying particles but very few nucleons [cf. e.g. *Alfvén and Elvius*, 1969].

However, since many details of the postulated early cosmogenic states involve imperfectly understood or entirely unknown physical factors, several possibilities could be said to obtain. It is thus uncertain whether antimatter is present in some regions of our galaxy, or whether some galaxies consist entirely of antimatter and others entirely of koinomatter.

In this respect, investigators at the Max-Planck-Institut für Kernphysik noted that under particular energy conditions, called 'resonances', koinomatter and antimatter may co-exist without annihilation, becoming separated by a 'superheated separation layer' ('*superheisse Trennschicht*') leading to a final disjunction of the two sorts of matter [cf. *Hintsches*, 1977a].

Galaxies pertaining to a cluster move about inside the cluster and may collide with each other. Because of the very large interstellar distances this does not mean that the stars of one galaxy actually hit those of the other. The free interpenetration of the stars, however, does not hold for the intragalactic gas clouds, whose collision results in violent energy emission, particularly in the radio frequencies. Such a powerful radio emission has been observed from two very distant galaxies in the constellation of *Cygnus*. Quite evidently, the results of such collisions would be particularly violent if one galaxy should consist of koinomatter and the other one of antimatter.

Be that as it may, the hypothesis of the primordial explosion or primeval fireball is, at the time of this writing, accepted as most likely by competent astronomers and cosmologists [e.g. *Oort*, 1970, 1975; *Unsöld*, 1975].

If one adopts causal thinking, which requires an uninterrupted sequence of determining changes, without beginning or end, one might then ask: what preceded the primordial explosion? This question can evidently be answered by postulating a gravitational collapse of the entire universe, followed by a rebound. There is indeed some evidence that the expansion of the universe is slowing down [cf. *Singh*, 1961]. The gravitational collapse displayed by the presumptive black holes possibly may be related to this general phenomenon of contraction, and the model of an oscillating universe with a duration[30] of perhaps approximately 15 or 16 Aeons for a periodic phase from explosion to collapse can be accepted as being rather probable. It would reasonably well conform to important aspects of *Einstein's* general relativity.

It is, moreover, of interest that *Schopenhauer*, in volume 1 of his '*Welt als Wille und Vorstellung*', brings the following three comments concerning the collapse of the physical universe.

With regard to 'attraction' and 'repulsion' he stated: '*Abstrahieren wir von aller chemischen Verschiedenheit der Materie, oder denken uns in die Kette der Ursachen und Wirkungen soweit zurück, dass noch keine chemische Differenz da ist; so bleibt uns die blosse Materie, die Welt zu einer Kugel geballt, deren Leben, d.h. Objektivation des Willens, nun jener Kampf zwischen Attraktions- und Repulsionskraft ausmacht, jene als Schwere, von allen Seiten zum Centrum drängend, diese als Undurchdringlichkeit, sei es durch Starrheit oder Undurchdringlichkeit jener widerstrebend*' ... (vol. 1, pp. 210–211).

'*Denn wäre auch, nach ihrem Willen, alle existirende Materie in einen Klumpen vereinigt; so würde im Inneren desselben die Schwere, zum Mittelpunkt strebend, noch immer mit der Undurchdringlichkeit, als Starrheit oder Elastizität, kämpfen.*'

'*Jedes erreichte Ziel ist wieder Anfang einer neuen Laufbahn, und so ins Unendliche*' (vol. 1, p. 228).

'*Wir sehen dies an der einfachsten aller Naturerscheinungen, der Schwere, die nicht aufhört zu streben nach einem ausdehnungslosen Mittelpunkt, dessen Erreichung ihr und der Materie Vernichtung wäre, zu drängen, nicht anfhört, wenn auch schon das ganze Weltall zusammengeballt wäre*' (vol. 1, p. 400). Substituting here 'action' for *Schopenhauer's* 'will', these comments by the cited author are rather remarkable and would well agree with the concept of an endlessly pulsating universe.

Speculative cosmologies of various types have been elaborated by *Bondi, de Sitter, Eddington, Einstein, Friedman, Hoyle, Jeans, Milne, Tolman*, and others [cf. e.g. *Hoyle*, 1955; *Singh*, 1961; *Whittaker*, 1948]. *Hoyle's* original but

---

[30] As regards physical time, *Milne* distinguished ephemeral or dynamical time τ, recorded by a molar timekeeper such as the chronometer or the rotating earth, and absolute or kinematic time t, which is the time recorded by a timekeeper based on atomic processes, such as a radioactive clock. The relationship between τ time, namely the time of *Newtonian mechanics*, and the t time of atomic respectively subatomic events, as well as additional considerations derived from relativity theory involve difficult problems whose attempted mathematical solutions remain ambiguous and controversial (cf. also above fn. 28).

apparently now abandoned theory postulated a steady state universe with continuous creation from nothing[31] compensating for galactic and stellar evolution as well as for a continuous expansion. *De Sitter's model* likewise included runaway expansion correlated, as it were, with expanding empty space.

While physical time, in which the universe may oscillate, can easily be conceived as without beginning and without end, the concept of infinite space involves certain difficulties. As regards an infinite universe, there is the well-known *Olbers paradox*, pointed out by this author at about 1823 and previously already intimated by *Chéseaux* (ca. 1744), namely, why is the sky dark at night? Assuming an infinite number of stars, any line of sight would eventually meet one, and the whole night sky would be lighted, since no starless intervall could obtain.

Assuming such infinite universe, several explanations resolving the paradox were proposed. Thus, since the speed of light is finite, light originating at an infinite distance might not have reached us because, even in an infinite universe, the stars themselves cannot be considered eternal, but originate in time and are subject to decay. We would see only such light as, with finite speed, could have had the time to reach us. Other explanations were based on a weakening of the distant light due to various physical factors, particularly the absorbing effects of cosmic dust. On the other hand, it becomes evident that *Hubble's* expanding universe completely resolves *Olber's paradox* both due to the weakening of light by the red shift, and, moreover, by the presumably finite dimensions of the universe.

Although the question whether the universe is finite or infinite[32] was, to some extent, implied in the elaborations of preceding Greek philosophers, this

---

[31] Continuous creation of matter in the universe, originating from nothing, and appearing everywhere from nowhere was also postulated by *Bondi and Gold* [cf. *Singh*, 1961]. This matter is supposed to appear in the form of hydrogen atoms, representing the most common element in the universe. Prima facie, and assuming the principle of causality to be valid, such postulate would appear absurd. It contradicts the conservation principle, particularly elaborated by *Robert Mayer* (1814–1878) who stressed that *'aus nichts wird nichts'* (*ex nihilo nihil fit*). Yet, if physical space, respectively the vacuum is considered to be a plenum (cf. e.g. *Dirac's* 'sea of negative energy', p. 19 above), said postulate by *Hoyle*, *Bondi* et al. might at least appear 'logically' defensible, although one may not be inclined to accept it.

[32] *Hindu thought*, in the 5th century BC, was apparently also much concerned with infinitude, both in space and in time. This topic is repeatedly mentioned, but dismissed as irrelevant, in the sermons (sutras, Skr.; suttas, Pâli) of the *Buddha*, e.g. *Majjhima Nikayo* 1/63 and several others. The gist of these diverse statements may be rendered as follows: 'The world is eternal, the world is not eternal, the world is both eternal and not eternal, the world is finite, the world is infinite, the world is both finite and infinite, the Tathâgata exists after death, the Tathâgata does not exist after death, the Tathâgata both exists and does not exist after death: all this I have not taught. My teachings state: this is suffering, this is the cause of suffering and this is the way to extinguish suffering.'

problem was apparently first examined in a detailed and fairly rigorous manner by *Aristotle*, who maintained that, being spherical, the universe was necessarily finite (*De Coelo*, I, 5, also *Physica* IV, 1–5). *Giordano Bruno*, who opposed many of *Aristotle's* views,[33] believed in the infinity of the universe, as elaborated in his *Italian dialogue 'Del infinito, universo e mondi'* (translated by L. *Kuhlenbeck* [1904]: *Zwiegespräche vom unendlichen All und den Welten*) as well as in his *Latin* poem *'De Immenso et Innumerabili'*.

L. *Kuhlenbeck* [1904], however, while stressing the great advance in cosmological thought accomplished by *Bruno*, nevertheless pointed out that this philosopher's concept of infinity remained unconvincing: '*Man kann Bruno's Sieg über die Aristotelische scholastische Kosmologie vollauf würdigen und darf gleichwohl in der philosophischen Kritik der Unendlichkeitsidee eher dem Aristoteles, als dem Nolaner beipflichten.*'

Bochner [1969], a mathematician at Princeton university, in his attempt to describe the history of knowledge in terms of 'eclosion' and 'synthesis', likewise expressed his objections to *Bruno's* concept of the infinite, but added some gratuitous and crudely disparaging comments. According to said *Bochner, Bruno* was 'a raucous vulgarian who somehow managed to be canonized by a martyr's death' and is 'cast in the role of the Great Liberator in the battle for infinitude. Even philosophers of delicate sensibilities who would squirm at the thought of receiving a live *Bruno* in their drawing room eagerly acknowledge the leadership of the dead *Bruno*, who is safe and sainted.'

Paraphrasing the unjustified censure of *Schopenhauer* by the *Royal Danish Society* in 1840, one could here, but with full justifcation, comment as follows: Non reticendum videtur, *Jordanum Brunonem* summum philosophum tam indecenter commemorari, ut vaniloquus iste Bochnerus justam et gravem offensionem habeat.

It will be sufficient to point out that, with a recommendation by *King Henri III of France*, Bruno lived for 2 years (1583–1585) as a houseguest of the gentlemanly French ambassador *Castelnau de Mauvissière* in London, staying until the ambassador's recall to Paris. While in England, *Bruno* was a close friend of *Lord Sidney*. The influence of *Bruno's* writings on *Descartes*, *Spinoza*, *Leibniz*, *Goethe*, and *Schopenhauer* is well documented.[34]

---

[33] To some extent, *Bruno's* opposition to diverse *Aristotelian* views was provoked by their dominating influence on scholastic thought and their interpretation as elaborated by the scholastic philosophers. It should also be recalled that *Bruno*, in his concept of infinity, anticipated various aspects of *Cantor's* development of the mathematics of infinity [cf. *K.*, 1961, p. 92].

[34] Thus, several of *Goethe's* poems include literal translations of *Bruno's* sayings. Several lines of the poem *'Gott und Welt'* (*'Was wär ein Gott, der nur von Aussen stiesse'*, etc.), e.g. are, translated and versified into German, taken word for word from *Bruno's* prose commentary to *'De Immenso'*. As regards the raucous vulgarity imputed by *Bochner*, it may be recalled that, as a remnant of the Dark Ages, considerable crudity and vulgarity still generally prevailed and were

As regards the developments of cosmology, *Kepler* seems to have concluded that the universe is finite both with respect to space and matter. *Newton's* absolute space, taken as a construct representing the *Euclidean geometrical* substratum of the universe, is evidently infinite. *Newton* considered the celestial bodies to be located in an immense vacuum, but was apparently noncommittal concerning their finite or infinite number. In a letter to *Bentley* in 1692, however, he admitted, upon being pressed by a direct inquiry, that the universe was probably infinite[35] [cf. *Bochner*, 1969].

Fontenelle (1657–1757), in his '*Entretiens sur la pluralités des mondes*', and many others accepted the belief in the infinitude of the universe.

Kant (1724–1804), in his antimony of cosmology,[36] claimed that the controversies concerning the infinitudes were meaningless, since the following contradictory propositions could be stated with equally valid arguments: (1) the world has a beginning in time and is limited by a boundary; (2) the world is infinite in time and space.

There obtain, however, some doubts concerning logical validity of the diverse arguments here elaborated by *Kant*, as *Schopenhauer* pointed out in his critique of *Kant's* philosophy appended to volume 1 of '*Die Welt als Wille und Vorstellung*'.

In his theory of special relativity, *Einstein* showed that there obtains an

---

permissible in the 16th century. *Martin Luther* (1483–1546) a highly accomplished scholar, a composer of magnificent hymns, and a great religious leader, was quite outspoken in his famed table talks. Thus, e.g., the following sample may be quoted [ed. Reclam, n.d. p. 378]. '*Ich wollte nicht hunderttausend Gulden dafür nehmen, dass ich Rom nicht gesehen hätte; wiewohl ich die grossen, schändlichen Gräuel noch nicht recht weiss. Da ich's erst sah, fiel ich auf die Erde, hub meine Hände auf, und sprach: Sei gegrüsst, du heiliges Rom. Ja, rechtschaffen heilig, von den heiligen Märtyrern und ihrem Blut, das da vergossen ist; aber sie ist nun zerrissen, und der Teufel hat den Papst, seinen Dreck, darauf geschissen.*'

With regard to such literary crudities, some quotations from *Goethe* are appropriate:

'"So sei doch höflich" – höflich mit dem Pack?
Mit Seide näht man keinen groben Sack.'
'Auf groben Klotz ein grober Keil
Auf einen Schelmen anderthalbe.'

'Du, Kräftiger, sei nicht so still,
Wenn auch sich andre scheuen!
Wer den Teufel erschrecken will,
Der muss laut schreien.'

[35] It is most interesting that, in his letter, *Newton* suggested the gravitational instability respectively collapse of a finite universe resulting in one great spherical mass. He thereby anticipated, as it were, the contemporary theory of a collapsing universe.

[36] This antinomy is elaborated by *Kant*, with slightly different wording, in '*Kritik der reinen Vernunft*' [1781] and in '*Prolegomena zu einer jeden künftigen Metaphysik, die als Wissenschaft wird auf treten können*' [1783].

unchanged space-time extension of material objects, but with a projection of this extension to both space and time as a varying proportion dependent on the relative velocity of the object, such that a reduction in spatial extension appears as an increase in temporal extension. Although length x and time t are not invariant for all observers, the combination $x^2 - c^2t^2$ is invariant, such that $x^2 - c^2t^2 = x'^2 - c^2t'^2$. The velocity of light, c, allows the conversion of an interval of time into an interval of space, 1 sec of time being equivalent to 300,000 km of space.[37] This suggested to *Minkowski* [1908] his mathematical elaboration of the unified *four-dimensional space-time*.

Poincaré [1913a, 1963] likewise stated that everything happens as if time were a fourth dimension of space, and as if four-dimensional space resulting from the combination of ordinary space and of time could rotate not only around an axis of ordinary space in such a way that time were not altered, but around any axis whatever. For the comparison to be mathematically accurate, it would be necessary to assign purely imaginary values to this fourth coordinate in space. The four coordinates of a point in our new space would not be x, y, z, and t, but x, y, z, and t $\sqrt{-1}$. The essential thing, however, is 'to notice that in the new conception space and time are no longer two entirely different entities which can be considered separately, but two parts of the same whole, two parts which are so closely knit that they cannot be easily separated'.

This of course, seems quite evident if, as was repeatedly stressed [*K.*, 1957 et passim], consciousness represents a (private) space-time system characterized by its here and now contents (percepts, perceptions).

Figure 12a illustrates two examples of simplified (public) two-dimensional space-time systems, in which the space dimension is the ordinate, and the time dimension represents the abscissa.

Einstein's theory of general relativity, by introducing concepts of *Non-Euclidean* (*Riemannian*, elliptic) geometry, with curved geodesics, into the four-dimensional physical space-time system, made it possible to conceive the universe as unbounded, but closed and finite.

Matter (mass, inertia, and energy), space and time are thereby not independent, but represent a conjoint plenum. In other words, the geometry of space-time is determined by the presence of matter, that is to say space exists only where matter (mass and energy) are present, and time is merely the aspect of physical interactions as, e.g. manifested by the frequencies of cyclic processes.

In this respect, a true 'vacuum', entirely devoid of 'matter' in the form of electromagnetic or gravitational radiation, respectively of 'fields', would rep-

---

[37] It is here of interest to note that, in accelerating a body toward the boundary value c a progressively increasing inertia is manifested such that more and more of the required energy becomes converted into the body's mass [cf. e.g. *Davies*, 1977].

resent a fiction lacking 'reality'. A recent paper by *Greiner and Hamilton* [1980] discusses the problem 'Is the vacuum really empty?'. Although mathematically highly sophisticated, said paper ignores the epistemologic aspect of the problem at issue.

Empty as well as absolute space and time would have no existence, space being coincident with matter, and time with the succession of material events. An oscillating universe would thus not expand into empty space but would expand and contract the correlated space. It should here be recalled that *Schopenhauer*, although maintaining a differing, 'a priori' aspect of space and time, nevertheless already expressed concepts somewhat similar to those of *Einstein* and *Minkowski*. *Schopenhauer* stated that: '*Das Wesen der Materie in der gänzlichen Vereinigung von Raum and Zeit besteht*'. '*Innige Vereinigung von Raum und Zeit – Kausalität, Materie, Wirklichkeit – sind also Eines*' (Ed. *Grisebach*, vol. 1, p. 602).

In contradistinction to space, however, which can be conceived finite, physical time must be conceived without beginning and without end, if the postulate of causality is adopted, since this postulate implies an infinite regress and progress. A 'first cause' or a '*causa sui*' represent here a *contradictio in adjecto*.

Accepting the model of a pulsating universe as the most likely and suitable one for cosmology and cosmogony of the assumed physical world (cf. above p. 56), it can be seen that *Kant's* antinomy of cosmology (cf. above p. 59) does not hold, but must be answered by a third statement: the universe has no beginning nor end in time, but is finite in an unbounded *non-Euclidean* space which alternates between expansion and contraction.

With regard to the various theories of cosmogony mentioned above, there are of course several possibilities concerning space and time, of which the spatial ones shall be considered first.

(1) The stellar universe may be no more than a small island within an infinite empty space. 'Empty' has here the meaning 'devoid of mass', but not of 'energy', this 'empty' space being represented by the 'infinitely' expanding electromagnetic and gravitational 'waves' radiating from said 'island'. Quite evidently, with increasing distance, the 'infinite' or rather 'infinitely expanding' space would gradually become more and more 'tenuous'.

(2) The stellar universe may consist of an infinite number of stars and galaxies in infinite space.

(3) The universe is finite but unbounded such that proceeding along a geodesic one would ultimately return to one's point of departure, and no path whatsoever would lead out of this universe into an 'empty space'.

With respect to time it could be assumed:

(1) The universe started with a primordial explosion at zero time and from a zero state out of 'nothing'. It will finally expand into a state of

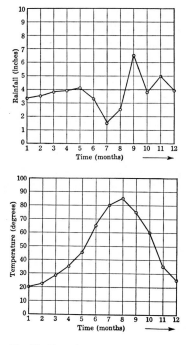

Fig. 12a. Two elementary graphs, illustrating events in a two-dimensional space-time. The ordinates represent the space dimension (depth of precipitation amount in top, hight of mercury column of thermometer in bottom), and the abscissae the time dimension. If the flow of time is reversed, symmetrical curves are obtained.

entropy,[38] as it were into an eternal state of heat (or rather cold) death according to the second law of thermodynamics. This would imply an infinitely expanding universe. A variant of this theory assumes that the 'singularity', that is to say the moment when the density of the universe was 'infinite' preceding the primordial fireball, resulted from an unexplained infinitely thin state an eternity ago, from which the universe contracted until it reached said maximum density [cf. *Gamow*, 1977]. Only two stages are thus presumed, namely, contraction out of figuratively 'nothingness' and unlimited as well as indefinite expansion into figuratively 'nothingness'.

(2) The universe pulsates in an endless cycle of recurring expansions and collapses.

---

[38] Entropy can be defined as a measure of energy, which due to an irreversible change, is not available to perform work in a thermodynamic system. It can also be conceived as irreversible degradation of energy, and as a measure of 'disorder'. Cf. also *K.* [1961, p. 343f.] concerning the application of the entropy and negentropy concepts to information theory.

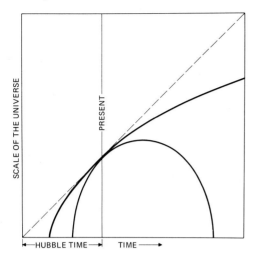

Fig. 12b. Three models of cosmic evolution based on concepts by *Friedmann* [from *Gott et al.*, 1977]. All three models must be consistent with the scale and rate of expansion observed today, so that all their curves must be tangent at the present moment. If the rate of expansion is unchanging (broken line) the age of the universe is *Hubble* time. Decelerating universes are younger, and both their history and their destiny depend on the magnitude of the deceleration. With modest deceleration the expansion continues indefinitely, albeit at an ever lower rate. Greater deceleration implies reversal of the expansion with final collapse. The infinitely expanding universe is said to be 'open' and the collapsing one 'closed'.

(3) The universe has always been and will always be as it is now, without beginning or end. This would for instance correspond to *Hoyle's* steady state universe with continuous creation out of 'nothing', but allowing for expansion and for evolution of galaxies and stars. The steady state theory with its diverse formulations qua details is, however, no longer in favor at present.

Figure 12b illustrates three models of cosmic evolution essentially based on the solutions of *Einstein's* cosmological equations provided by *Friedman*, who discovered an error, subsequently admitted by *Einstein*, in this latter's original proof for a static universe. Two of these models assume indefinite expansion in either *hyperbolic* space with negative curvature or *parabolic* (*Euclidean, flat*) space, and the third assumes final collapse in *elliptic* (*Riemannian*) space with positive curvature [cf. *Gott* et al., 1977].

The complex mathematics elaborated by the diverse cosmogonists remain quite unconvincing because the available knowledge concerning the nature of the universe still remains very incomplete, despite undeniable considerable progress. Thus, because of the constraints or parameters provided by numerous unknown boundary value conditions, impressive equations set up by mathematically proficient cosmologists may represent quite meaningless constructions.

Cosmologic and cosmogonic speculations are based on astronomy supplemented by extrapolations from physics, which latter, in turn, is based on terrestrial observations including laboratory experiments and on mathematics, both applied and 'pure'. The rationality and the logical foundations of the astronomic, physical, and mathematical principles thereby involved finally pertain to the domain of philosophy.

In this respect, and despite its apparent futility of endless cyclical repetitions, the model of a pulsating physical universe appears the least unlikely one. It is compatible with, although not necessarily required by, *Einstein's* concepts of relativity. The combined effects of the four main physical interactions, namely gravity, electromagnetism, strong, and weak particle interactions would result in transitory states of negentropy, that is of transient order out of disorder occurring in a strictly causal cosmic game of chance with 'loaded dice'. Gravitation plays here a role of both 'midwife' and 'undertaker' [*Davies*, 1977] in birth and death of a temporary universe. Again, in each newly born universe, its ultimate size and lifetime could be determined by random yet causal processes which might or might not be suitable for the evolution of life as obtaining in our present one. Finally one could ask whether these endless repetitions of combinations and permutations involving a presumably finite number of still unknown 'elementary particles' might swing back into a closed but random complete cycle[39] which, although infinite qua repetitions, would include an extremely large but still finite number of possible states.

With regard to the theory of cyclic primordial explosions and subsequent gravitational collapses of the universe it has been pointed out that this requires a sufficient amount of mass to overcome the outward expansion. According to some estimates, the mass in all the galaxies is said to be insufficient, but the additional mass in the intergalactic clouds has been assumed to provide all the required mass amount. This again has been questioned on the basis of X-ray recordings by a satellite (named *Einstein*), and some cosmologists therefore

---

[39] Thus, as in the case of a finite but unlimited space, an unlimited but finite conceptual time could be postulated, in which the 'future' extends into the 'past'. Mystics, such as *Nietzsche* ('*Ewige Wiederkunft*') and *Lafcadio Hearn*, have elaborated upon this concept. *Hearn* [*Gleamings in Buddha-Fields*, 1910] writes: 'Could you have looked back incomparably further than your power permitted, then the Past would have become for you the Future. And could you have endured even yet more, the Future would have orbed back for you into the Present.'
   'Yet why?' I murmured marvelling ... 'What is the Circle?'
   'Circle there is none', was the response; – Circle there is none but the great phantom-whirl of birth and death to which, by their own thoughts and deeds, the ignorant remain condemned. But this has being only in Time; and Time itself is illusion.'

assumed the probability of indefinite expansion. This, however, would imply a unique primordial explosion 'out of nothing', which involves greater 'logical' difficulties than the 'cyclic theory'. In favor of the latter it could be replied that all estimates qua mass of galaxies and amount of extragalactic gas clouds still remain very uncertain. In particular, the role played by neutron stars, black holes, quasars and related phenomena including the significance of the curved *Riemannian space-time* seem still poorly understood. Again, the very high velocities of the outward expansion indicated by the *Hubble constant* for the most distant galaxies refer to events more than a billion (10^9) years ago, and might well have considerably slowed down since that time.

Because of the numerous uncertainties, cosmologists will select as 'most probable' those models that appeal to them for other than purely 'logical' or 'scientific' reasons,[40] namely for esthetic, emotional, moral, and even 'metaphysical' or 'religious' reasons, which depend on mental attitudes conditioned by the cerebral mechanisms of affectivity.

Turning now from the evolution of the universe to that of our solar system with its planets, asteroids and comets, it could be said that present-day views represent modifications of the well-known *Kant-Laplace theory*, assuming a rotating hot gaseous mass. This theory was first suggested by *Kant* and subsequently elaborated in more rigorous mathematical terms by *Laplace*, but later was found to be deficient. It was then replaced by catastrophic tidal and planetesimal theories adapted from *Buffon's* earlier collision theory. More recently, however, *Alfvén, Kuiper, Lyttleton, McCrea, TerHaas, Weizsäcker, Woolfson*, and others have revived the notion of planets generated by a primordial sun condensing out of a gas cloud [cf. e.g. *Singh*, 1961; *Alfvén*, 1971; *McCrea*, 1975].

The rotating condensed sun remained surrounded by a perhaps cold solar nebula. In a sequence of electromagnetic interactions, turbulences and condensations, protoplanets of different sorts, breaking up into planets, satellites, and asteroids resulted. These latter, together with meteorites and comets, perhaps also some small satellites like those of *Mars* might represent what could be called 'cosmic debris'.

As regards the details, diverse, but not generally accepted theories of planetary evolution have been elaborated by the above-mentioned and other authors.

Protoplanets might be of a type generating planets of 'terrestrial type' such as *Mercury, Venus, Earth, Mars*, or of a type generating planets such as *Jupiter* and *Saturn*, these types differing in relative amount of heavy atoms and of light ones (*hydrogen* and *helium*).

---

[40] Cf. the discussion by *Singh* [1961, p. 9].

The relevant physical processes include condensation of dust from gas, gas turbulences, sediment formation, separation of different sorts of atomic matter, rotational variations and rotational instability. Depending on a diversity of factors, such events, which originated sun and planetary system, could also originate double stars and diverse sorts of rapidly rotating stars. Altogether, the planetary conditions suitable for origin of rudimentary organic life, not to speak of advanced, intelligent life such as displayed by Man, are considered by *McCrea* [1975] to be 'extremely rare'. This is also evidenced by our Solar system in which advanced forms of organic life are restricted to our own planet. Whether some rudimentary forms of life occur or have occurred on Mars is still a moot question at the time of this writing.[41] Likewise, although conditions suitable for life do not seem to obtain on Venus, the question remains whether some sort of life could not originate on that planet in the very distant future following cooling and appropriate chemical atmospheric changes. By that time, however, the Sun might already have reached its red giant stage and engulfed Venus.

Assuming an age of about 8 AE for our Universe in accordance with the relativistic and expanding model of the Cosmos, *Unsöld* [1975] assumes an age of about 4.5 AE for our planetary system whose early formative phase involved only a few million years.

The primordial Earth is supposed to have lacked oceans and atmosphere because of high temperature. On the Moon, a crust began already to form at 4.5 AE, while the first terrestrial crust dates back to only 3.7 AE, presumably because of the Earth's larger size. The earlier extremely heavy bombardment with large meteorites, some of which had a diameter of more than 100 km, that formed the craters displayed by Moon,[42] Mercury and Mars, did thus not

---

[41] The results of the experiments performed on *Mars* by the two Viking robot landers in 1976 remained inconclusive. While not definitely excluding a remote possibility that some primitive form of organic life occurs on that planet, the result of these experiments did not provide any proof for the occurrence of biologic processes. The areas on *Mars* examined by the two robot spacecrafts do not seem to be habitats of life [cf. e.g. *Horowitz*, 1977]. The very small amount of water observed on that planet suggests a lifeless *Mars*. However, it seems that, at an earlier time, flowing water may have been present and some organic life might have then occurred. Future explorations should provide more data concerning these questions.

[42] At the beginning of the century, astronomers and geologists were generally in favor of the view that the craters of the Moon were results of a great volcanic activity in former age, which had now ceased entirely [cf. *Baker*, 1932]. *Neumayr* [1920] supported '*Die Auffassung des Mondbildes als Ausdruck eines grossartigen Entgasungsvorganges*'. A few authors, however, suggested an origin of the craters from impact. By now, it is widely agreed that many, if not all the craters were formed by objects that struck the moon from the outside [*Hoyle*, 1975a]. This seems also to be the case for *Mercury*, whose surface is strikingly similar to that of the Moon, and to some extent also for the somewhat less Moon-like surface of *Mars*. This latter planet, however, appears to display a number of true (but perhaps extinct?) volcanoes.

leave its permanent trace on Earth. Here, the oceans and a primitive atmosphere, still lacking oxygen, gradually resulted from volcanic activities, and prebiotic systems (primitive Procaryotes) presumably originated about 3 AE ago. The nature, origin, and evolution of organic life shall be considered further below, following some comments on causality.

Figures 13a–c and 14a–d illustrate, with respect to size and time measurement, significant magnitudes obtaining in the assumed physical world as discussed in the present section. It should be emphasized that all spatial and temporal magnitudes are relative, that is to say are expressed as relationships in comparison with arbitrarily assumed standards. As *Berkeley* justly stressed, there is no 'absolute' or 'true' magnitude respectively 'size' of an object. In this connection it is of interest that Man, with regard to his size, stands, very roughly speaking, midway between the size of the known universe and that of the inferred smallest particles (cf. fig. 13c). Although measurements of size are generally based on the metric centimeter-gram-second system, Man's perceptual appreciation of size is evidently based upon the size relationships of his own body and nervous system to environmental magnitudes.

Relativity concepts, apparently first clearly discussed by *Berkeley* and subsequently elaborated by numerous authors particularly including *Mach* and *Poincaré*, became further expanded and rigorously formulated in the special and general relativity theories of *Einstein*, which completely eliminated *Newton's* concepts of absolute space and absolute time, implying, moreover, *Minkowski's* concept of four-dimensional space-time.

It is of interest, however, that *Newton* clearly recognized the significance of relative motion. He maintained, nevertheless, that 'absolute' motion could be distinguished from relative one by the detection of 'forces' (*vires impressae*), resulting in acceleration. In circular motion, there result centrifugal forces (*vires recedendi ab axe motus circularis*). The *Newtonian* system does indeed provide a means for determining what was considered 'absolute' acceleration of a body, since the force ($F = ma = g \times cm \times sec^{-2}$) acting on such body can be measured or calculated. Acceleration, however, is merely a measure of the change of velocity or position of a body, and does not determine its velocity or position in an absolute space. In accordance with *Einstein's* principle of equivalence, it is impossible to distinguish between the effects of accelerated motion and the effects of a gravitational field.

Mach's principle, claiming that the inertia displayed by a body (i.e. mass) is somehow due to the presence of other masses in the universe, has been supported by highly unconvincing and artificial reasoning. The flattening of the rotating earth resulting from the inertial tendency to fly off at the equator, that is through the action of centrifugal force, is supposed to be also displayed in a reference frame assuming a stationary earth at the center of a rotating universe. While such reference frame is theoretically admissible from the

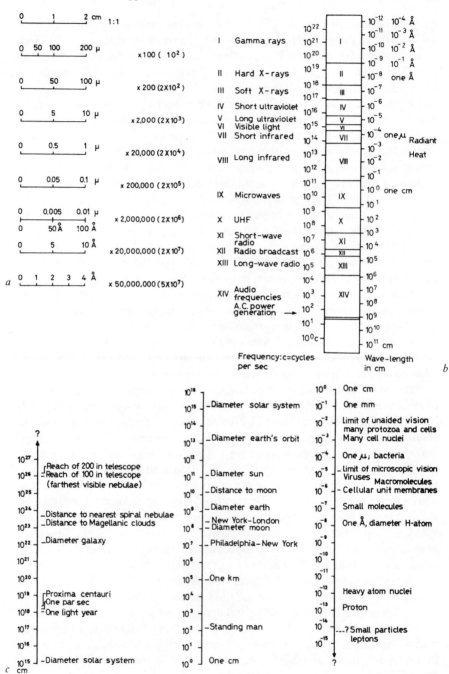

0   1   2 cm   1:1

0   50 100   200 μ   x100 (10²)

0   50   100 μ   x 200 (2X10²)

0   5   10 μ   x 2,000 (2 x 10³)

0   0.5   1 μ   x 20,000 (2 X 10⁴)

0   0.05   0.1 μ   x 200,000 (2X10⁵)

0   0.005   0.01 μ   x 2,000,000 (2X10⁶)
0   50 Å   100 Å

0   5   10 Å   x 20,000,000 (2X10⁷)

a   0   1   2   3   4 Å   x 50,000,000 (5X10⁷)

I	Gamma rays	10^{22} 10^{21} 10^{20}	I	10^{-12} 10^{-4} Å 10^{-11} 10^{-3} Å 10^{-10} 10^{-2} Å

I   Gamma rays 10^{22} / 10^{21} / 10^{20} I 10^{-12} 10^{-4} Å / 10^{-11} 10^{-3} Å / 10^{-10} 10^{-2} Å

10^{19} 10^{-9} 10^{-1} Å

II   Hard X-rays 10^{18} II 10^{-8} one Å

III   Soft X-rays 10^{17} III 10^{-7}

IV   Short ultraviolet 10^{16} IV 10^{-6}

V   Long ultraviolet 10^{15} V 10^{-5}
VI   Visible light   VI
VII   Short infrared 10^{14} VII 10^{-4} one μ Radiant

VIII Long infrared 10^{13} VIII 10^{-3} / 10^{-2} Heat
                           10^{12}
                           10^{11} 10^{-1}

IX   Microwaves 10^{10} IX 10^{0} one cm
                           10^{9} 10^{1}

X   UHF 10^{8} X 10^{2}
                           10^{7} 10^{3}
XI   Short-wave radio   XI 10^{4}
XII   Radio broadcast 10^{6} XII
XIII Long-wave radio 10^{5} XIII 10^{5}

                           10^{4} 10^{6}
                           10^{3} XIV 10^{7}
XIV   Audio frequencies
      A.C. power generation → 10^{2} 10^{8}
                           10^{1} 10^{9}
                           10^{0} c 10^{10}
                                               10^{11} cm

Frequency: c = cycles per sec   Wave-length in cm   b

10^{16}
10^{15} – Diameter solar system 10^{0} – One cm
10^{14} 10^{-1} – One mm
                                           10^{-2} – Limit of unaided vision
10^{13} – Diameter earth's orbit   many protozoa and cells
                                           10^{-3} – Many cell nuclei

? ↑
10^{27} 10^{12} 10^{-4} – One μ; bacteria
10^{26} – ⌐ Reach of 200 in telescope
         ⌐ Reach of 100 in telescope 10^{11} – Diameter sun 10^{-5} – Limit of microscopic vision
           (farthest visible nebulae)   Viruses
10^{25} 10^{10} – Distance to moon   Macromolecules
                                                            10^{-6} – Cellular unit membranes
10^{24} – Distance to nearest spiral nebula 10^{9} – Diameter earth 10^{-7} – Small molecules
10^{23} – Distance to Magellanic clouds 10^{8} – New York–London
                                                – Diameter moon 10^{-8} – One Å, diameter H-atom
10^{22} – Diameter galaxy 10^{7} – Philadelphia–New York 10^{-9}
10^{21} 10^{6} 10^{-10}
10^{20} 10^{5} – One km 10^{-11}
10^{19} – ⌐ Proxima centauri 10^{4} 10^{-12} – Heavy atom nuclei
         ⌐ One par sec
10^{18} – One light year 10^{3} 10^{-13} – Proton
10^{17} 10^{2} – Standing man 10^{-14}
10^{16} 10^{1} 10^{-15} – ...? Small particles
10^{15} – Diameter solar system 10^{0} – One cm   leptons
c cm   ?

viewpoint of pure kinematics in accordance with the theories of relativity, it is, nevertheless, entirely ruled out from a valid viewpoint of dynamics. It would presuppose fantastic circular velocities far beyond the constant c for said 'rotating universe'.

It is then further argued that if fewer bodies were present in the 'rotating universe', the earth would become less flattened. Returning to a reference frame assuming a rotating earth in an 'empty universe', the earth would furthermore not be flattened at all.

However, since the inertia of a body depends upon its energy content, a rotating earth in a fictional 'empty universe' can still be assumed to display typical flattening by centrifugal forces and to manifest the *Foucault* pendulum phenomenon. The rotation of such earth would take place in a reference frame with respect to orbiting and spinning intra-atomic motions of its own interior. One might ask, moreover, how, since any external object would be lacking in an 'empty universe', a rotating earth would otherwise at all be distinguished from a stationary one. This question, however, can be answered by pointing out the displacement of the rotating earth's surface to the direction of electromagnetic quanta (e.g. 'heat' or 'light') emitted from that surface, but this would require an external observer stationary with respect to the earth's rotation.

With regard to numerical magnitudes, it is of interest that several authors, notably *Eddington* [1928, 1929, 1939] and *Dirac* [1963 et passim], have constructed a series of dimensionless numbers from diverse primitive constants of physics. *Eddingtons* 'fine structure constant',

$$\frac{hc}{2\pi e^2}$$

Fig. 13a. Scales, beginning with a standard metric scale displaying centimeters in natural size, superposed to illustrate orders of magnitude up to a linear magnification of 5×10^7 (50 million). An ångström (Å) roughly corresponds to the diameter of a hydrogen atom. The scales are approximate, i.e. not rigorously 'accurate' but should give a correct idea of the orders of magnitude involved at different levels of optic or ultrastructural resolution [from *K.*, 1970].

Fig. 13b. Scales in power of 10, approximately correlating frequency and wavelength of electromagnetic radiation phenomena. The 'dualistic' nature of electromagnetic radiation is such that, within the region of long waves, the 'wave-like' characteristics are strongly predominant, while in the short-wave region, such as pertaining to X-rays, the 'corpuscular' characteristics, displayed by 'photons', are more obvious. This, of course, is related to the increase of energy concomitant with increasing frequency and decreasing wavelength [from *K.*, 1970].

Fig. 13c. Scales in power of 10, approximately indicating, with respect to the g·cm·sec system, a number of significant magnitudes pertaining to the physical world. The notation is not logarithmic, but roughly involves multiples from 1 to 9.9, of integer powers of ten [from *K.*, 1970]. Read parsec instead of par sec.

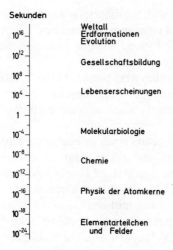

Sekunden

10^{16}	Weltall Erdformationen Evolution
10^{12}	Gesellschaftsbildung
10^{8}	
10^{4}	Lebenserscheinungen
1	
10^{-4}	Molekularbiologie
10^{-8}	Chemie
10^{-12}	
10^{-16}	Physik der Atomkerne
10^{-18}	
10^{-24}	Elementarteilchen und Felder

Fig. 14a. Time scale in seconds, indicating duration of a variety of events, as well as 'age' of certain states, stages, happenings, configurations or systems which provide assumed characteristic reference data ('*Fixpunkte*' according to *Eigen*) of our experiences, i.e. phenomena and inferred interphenomena [after *Eigen*, 1966, from *K.*, 1973a].

Periode	Sekunden	Lebensdauer
	$-10^{16}-$	^{238}U
	$- \quad -$	
Erdpräzession	$-10^{12}-$	
	$- \quad -$	^{14}C
Erdumlauf	$-10^{8}-$	
Mondumlauf	$- \quad -$	
Erddrehung	$-10^{4}-$	
	$- \quad -$	Neutron
	$-10^{0}-$	
	$- \quad -$	
	$-10^{-4}-$	
	$- \quad -$	Myon (μ^-)
Kernpräzession	$-10^{-8}-$	Mesonen ($\pi^+_,\pi^-_,K^+_,K^-$)
(bei 10^4 Gauß)	$- \quad -$	Hyperonen
	$-10^{-12}-$	($\Lambda,\Sigma^+,\Sigma^-,\Xi^-$)
Molekülschwingung		
Atomschwingung	$-10^{-16}-$	π°-Meson
	$- \quad -$	
	$-10^{-20}-$	
Kernschwingung	$- \quad -$	
	$-10^{-24}-$	???

Fig. 14b. Time-constants of physics, including nuclear and astronomic events. The term '*Lebensdauer*' refers to the 'half-life' of radioactive substances referred to above on page 15 [after *Eigen*, 1966, from *K.*, 1973a].

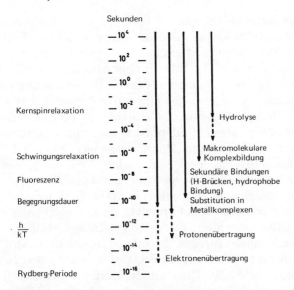

Fig. 14c. Time constants of some chemical reactions compared with a few periods significant for small-scale physical events. The suffix 'relaxation' refers to time constants based on the exponential law [after *Eigen*, 1966, from *K.*, 1973a].

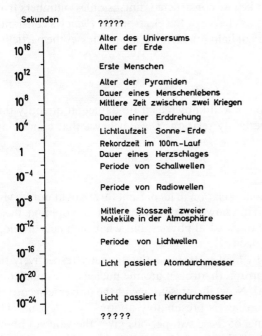

Fig. 14d. Time constants significant for cosmic evolution [after *Eigen*, 1966, from *K.*, 1973a].

derived from *Planck's* constant h, the speed of light, c, and the charge of an electron (e) is a 'pure number' which has the value of approximately 137. The so-called 'force constant' is the ratio of electrical and gravitational forces between an electron and a proton. Its value is approximately 2.3×10^{39}. Another such number is the cosmical number N purporting to represent the total number of elementary particles in the universe and estimated at approximately 1.4×10^{79}. It is presumed that, in terms of such 'pure numbers', of which *Eddington* introduced about 16, all physical facts can be expressed. Some cosmologists, e.g. *Whittaker* and *Milne*, were much impressed by *Eddington's* elaboration and considered said author to be a 'modern Archimedes'. For others, however, *Eddington's* attempt to establish the constants of nature by pure calculation, carries no conviction. Thus, the derivation of the 'fine structure constant' fails to provide any new elucidation of electron-photon interaction. Moreover, *Eddington's* deduction, from his 'a priori' principles, of the observed speed of the galactic recessions, yielded a figure close to the earlier erroneous values calculated by *Hubble* and subsequently greatly reduced by *Baade*. There are therefore good reasons for questioning the significance of the *Eddington* numbers, despite the diverse strange coincidences, in several instances, between their deduced and the actually observed values.

Dirac [1963 et passim] likewise constructed dimensionless numbers from fundamental constants such as charge of the electron (e), *Planck's* constant h divided by 2, and the velocity of light (c). Here, he again stresses the particular value

$$\frac{hc}{2\pi e^2}$$

close to 137. This expression is well known as a fundamental quantity that occurs in *Heisenberg's* uncertainty relation. *Dirac* believes that c and e are fundamental, but that

$$\frac{hc}{2\pi e^2}$$

is derived. Thus, the uncertainty relation in its present form might not survive in the physics of the future. This, however, does not, in *Dirac's* opinion, mean a return to the determinism of classical physics, but what such new developments will be, *Dirac* leaves open.

Again, the time taken by light to traverse the diameter respectively the radius of an electron or a proton (hydrogen atomic nucleus) is estimated at about 10^{-23} sec (cf. fig. 13a). Now, the present age of the universe according to *Hubble's* revised recession law is presumably about 7×10^9 years. The ratio, in atomic units of time, of these two periods gives the value of about 2.4×10^{39}, which is one of the *Eddington* numbers mentioned above. There is, moreover, indeed a remarkable coincidence between large dimensionless numbers of the order of magnitude 10^{39} and 10^{79}, but *Dirac* infers that these numbers vary with the epoch of their observation and assumes that the constant of gravitation varies inversely with the age of the universe. This, however, leads to substantial difficulties and may not agree with better supported contradictory evidence.

Considerable scepticism concerning the significance of these pure numbers and of their interrelationships seems advisable. Dimensional analysis and the concept of 'dimensionless numbers' were briefly discussed from an elementary viewpoint in volume 1, page 285 of the present authors series on *The Central Nervous System of Vertebrates* [*K.*, 1967a]. Much the same could be said about the outlandish results of various mathematical speculations attempting to describe events in 'black holes' and their immediate neighborhood. The publication by *Davies* [1977] contains lengthy accounts of several such attempts. It is evident that no observational data are available concerning details of the behavior of matter (mass and energy) at these superdense states. This lack of data precludes meaningful mathematical formulations. Constructs such as a 'singularity', referring to a 'single mathematical point of infinite density' can be evaluated as mathematical gobbledygook.

With regard to cosmology and cosmogony, two appropriate postulates are usually made, which are known as 'cosmologic principles'. The first one holds that the same physical laws obtain everywhere and at all times in the universe. Although not rigorously provable and questioned by some, this principle appears strongly supported by the data of spectroscopy which disclose the same sort of physical matter (atoms, etc.) in the entire astronomically observable universe. Since, in the aspect under consideration, organic life is also a physical (physicochemical) phenomenon, the same biological laws, discussed in section 3, p. 101f. of the present chapter, could likewise be presumed to obtain in all regions of the universe where the necessary conditions for origin and evolution of life become realized. The second cosmologic principle assumes that the large-scale structure of the universe is the same in all directions (*isotropic*) and also the same when seen from different localities (*homogeneous*).

2. Causality

Stripped of all mathematical details, the physical world is now conceived as consisting of highly abstract, as it were 'empty' movable magnitudes and magnitudes of motion in a space-time system. Some of these magnitudes have a property measurable as mass, others a property measurable as energy, the two being convertible into each other. Energy and mass are likewise highly abstract quantities whose mode of change of distribution is subject to formulated laws: mass as a movable magnitude in terms of magnitude of motion and energy as a magnitude of motion in terms of movable magnitudes. The magnitudes are unevenly distributed in space; small regions contain great amounts of magnitudes, again absorbing or emitting magnitudes. In addition, this distribution displays an order of significant patterns, leading to the concept of fields as well as to the concepts of particles, atoms, and molecules. A large number of complicated periodic processes[43] can be inferred and formulated in mathematical terms. In general, as regards magnitudes, quantitative, that is numerical statements can be made, and as regards patterns, topologic and qualitative assertions are possible, which do not always necessarily involve particular numbers. Above a certain level of magnitude the orderliness of the physical world can here be described as strictly determined in accordance with the law of causality.

Causality may be defined as an expression of the orderly succession of events in the physical world, such that in a system of related states involving mass, force, or energy, all changes are characterized as events manifesting certain invariants expressible as 'rules', 'laws', or 'norms' and thereby follow one another in a constant, rigidly determined fashion. Since this occurs in time which has a direction or vector property, it is possible to fractionalize the occurrence in an arbitrary manner, as it were by a '*Dedekind cut*' separating cause and effect, thereby assuming that any state represents an effect preceded by another state as a cause. Any effect is, upon its occurrence, a change and implies as its cause a previous change which in turn is the effect of an earlier change.[44] These connections can be designated as a causal chain or causal line which implies spatial and temporal continuity. The requirement of spatial continuity thus excludes the notion of 'action at a distance'.[45] There is no logical limit to causal succession upstream or downstream the flow of time.

---

[43] It is of interest that *Descartes* (1596–1650), in his attempts at reducing all physical phenomena to mechanics, eliminating action at a distance, correctly although rather vaguely, anticipated present-day atomic concepts by his theory of vortices. Quite evidently, the various orbiting, spinning and other periodic processes characterize, figuratively speaking, atoms and particles as whirling vortex rings. This was also, about 1867, suggested by *William Thomson* [cf. *Whittaker*, 1948]. *Descartes* particularly made use of the vortex theory in attempting to explain gravitation. Generally speaking, the vortices of *Cartesian* physics represent whirling figures presumed to explain the differentiation, on geometrical and mechanical principles, of pure extension into various kinds of bodies.

[44] A cause might thus also be conceived as a change in a variable or parameter in accordance with *Ashby's* [1952] terminology.

[45] In *Newton's* system, gravitation apparently implied 'action at a distance', but *Newton* himself denied the possibility of such action. In a letter to *Bentley* he stated: 'that gravity should be innate, inherent, and essential to matter, so that one body may act upon another at a distance

Again, with reference to this vector property, it is easier to predict the effect of a cause than to infer the cause from an effect, since identical or closely similar states (effects) may result from different causes, while in a system of definite variables a cause (definite change) will have only one definite (simple or complex) effect. In our interpretation against the direction of the temporal flow we are thus faced with possible dichotomies of the causal lines, as *J. S. Mill* emphasized in his doctrine of the plurality of causes. This is not the case in the direction of the flow, if all significant variables of the initial state are known. Added difficulties, besides uncertainties concerning the initial states as well as inferences against the direction of temporal flow, are inherent in the multiplicity of events in a system, resulting in multiple causality involving contributory and jointly effective conditions or changes. There are thus not only dichotomies but actually multiple intersections of interweaving causal lines. Thus, in *Ashby's* terminology, an effect would represent a transform which does not necessarily indicate an unique operand.

In mathematical formulation, causal sequences can be conceived in terms of differential equations which express the relation between two states following each other at an 'infinitesimal' (i.e. negligible) separation in time:

$$\frac{dx}{dt} = \text{the limit of } \frac{x_2 - x_1}{t_2 - t_1} \text{ for } t_2 - t_1 \to 0.$$

This may be called the *Newtonian concept of causality* which implies predictability as a significant aspect. Many physicists have therefore emphasized predictability as the essential feature of causality. This is indeed the case in the direction of the temporal succession, if all significant variables of the initial state would be known. In many instances, however, unknown variables, factors, or parameters obtain. There is thus no justification to consider unpredictable events as not caused, or to equate predictability with causality.

In the succession of events many recurrent states, characterized by invariants, ensue. The concept of causality is thus confirmed and strengthened, but this concept does by no means refer only to such recurring states.

---

through a vacuum, without the mediation of any thing else, by and through which their action and force may be conveyed from one to another, is to me so great an absurdity, that I believe no man, who has in philosophical matters a competent faculty of thinking, can ever fall into it' [quoted after *Cajori*, in *K.*, 1961, p. 151, fn.9]. In contemporary physics, gravity is either, *qua* kinematics, a geometrical property of the space-time plenum (*Einstein*), or *qua* dynamics, is presumably mediated by energy quanta (gravitons) with the speed c. Some recent authors [cf. *Kolata*, 1977b] have confused alleged 'action at a distance' in DNA molecules with the transmission of an effect along a molecular strand, such that, as here naively expressed, one of the molecules 'knows' what is happening at the other end. Less naively, it should have been said that one end of the molecule can register what is happening at the other end.

It will be seen that the here adopted definition, according to which a cause represents a change in a physical state [*Schopenhauer*, 1847], refers exclusively to the third of the four classical causes expounded by *Aristotle* and the *Scholastics*, and enumerated as material, formal, efficient, and final.

Necessity or *determination* of a physical event is the relationship of that event to its causal chain. *Chance* is a negative term with several denotations and connotations, thereby involving considerable ambiguity and vagueness. Its two main meanings are (a) lack of a causal connection, and (b) lack of purpose, (a) being thus 'objective', and (b) 'subjective'.

With respect to (a), the lack of a causal connection (i.e. of a cause) may either be true, which does not seem likely if the principle *ex nihilo nihil fit* is valid for the physical world, or may merely be apparent, because the causal data remain unknown.[46] Events are simultaneously determined and chanced: determined in relation to their significant cause, and chanced in respect to other, not directly related events. This was expressed by *Schopenhauer* as '*Einheit des Zufälligen und des Notwendigen*'.

Mach [1896] justly stated that '*wenn wir die Tatsachen in Gedanken nachbilden, so bilden wir niemals die Tatsachen überhaupt ab, sondern nur nach jener Seite, die für uns wichtig ist; ... unsere Nachbildungen sind immer Abstraktionen*'.

'*Wenn wir von Ursache und Wirkung sprechen, so heben wir willkürlich jene Momente heraus, auf deren Zusammenhang wir bei Nachbildung einer Tatsache in der für uns wichtigen Richtung zu achten haben*'. This is known as '*der denkökonomische Ursachenbegriff*' [cf. also *Winterstein*, 1928].

One could also conceive '*chance*' as the intersection of two or more separate or different causal lines. Thus, if a workman, repairing a roof, through a misjudged movement drops a tile, which accidentally happens to hit a person who steps out of the house door at that moment, such intersection of causal lines obtains. Yet, all thereby involved events can be regarded as strictly causal, although unpredictable in the relevant aspects under consideration. It could also be said that the accident was fortuitous, occurring by chance without intent, purpose, or design. Besides '*fortuitous*', the terms '*haphazard*', and '*random*' are related to 'chance' and especially denote lack of particular plan, of definable order, of definable pattern, of definable direction, and of purpose. The term '*happen*' may also signify 'occurring by chance', but, since 'happen' does also mean 'to come into being', one can, on the other hand, refer to 'causal happenings'.

---

[46] *David Hume* (1739) justly remarks 'that what the vulgar call chance is nothing but a secret and concealed cause' (I, e, Section XII: 'Of the probability of chance'). This is said to be properly understood ('commonly allowed') by philosophers.

Chance, again, is related to *possibility* and *probability*. Both these latter terms involve *uncertainty*, that is to say lack of 'complete' or sufficient knowledge (information) in the particular aspect under consideration.

Given a set of rules obtaining for a certain domain of events, any event can be considered possible, if the assumption of that event does not contradict the postulated rules, or, in other words, if that event would occur in accordance with the postulated orderliness. One might also use the term 'permissible' in characterizing the assumption of a possible event.

It is much more difficult to define probable and probability. These concepts imply, in *Craik's* [1943] phraseology, 'a curious combination of psychological and mathematical and empirical conditions'. Probability, inter alia, involves 'expectation'. Tentatively, we might also say that probability involves extrapolation, namely the determining, in conformity with the orderliness assumed in a domain comprising presumably known events, of events outside that domain. Some such events may be expressed in terms of numerical value. In this latter instance it is customary to measure probability on a scale marked zero at one end, and unity at the other: $p = 0$, and $p = 1$. Unity represents complete or absolute probability which, as the limit is approached, merges with what might (perhaps wrongly) be called 'absolute certainty'. As the limit zero is reached, we have here 'absolute improbability', merging with what could be called 'absolute impossibility'.[47]

In discussion of elementary probability problems, the tossing of a coin is a traditional model. It is assumed that, in the aspect under consideration, a tossed coin must come to rest on one of its surfaces, and it will be designated, by its free surface, as either head (H) or tail (T). It is next assumed that these two different events are equally probable (or equiprobable). What does this mean? That, in the conceptual model, we do not postulate a sufficient reason for the occurrence of either H or T, although one of the two must necessarily result. In other words, as regards H or T, *non datur ratio cur potius sit*, quam non sit. It is interesting to note that we have here introduced the principle of nonsufficient reason. This represents, in the case under consideration, merely a lack of knowledge or of information. It is, moreover, evident that this traditional model excludes unnecessary complicating parameters. The tossed coin must come to rest on an even, horizontal surface. Quite obviously, if the surface is irregular, e.g. with narrowing channels of a certain depth, the tossed coin might roll into such a channel and come to rest on its edge.

In numerical terms, we have here the probabilities H 0.5 and T 0.5, adding up to 1. *Mutatis mutandis*, in the case of a die, we have six surfaces (1–6), upon one of which, following a throw, it will come to rest. Assuming equiprob-

What is the probability that Jesus walked on water? rose from the dead?

---

[47] Further elaborations on chance and probability with regard to relevant epistemological aspects are given in §65–70, pp. 303–399 of the author's monograph *Mind and Matter* [K., 1961].

ability, the probability of any upper surface will be 1/6, again adding up to 1. Thus, the probability of throwing a six will be 1/6, and that of not throwing a six will be 5/6. If the die is 'loaded', the probabilities will be altered in favor of the upper surface opposite to the 'loaded' one, and can be ascertained by observation and averaging of repeated trials, but will still add to 1.

Again, the tossing of a coin or the throwing of dice can be considered strictly causal events in accordance with the 'laws' of classical mechanics, although relevant details of these events remain unascertainable. Yet the outcome of these uncertain events remains statistically predictable in terms of probabilities whose numerical aspects (2 respectively 1/2 in case of the coin, 6 respectively 1/6 in case of the die) are determined by the obtaining constraints or parameters. Thus, in cases such as coins and dice, probabilities are calculated on the basis of rather exact knowledge concerning type and number of possible but random events. Such events involving 'chance' or 'probability' are also designated as *stochastic*.

If relevant knowledge concerning number, 'degree of freedom', type or other details concerning possible events does not obtain, diverse other procedures for the determination of probabilities become necessary. Thus, numerical data on probabilities which cannot be calculated 'a priori' may be empirically ascertained by registration, recording, and averaging a large number of instances concerning group phenomena, as e.g. in actuarial life expectancy tables based on vital statistics,[48] or in predicting the approximate number (i.e. its order of magnitude) of fatal traffic accidents over an American holiday weekend.

The '*law of large numbers*', which is still poorly understood, plays an important role with regard to probabilities and statistics. It states that the deviations from a mean or average ('*Streuung eines Mittelwertes*') decrease with increasing number of elements (or increasing size of the sample). The best known formulation of that 'law' is given by *Bernoulli's theorem* which can be expressed as follows. Let p be the probability of the event A on a trial, and m/n the observed proportion of the event in n trials, then the probability that

$$\left[\frac{m}{n} - p \right] < \varepsilon$$

has a limit of one as n $\rightarrow \infty$ for any arbitrary ε. A slightly different but essentially similar formulation is expressed in *Tchebycheff's theorem*, whose details can here be omitted.

---

[48] Cf. the discussion of statistics in §65–70 of *K*. [1961] mentioned in the preceding footnote. Among the problems there considered are binomial distribution, *Gaussian* curve, random walk, disorderly motion including *Brownian* motion, *Buffon's* needle problem, ergodic processes, entropy and negentropy, moreover cryptography and cryptanalysis.

The '*law of large numbers*' is a purely empirical one, and leads to a *circulus vitiosus* if an attempt is made to define by it probabilities which, in turn, are the presupposition for the validity of the mathematical theorem [cf. e.g. the comments by *Jaffé*, 1954].

An important application of the 'law of large numbers' is implied in the *kinetic theory of gases*, which 'explains' the mechanical and thermodynamic properties of an 'ideal' gas from the average behavior of its molecules. This involves the so-called '*principle of molecular chaos*' such that in absence of external forces all positions and all directions of velocity of the molecules are equally probable. It is here convenient to use *Hamilton's* formulation of *Newton's* laws. This concerns a system of particles described by any coordinates $q_1, q_2, \ldots$; then, the potential energy is a function of these, $V(q_1, q_2, \ldots)$ or short Vq, and the kinetic energy T is a function of both the coordinates and the generalized velocities $\dot{q}_1, \dot{q}_2, \ldots$ T. The generalized momenta are defined as

$$p_\alpha = \frac{\partial T}{\partial \dot{q}_\alpha}$$

and the total energy $T + V$ becomes a function of q_α and p_α. This function $T + V = H(q, p)$ is designated as the *Hamiltonian*. The equations of motion assume the 'canonical' forms

$$\dot{q}_\alpha = \frac{\partial H}{\partial p_\alpha}, \quad \dot{p}_\alpha = -\frac{\partial H}{\partial \dot{q}_\alpha}$$

from which one reads at once the conservation law of energy

$$\frac{dH}{dt} = 0, \quad H = \text{const.}$$

As regards the above-mentioned 'molecular chaos' the statistical behavior of any future state is then completely determined by the laws of mechanics. This is in particular the case for 'statistical equilibrium', where the equation of motion in Hamilton's 'canonical form' can be used. The distribution is described by a function $f(t, q_1, q_2, \ldots q_n, p_1, p_2, \ldots p_n)$ of all coordinates and momenta, and of time, such that fdpdq is the probability for finding the system at time t in a given element.

Boltzmann, in elaborating on the statistics of molecular collisions, used the term '*Stosszahlansatz*' anent the assumption of 'molecular chaos' and adopted the H-theorem in a modified form, where H is not the *Hamiltonian* of the whole system but that of a single molecule. The resulting averaging is the expression of our ignorance of the actual microscopic situation. *Boltzmann's theorem* claims that his equation, mixing mechanical knowledge with ignorance of details, leads to irreversibility. This latter is related to the second law of thermodynamics where the degree of irreversibility or 'degradation' can be expressed in terms of entropy[49] which also involves the concept of a 'closed system'.

There are, moreover, numerous still open and controversial questions concerning neglected parameters and various objections to mathematical aspects involved in the kinetic theory of gases and its extension to statistical mechanics in general. The interested reader with adequate mathematical training may be referred for further details to *Born's* [1964] treatise, use of which was made by the present author as regards diverse points of the preceding discussion. In nonmathematical terms, these questions are also ably discussed in *Jaffé's* [1954] publication.

Brief mention also should be made here of the '*ergodic*' hypothesis concerning the behavior of such mechanical systems which have the property that each particular motion, when continued indefinitely, passes through every configuration and state of motion of the system, compatible with the value of the total energy. The probability that any state will never recur is thereby given as zero. Yet, several meanings and interpretations of the ergodic concept can be maintained or disputed.

Reverting now to the relationship of 'chance' to 'causality', we may have two different, spatially separated causal sequences whereby one of the effects follows that of the other such that no causal line interconnects their sequence. Thus, in the two clocks of *Geulinx*, one strikes the hour exactly before the other does, whereby the circumstance *post hoc sed non propter hoc*, is displayed. It has therefore been pointed out that, when two events have a space-like interval not traversed by force respectively energy transmission, there can be no direct causal relation between them. This is doubtless partly true, but appears as a questionable generalization. All events in a universe representing a system or set can furthermore be presumed to be connected by common causal ancestors. We might therefore also define causality as the orderly interaction of spatially related events.

As a preliminary summary, the following statements seem appropriate:

(1) '*Causality*' postulates that there are 'laws' according to which the occurrence of a physical 'event' or 'state' B of a certain class depends on a *previous change* manifested by a physical event A which, in this respect, may pertain to another class.[50] A is called the *cause*, B the *effect*.

---

[49] Cf. the references given in the preceding footnotes 47 and 48.

[50] May, but not must. In acceleration as e.g. 'caused' by the interaction of gravity, A is of the same 'class' as B, namely the additional 'impact' of 'gravitons', expressed by change in the parameter time. In the firing of a gun, the mechanical impact (cause) pertains to another 'class' than the triggered explosion (effect) manifested by release of potential chemical energy. We have here a 'step function' in *Ashby's* sense, related to the recent mathematical concept of so-called 'catastrophe theory' briefly discussed further below, p. 90.

(2) '*Determinism*' postulates that physical events at different times are connected in such a way that these events are '*necessary*', that is to say are as they are and could not be or have occurred otherwise, in accordance with the 'law of causality'. This involves the possibility, by extrapolation from the present, of *prediction* of future events, and of cognizance of past events if, but only if, the relevant causal data are known.

(3) *Antecedence* postulates that the cause must be prior to the effect. In case of continuous interaction which gives the impression that cause may be simultaneous with effect, antecedent cause and subsequent effect in the continuous sequence of events can still be separated by a '*Dedekind cut*'.

(4) *Contiguity* postulates that cause and effect are in spatial contact or connected by a chain of intermediate physical events ultimately involving contact.[51]

Causality is, moreover, the application of the principle of sufficient reason to the interpretation of events in the physical world. This principle is in its generalized form a statement of universal orderly relationship whose applications were first systematically examined by *Aristotle*; as reformulated by *Christian Wolff* and subsequently analyzed by *Schopenhauer* [1847] it was expressed as follows: '*Nihil est sine ratione cur potius sit, quam non sit.*' It is an axiomatic truth which cannot be proved, since this would lead to the circulus vitiosus of requiring a proof for the requirement of a proof.[52]

Since, in the present context, the discussion is essentially restricted to causality, the diverse other applications and the overall significance of the principle of sufficient reason shall be considered further below, at the end of the present chapter II. However, it will here be appropriate to mention, for a preliminary approach, the four applications of this principle distinguished by *Schopenhauer*, whose treatise '*Über die vierfache Wurzel des Satzes vom zureichenden Grunde*' [1813, 1847] remains of fundamental importance despite several weaknesses and some instances of faulty reasoning as shall be pointed

---

[51] These definitions of causality, determinism, antecedence, and contiguity are modified after those given by *Born* [1964, p. 9], who apparently was not acquainted with *Schopenhauer's* treatise on the principle of sufficient reason and thus failed to emphasize cause as a change; he thereby included 'objects', which, *per se*, are not changes, wrongly as causes. *Born*, moreover, equates determinism with predictability. This represents both a semantic and logical weakness if not outright error.

[52] *Schopenhauer* [ed. *Grisebach*, vol. 3, p. 173] states: '*Denn der Satz vom zureichenden Grunde ist das Prinzip aller Erklärung; eine Sache erklären heisst ihren gegebenen Bestand oder Zusammenhang zurückführen auf irgendeine Gestaltung des Satzes vom Grunde selbst, der gemäss er seyn muss wie er ist. Diesem gemäss ist der Satz vom Grunde selbst, d.h. der Zusammenhang, den er, in irgend einer Gestalt ausdrückt, nicht weiter erklärbar; weil es kein Prinzip gibt, das Prinzip aller Erklärung zu erklären*'. In volume 5, page 442 *Schopenhauer* refers to the '*Leitfaden des Satzes vom Grunde, diesem Element der Relationen*'.

out below. Much of the confusion, noticeable to the competent and critical reader, which is evident in present-day writings on causality, determinism, indeterminism, chance and necessity can be traced to the fact that such writers were unacquainted with, or failed to understand, the cited basic treatise.

The four applications of the principle of sufficient reason pointed out by *Schopenhauer* are: (1) to physical events, as causality; (2) to logical processes as ground of knowledge or reason; (3) to formal (conceptual) space-time relationships as topological, geometric, arithmetic and algebraic orderliness; and (4) to conscious, intended action as motivation. In latinized formulation, this classification is given as: *principium rationis sufficientis fiendi, cognoscendi, essendi, agendi*. The merits of this classification lie in the clear distinction between the reason for a logical conclusion or valid inference, and the cause of an event. It prevents such legerdemain as '*causa sive ratio*' (related to the ontologic argument), and indicates the fallacies of such notions as '*causa sui*' and '*first cause*' related to the cosmologic argument. Following *Kant*, the concept of a priorism is stressed, but cannot be upheld.

The scepticism of *Hume* [1739, 1748], directed against many ambiguities and contradictions in ordinary thinking, greatly contributed to the subsequent advances in philosophy. *Hume* clearly showed that our 'idea of causation' is derived from experience and involves both contiguity and succession. That a particular cause must necessarily have a particular effect is inferred from their constant conjunction and it is thereby concluded that such particular causes must necessarily have such particular effects. 'We suppose, but are never able to prove, that there must be a resemblance betwixt those objects of which we have had experience, and those which lie beyond the reach of our discovery'.

'We have no other notion of cause and effect, but that of certain objects, which have been always conjoined together, and which in all past instances have been inseparable. We cannot penetrate into the reason of the conjunction.'

The weaknesses in *Hume's* highly important and essentially valid argumentation on causality concern three main points.

(1) *Hume* speaks of 'objects' as 'causes'. He failed to realize that causal sequences represent successions of events[53] and that, as *Schopenhauer* subsequently pointed out, a cause should be conceived as a change, but not as an 'object'.

---

[53] *In Schopenhauer's* phraseology: '*Ursache ist stets ein Vorgang, niemals ein Gegenstand als solcher.*' While a 'force' ('*Naturkraft*') such as gravitation may be considered the 'cause' of acceleration (cf. above footnote 50), *Schopenhauer* emphasizes that such force may not necessarily be considered a 'cause', this latter being rather the particular 'change' which results in the manifestation of a given '*Naturkraft*' (e.g. a fall being not 'caused' by gravitation but by the 'change' – such as withdrawing of support – initiating the manifestation of gravity in the free fall

(2) *Hume* failed to point out that, from experience and reasoning (by analytical thought), all causal events can be recognized as being physical interactions involving 'force' or 'energy', and 'mass' all of which allow for a practical, operationally valid mathematical formulation and numerical definition. *Whitehead* [1925, 1948] has maintained that if we are to get out of *Hume's* difficulty, the solution is not to be found in the accumulation of instances, but in the intrinsic character of each instance. 'When we have found that, we will have struck at the heart of *Hume's* argument'. Now, this 'intrinsic character', looked for by *Whitehead*, is evidently provided by what is called 'force' and 'energy' in classical and even in quantum physics. Nevertheless, *Hume* remains doubtless right when he claims that our 'idea of causation' is derived from the experience of succession,[54] moreover also that 'the ultimate force and efficacy of nature is perfectly unknown to us, and that it is vain we search for it in all the known qualities of matter'. *Hume* stresses 'that the terms efficacy, agency, power, force, energy, necessity, connection and productive quality, are all nearly synonymous, and therefore it is an absurdity to employ any one in defining the rest'. Yet, this may be qualified by accepting the formulations of physics qua force, energy and mass as fictions with considerable practical operational validity. It will be recalled that, in the mechanistic concept of *Descartes*, the best understood aspect of causation is our acquired experience of push and pull, which latter could be conceived as a mere sort of pull, e.g. by a hook. Push and pull, of course, imply the so-called 'primary quality' of 'solidity' respectively 'impenetrability' of 'matter'. Yet, 'matter' must now be conceived as essentially empty space characterized by exceedingly rapid 'orbital events', comparable to gyroscopic motion respectively to the motion of spinning tops.

---

of an object). *Schopenhauer's* '*Naturkräfte*' are abstractions of a particular sort of interactions (e.g. at present gravity, electromagnetism, strong and weak particle interactions). His '*Naturgesetze*' are abstractions of the 'norms' which a '*Naturkraft*' displays within the chains of causal interactions. '*Ursache*' and '*Wirkung*' are the concrete (actual) changes which can be detected in said causal chains, such that the 'cause' represents the dynamic factor which is arbitrarily emphasized in the particular aspect under consideration (cf. *Mach's* remark quoted above on p. 9).

[54] *Schopenhauer* vainly tries to disprove *Hume* by citing the well-known succession of day and night, in which the preceding day cannot be considered the cause, and the succeeding night the day's effect. *Schopenhauer* forgets here his own definition of cause, namely that, in this improper formulation, 'day' does not represent a change but a continuous state. However, taking 'day' as corresponding to a certain course of the sun, we have then, in a proper formulation, a succession leading to sunset, which provides the required change, causing night as its effect. In other words, the succession must be described in appropriate terms involving force or energy, in this case the transmission of sunlight. It can be seen that, in discussing a given problem, the appropriate semantic formulation of the relevant propositions is a logical requirement.

Push and pull effects must therefore be explained, i.e. described in terms of other interactions (electromagnetic, gravitational, weak and strong atomic respectively subatomic interactions). The 'explanation' of cohesion and adhesion likewise involves considerable difficulties. 'Impenetrability', as the assumed condition of matter in the core of the earth, in the interior of stars, in white dwarfs, in neutron stars or in the presumed 'black holes' indicates, is thus quite relative. Yet, there may be an ultimate limit, preceding the presumed 'rebound' resulting in the primordial explosion originating a new expanding universe following the collapse of the antecedent one.

The term 'push-pull causality' has been used in a derogatory sense to characterize the causality concept as such. Yet, it should be pointed out that all material (physical) changes involve interactions of mass and energy based on repulsion and attraction, i.e. on 'push and pull'. This applies as well to the impact of billiard balls in terms of classical mechanics as to the complex interactions described in the new physics.

With regard to repulsion and attraction, it is evidently easier, because of the macroscopic aspect characterizing our senses, to 'understand' or 'explain' repulsion ('push'). It is much more difficult to 'understand', 'explain', or 'describe' how two 'masses', separated by a space, 'attract' each other, either by 'electromagnetism' or by 'gravity', even if we assume a continuity of energy transmission, thereby excluding action at a distance. However, regardless of the thereby involved insufficiently elucidated mathematical details, it should be recalled that gyroscopic motion, such as manifested by 'matter', does give to 'material entities' curious properties of elasticity, repulsion and attraction [cf. e.g. *Perry*, 1957]. One could here add that the *Cartesian* theory of vortices, mentioned before in footnote 43, was, after all, not entirely unjustified if considered to be a forerunner of present-day theories conceiving 'matter' as a hierarchy of complex orbiting patterns involving mass, energy, and electric charges in the most diversified combinations.

(3) *Hume* failed to take into sufficient consideration the mechanisms of the brain which result in our experiencing significant relatedness in the sequence of perceived events. Although our (conscious) formulated 'knowledge' of causality and our (likewise conscious, but 'sphairal') vague intuition assuming causal events are indeed based on actual experience gradually unfolding in postnatal life, both are also based on the given *modus operandi* of the cerebral mechanisms. This modus, at most, would be a component of our causal thinking which would, with a modicum of justification, be designated as 'a priori'. Yet, it can be maintained that both the formal and the vague, 'intuitive knowledge' of causality are, in all relevant respects, based on experience acquired in the course of postnatal ontogenetic development.

It should, moreover, be pointed out that *Hume*, despite his scepticism, as qualified further below, does not question, but on the contrary strongly upholds the concepts of causality and necessity.[55] In this respect, his sceptical inquiry is merely directed at the logical foundation upon which these concepts are based, or, in other words, at their origin and derivation from experience.

With respect to extreme scepticism[56] such as is often wrongly imputed to *Hume* (cf. the preceding footnote 55) this author stated: 'When I reflect on the natural fallibility of my judgment, I have less confidence in my opinions than when I only consider the objects concerning which I reason; and when I proceed still further, to turn the scrutiny against every successive estimation I make of my faculties, all the rules of logic require a continual diminution, and at last a total extinction of belief and evidence.'

'Should it here be asked me, whether I sincerely assent to this argument, which I seem to take such pains to inculcate, and whether I be really one of those sceptics who hold that all is uncertain, and that our judgment is not in any thing possessed of any measures of truth and falsity; I should reply that this question is entirely superfluous, and that neither I, nor any other person, was ever sincerely and constantly of that opinion. Nature, by an absolute and uncontrollable necessity, has determined us to judge as well as to breathe and feel; nor can we any more forbear viewing certain objects in a stronger and fuller light, upon account of their customary connection with a present impression, than we can hinder ourselves from thinking, as long as we are awake, or seeing the surrounding bodies, when we turn our eyes towards them in broad sunshine.' [57]

'Whoever has taken the pains to refute the cavils of this *total* scepticism, has really disputed without an antagonist, and endeavored by arguments to establish a faculty, which nature has antecedently implanted in the mind, and rendered unavoidable'.[58]

'My intention then in displaying so carefully the arguments of that fantastic sect, is only to make the reader sensible of the truth of my hypothesis, *that all our reasonings concerning cause and effect, are derived from nothing but*

---

[55] *Heisenberg* [1958] comments on the 'extreme scepticism' of *Hume*, 'who denied induction and causality and thereby arrived at a conclusion which if taken seriously would destroy the basis of empirical science'. It is here evident that *Heisenberg* completely failed to understand *Hume's* elaboration on this topic.

[56] *Craik* [1943] similarly commented that scepticism 'either assumes the validity of verbal or other symbolism, in which case the symbolization and discussion of external events is also legitimate, or it denies the possibility of symbolism at all, in which case it is reduced to silence and cannot express any meaning in any way'.

[57] This sentence is a close paraphrase of a similar statement by *Berkeley* in his treatise concerning the principles of human knowledge [1710, Section XXIX]: 'When in broad daylight I open my eyes, it is not in my power to choose whether I shall see or no' etc. It should be added that *Hume* greatly admired *Berkeley*.

[58] This 'antecedently implanted' evidently applies to the '*a priori*' component mentioned above on page 84.

custom; and that belief is more properly an act of the sensitive, than of the cogitative part of our nature.' [59]

Schopenhauer, in his critique of both *Hume's* and *Kant's* derivation of causality, states that *Kant 'in seinem Beweise ist in den, dem des Hume entgegengesetzten Fehler gerathen. Dieser nämlich erklärte alles Erfolgen für blosses Folgen: Kant hingegen will, dass es kein anderes Folgen gebe, als das Erfolgen'.* In contradiction to *Schopenhauer*, however, it could be maintained that both *Hume* and *Kant* are right, and that the apparent discrepancy in their opinions is merely based on incomplete semantic formulation. Quite evidently all causal events are successions in agreement with *Hume*, and all successions of events are causal sequences in agreement with *Kant*. Thus: *alles Erfolgen ist ein Folgen und alles Folgen ist ein Erfolgen.* The qualification required for this statement should add that it applies to an assumed totality (*'alles'*) of causal lines. All events in a particular given causal line are sequences of cause and effect. The German term *'Zufall'* for 'chance' (in one of its several denotations) correctly indicates the coincidence (*Zusammentreffen, Zusammenfallen des nicht verknüpften*) displayed by the intersection or interweaving of different and separate causal lines, such that an event pertaining to one causal line follows an event pertaining to another causal line, whereby the succession of these two events does not involve cause and effect. The coincidence concerns here the occurrence of a sequence *post hoc sed non propter hoc*.

Although *Schopenhauer* recognized and emphasized that the principle or 'law' of causality is incapable of being proved, he attempted, nevertheless to prove that said principle represents a knowledge 'a priori' in *Kant's* sense. He analyzed and rejected the evidently faulty proof given by *Kant* and claimed that his own proof was the only valid one. [60]

Schopenhauer's lengthy 'proof' can be concisely rendered as follows. In seeing, the directly given events are represented by the sensations of the retina, namely light, darkness, and colors. These sensations are entirely 'subjective', within the organism and under the skin. It is the 'understanding' (*'Verstand'*), who, referring these 'sensations' to their causes by several unconscious operations, [61] constructs the external world of sight. Therefore, in order to perform these *'Verstandesoperationen'*, the 'understanding' or 'intellect' must, prior to all experience, be endowed with the 'forms' of space and time as well as with an unconscious 'knowledge' of causality. Comparable operations are performed

---

[59] In other words, belief pertains to the 'irrational' mental component represented by 'affectivity' as much and sometimes more so than to the 'rational' component of reason.

[60] *'Den allein richtigen Beweis der Apriorität des Kausalitätsgesetzes habe ich in §21 gegeben'* [*Schopenhauer*, vol. 3, p. 107. He refers here to §21 of his treatise on the principle of sufficient reason].

[61] The interesting details of these 'operations', which include important concepts of sensory physiology, shall be considered in volume 2, chapter IV with respect to localization.

by the 'understanding' as regards the sense of touch. The critical and competent reader will notice in *Schopenhauer's* 'proof' a number of weaknesses, inconsistencies and instances of false reasoning.

(1) The assumption of 'retina', 'skin', and 'organism' represents here a petitio principii and ὕστερον πρότερον. If an eye with retina and a body are given, upon which 'sensations' become 'caused', then a material world is already taken to exist independently of the 'understanding' that does not construct, but merely, by unconscious reference from effect to cause, reproduces said independently existing external world, which, therefore could not be merely appearance (*Vorstellung, Erscheinung*). Yet, *Schopenhauer* quite rightly, in accordance with *Berkeley*, *Hume*, and *Kant*, denies the independent existence of such physical world and conceives the experienced world as a mental phenomenon, that is to say as '*Erscheinung*' or '*Vorstellung*'.

(2) It seems, moreover, well established that no 'sensations' occur in the retina or at the sensory endings, which merely '*register*' physicochemical events in a manner not essentially different from the performance of a recording instrument.[62] '*Sensations*' can only be conceived as aspects of consciousness, and consciousness must be regarded as a 'function' of the brain, more particularly (in Man and presumably in most or all Mammals) of certain corticothalamic events, and not as 'functions' of the sensory endings or of the sense organs. It is also evident that *Schopenhauer* was not aware of the *brain paradox* (to be discussed further below) nor of the implications of said paradox.

(3) Granted, for argument's sake, that the 'understanding' refers the retinal sensations etc. as effects[63] to their external causes and thereby 'locates' or 'localizes' them in space-time, which, however, is supposed to be exclu-

---

[62] It should here also be pointed out that *Haeckel* [1898], in his '*Welträthsel*', assumes 'unconscious sensations' ('*unbewusste Empfindungen und Vorstellungen*') which he considers to be 'psychic processes' or elementary aspects of the 'soul' ('*Psyche*'). He thus attributes 'psychic processes' to individual cells ('*Zellseele*') and even to atoms, with the qualification that such 'psychic processes' are unconscious. Consciousness is assumed by *Haeckel* to be merely the highly stage of the '*Psyche*': at this stage '*entwickelt sich durch Spiegelung der Empfindungen in einem Centraltheile des Nervensystems die höchste psychische Funktion, die bewusste Empfindung: so beim Menschen und den höheren Wirbelthieren, wahrscheinlich auch bei einem Theile der höheren wirbellosen Thiere, besonders der Gliederthiere.*' Quite apart from the meaningless concept of '*Spiegelung*' it should here again be emphasized that an unconscious sensation or an unconscious psyche involve a *contradictio in adjecto* ('unconscious consciousness') if, in accordance with rigorous semantic procedure, sensation, perception, mind and psyche ('soul') are considered synonymous with consciousness. *Sherrington's* [1950] relevant dictum: 'most life is, I imagine, mindless' should again be stressed.

[63] *Brain* [1959] justly states that we do not normally experience e.g. seeing a tree as an 'effect', although we can, in scientific thinking, describe it as related to an effect of a series of events ending in the brain and resulting in the experience of seeing. Yet the conscious event of 'seeing' cannot be properly described as 'caused' by physical events involving mass or energy transformations in terms of physical science respectively behavioristic physiology.

sively a '*form a priori*' of the 'understanding' (cf. the petitio principii pointed out above under 1), such unconscious application of the principle of causality by the 'understanding' could hardly be called '*knowledge a priori*'. *Schopenhauer* admits that such seeing is, physiologically, '*eine Funktion des Gehirns, welches dieses so wenig erst aus der Erfahrung gelernt, wie der Magen das Verdauen*'. What *Schopenhauer* thereby states is merely the uncontestable fact, also fully recognized by *Hume*, that physical (including physiological) events are causal occurrences. But this does not imply that we have '*knowledge*' (in the accepted sense of this word) of causality prior to relevant (conscious) experiences.

Reverting to the processes of digestion, as mentioned by *Schopenhauer*, the secretion of digestive juice by the pancreas occurs if the duodenal lining, stimulated by acid gastric contents, produces an hormone called secretin which reaches the pancreas by way of the blood stream. We have here a strictly causal process, but it could hardly be said that the pancreas has '*knowledge*' (implying conscious reasoning or at least sphairal conscious intuition) of the acidity in the duodenum and still less that the pancreas has a priori '*knowledge*' of its own mechanisms or of '*causality*', although its mechanisms are evidently genetically predetermined and thus at least in part 'prefunctional'. Neither the Human body as a whole, nor the reasoning, conscious Human mind as a brain function do have a priori 'knowledge' of said aspects of digestive events, nor, for that matter, of the other multitudinous causal body mechanisms. Such knowledge, as far as it is available, was obtained quite *a posteriori* on the basis of repeated experimentation and lengthy reasonings.[64] *Mutatis mutandis*, by unconscious and subconscious (sphairal) thought processes as well as by the subsequent formal logical reasoning, but strictly on the basis of events registered and experienced by the brain, a posteriori knowledge of causality, leading to the causality concept, is obtained, as *Hume* rightly concluded.

(4) *Schopenhauer* tends to hypostatize or reify what he calls '*Verstand*' (understanding) and '*Vernunft*' (reasoning)[65] and thereby weakens his argumentation by what *Whitehead* calls' 'the fallacy of misplaced concreteness', whereby objects and events are given a precision in words which they do not in

---

[64] Thus, although for millions of years the causal pancreas-duodenum interactions were taking place, knowledge of these mechanisms was first obtained through the studies of *Bayliss* and *Starling* at about 1902.

[65] It is here of interest to note that, because of their semantic vagueness, the terms '*Vernunft*' and '*Verstand*', i.e. 'reason' and 'understanding', are used with almost reversed meanings by *Kant* and by *Schopenhauer*. *Kant* defines '*Verstand*' as '*das Vermögen der Begriffe*', '*Vernunft*' as '*das Vermögen der Prinzipien*', and '*Urtheilskraft*' as '*das Mittelglied*' between '*Verstand*' and '*Vernunft*'. According to *Schopenhauer*, however, '*das subjektive Korrelat der Materie oder der Kausalität, denn beide sind eines, ist der Verstand und er ist nichts ausserdem*'. '*Für das Vermögen der Begriffe habe ich die Vernunft erklärt.*' He defines '*Urtheilskraft*' as '*die Fähigkeit, die*'

fact possess.[66] It seems evident, that, at best, *'Verstand'* *'Vernunft'*, and *'Urteilskraft'* (judgment) merely represent poorly definable aspects of the cortical brain mechanisms related to the likewise vague capacity or ability called *'intelligence'* [cf. *K.*, 1965a].

As regards the *principle of causality*, *Schopenhauer* distinguishes three different sorts of manifestations, namely (1) as *cause sensu strictiori* in the anorganic (i.e. non-living) world, (2) as *stimulus* ('Reiz') in plants and vegetative functions of animals, and (3) as *'motive'* in conscious animal activities, mediated by the *'intellect'*.

In anorganic *causality sensu strictiori* (1) cause and effect are conceived as corresponding to each other in *Newton's* sense, such that action and reaction are equal. A *stimulus* (2), however, characteristic for organic life, is conceived as a cause whose effect does not correspond to the magnitude or strength of the cause.[67] *Motives* (3) are said to represent the causality regulating animal life in the strict sense: *'also das Thun, d.h. die äussern, mit Bewusstseyn geschehenden Aktionen aller thierischen Wesen. Das Medium der Motive ist die Erkenntniss: die Empfänglichkeit für sie erfordert folglich einen Intellekt. Daher ist das wahre Charakteristikon des Thieres das Erkennen, das Vorstellen. Das Thier bewegt sich allemal nach einem Ziel und Zweck: diesen muss es demnach erkannt haben: d.h. derselbe muss ihm als ein von ihm verschiedenes, dessen es sich dennoch bewusst ist, sich darstellen. Demzufolge ist das Thier zu definiren "was erkennt": keine andere Definition trifft das Wesentliche.'*[68]

---

anschauliche Erkenntnis in die abstrakte zu übertragen und diese wieder richtig auf jene anzuwenden'. In this respect, there is at least partial agreement between *Schopenhauer* and *Kant* concerning *'Urtheilskraft'*.

[66] It should be emphasized, however, that this criticism does by no means apply in some particular degree to *Schopenhauer* alone, but rather to most if not all philosophical and scientific authors.

[67] *'Ich nenne nämlich Ursach, im engsten Sinne des Worts, denjenigen Zustand der Materie, der, indem er einen anderen mit Nothwendigkeit herbeiführt, selbst eine ebensogrosse Veränderung erleidet, wie die ist, welche er verursacht, welcher durch die Regel "Wirkung and Gegenwirkung sind gleich" ausgedrückt wird.' 'Ich nenne Reiz diejenige Ursach, die selbst keine ihrer Wirkung angemessene Gegenwirkung erleidet, und deren Intensität durchaus nicht dem Grade nach parallel geht mit der Intensität der Wirkung, welche daher nicht nach jener gemessen werden kann: vielmehr kann eine kleine Vermehrung des Reizes eine sehr grosse in der Wirkung veranlassen oder auch umgekehrt die vorherige Wirkung ganz aufheben usw.'* [*Schopenhauer*, vol. 1, p. 169].

[68] From a viewpoint of biology, one must obviously disagree with *Schopenhauer's* definition. Not all animals possess a nervous system needed for *'Erkennen'*, and it is furthermore doubtful whether the most primitive nervous systems (e.g. Hydra) imply the occurrence of consciousness. Moreover, below the metazoan level, it is evidently very difficult to distinguish, by definition, plants from animals at the protozoan and protophytan prokaryote and eukaryote level, where the concepts of plants and animals seem to overlap. At the metazoan level, however, the gastrula stage unequivocally characterizes animals, which above the Porifera level, display a nervous system [cf. *K.*, 1967, vol. 1, pp. 41–43, vol. 2, pp. 5–8; 1973, vol. 3/II, pp. 20–23].

Despite *Schopenhauer's* uncontestable merits in providing a first systematic attempt at analysis and classification of causality and (following *Aristotle*) of the principle of sufficient reason in general, pointing out the problems at issue, and leading to a first approximation, that author's formulation of causality displays considerable weaknesses.

As regards (1) *Schopenhauer* entirely forgets physical *'trigger-actions'* in which a relatively weak causal event, by releasing potential mechanical, chemical or electromagnetic energy, results in a much stronger effect such as the toppling of a large mass in labile equilibrium, or the firing of a gun by slight mechanical pressure, or the firing of a mine. Again, a relatively weak causal action can, as its effect, stop or inhibit the flow of considerable energy (e.g. by opening a closed switch). In *Ashby's* [1952] terminology, we have here sudden changes in a 'field' related to the change of value of a *'step-function'*. More recently, the mathematician *René Thom* at the French *'Institut des Hautes Études Scientifiques'* has introduced the term 'catastrophe theory' for a mathematical formulation showing that discontinuities can arise as a result of continuous changes. When certain parameters vary, the solutions in a system of equations display 'jumps' from one value to the next. These 'jumps' or 'discontinuities' are designated as *'catastrophes'*. Such discontinuous phenomena, corresponding to the above-mentioned 'field changes' related to 'step-functions' indeed lend themselves to descriptions in the mathematical terms of 'catastrophe theory'. However, the application of said theory, which, more often than not, represents a triviality or platitude expressed by a redoubtable notation, has been greatly exaggerated and therefore became the target of harsh criticism summarized by the quip: 'catastrophe theory: the emperor has no clothes' [*Kolata*, 1977a; cf. also *Sussmann and Zahler*, 1977, who point out to 'mathematics misused'].

More important causal concepts than 'catastrophe theory' which was already, in the aspect here under consideration, adequately included in *Ashby's* step-function formulation, are the engineering concepts of *feedback*, *servomechanisms* and *transducers*. In *feedback*, either positive or negative, control is actuated by a quantity which is in turn affected (either increased or decreased) by the result of a physical (including organic) system's output, such that aspects of the output are fed back into the system as part of the system's input. A *servomechanism* has the characteristic of imposing upon the output signal y (t) the same functional form as the input signal x (t), subject to the restriction that the energy associated with y (t) shall be provided by the system, and shall not be furnished directly by the input signal [*MacColl*, 1945]. A *transducer* is a device which converts energy from one form into the other, e.g. electrical energy into sound energy or vice versa. Such device makes possible the conversion of any physical or chemical phenomenon into a mechanical, electrical or chemical signal for transmission. The energy of the transform, namely of the signal emitted by the detecting transducer, is generally not provided by the detected energy, but derived, as in servomechanisms, from the system to which transducer and transduced effect pertain. In a transmitting transducer, the signal transmitted by this latter triggers energy pertaining to the system receiving the signal. There are, accordingly, input transducers, output transducers, and control transducers, which may be linked together. Among input transducers are sensing elements or sensors (better: *'registering'* devices, since 'sensing' could wrongly be interpreted as implying 'sensation', i.e. consciousness), pick-ups, detectors, and probes [cf. e.g. *Berkeley*, 1962].

With regard to (2) *Schopenhauer* justly distinguished 'stimulus' (*'Reiz'*) as a sort of causality pertaining to living organisms and differing from the manifestations of causality in non-living systems. He failed, however, to realize both the similarities and the differences between vital and nonvital manifestations of causality.

As regards the similarities, a stimulus (cause) and its effect merely represent a trigger mechanism whereby potential energy is released or a flow of energy is inhibited. As regards the differences, the released or inhibited 'vital' energy is that provided by the metabolism of the living substance, that is to say by a system of cyclic processes liberating energy and representing one of the fundamental characteristics whereby organic life ('living matter') differs from lifeless matter. This topic, including a pertinent definition of 'life', shall be discussed further below in the present chapter's next subsection.

Thus, a *'Reiz'* (stimulus) can be defined as any change (cause) acting upon 'living substance' such that the latter 'reacts' with a change in its vital activities, said change being an effect. Such stimulus is commonly conceived as an 'external change' acting upon a living system (e.g. upon a region or the whole of its 'surface membrane'). There are, however, also 'internal changes' within a living system which can be conceived as 'internal stimuli'.

Moreover, a distinction can be made between a 'local excitatory process' and the resulting 'propagated disturbance'. *Winterstein* [1929] accordingly distinguishes *'Reiz am Receptionsort'* and the resulting *'Erregung'* respectively *'Erregungsleitung'* (i.e. stimulus, excitation, and transmission of excitation, that is to say 'impulse' or 'conductivity'). The cited author also distinguishes *'Susceptionsort'*, where the stimulus is received and *'Receptionsort'* where the excitation results. In contradistinction to *'Erregungsleitung'* he defines *'Reizleitung'* (stimulus conduction) as *'Übertragung eines äusseren, physikalischen oder chemischen Reizes durch Teile eines lebenden Organismus ohne aktive Beteiligung desselben'*, namely *'Leitung eines Reizes vom Susceptionsort zum Receptionsort'*. This is for instance the case in the transmission of vibrations through middle and inner ear to the *'Receptionsort'* provided by the sensory cells of *Corti's organ*.

As regards *Schopenhauer's* third sort of causality, namely motive or motivations (3) which requires an 'intellect' restricted to animals, and characterized by '*Erkennen*', '*Vorstellungen*', '*Bewusstsein*', it seems evident that he means the activities of a nervous system. All relevant performances of a nervous system are reflexes, which indeed represent a special sort of causality differing from (1) and from (2), and in this respect he is doubtless right in making that distinction. He failed, however, to realize that (3) represents merely a special case of (2) provided by the phylogenetic origin of nervous tissue. In addition, he failed to take into sufficient account that most activities of a nervous system (as evidenced in Man) are unconscious and thereby do not involve '*Erkennen*', '*Vorstellungen*' and '*Bewusstsein*', but merely registration of input, processing of signals, storage, and output. In volume 5/II (chapter XV, pp. 321–324) of the present author's series on *The Central Nervous System of Vertebrates* it was pointed out, in agreement with several competent authors, that the reflex concept represents the basis of all relevant nervous functions, such that even the most complex activities differ from the simple ones merely by their much more complex synaptic arrangements and functional aspects including long-term storage, delay, as well as correlation with consciousness. Although not in essence, but merely *qua* intricacy, there are indeed differences, with many gradations and ill-defined boundaries, between relatively simple reflex activities and the most complex ones comprising conscious deliberation and difficult choices respectively decisions.

Thus, *Schopenhauer*, who included motivation under the *principium rationis sufficients fiendi* (causality), enumerates motivation again as a fourth aspect of the principle of sufficient reason, namely as '*Satz vom zureichenden Grunde des Handelns*' (*principium rationis sufficients agendi*). Quite evidently a motive in this sense is a complex of (conscious) percepts (which can 'emerge' from unconscious cerebration) with a relevant component of affectivity (e.g. 'will'), and resulting in an intended (conscious) action. *Schopenhauer* should have called his third sort of causality (3) *reflex*, and entirely reserved motivation for the complex, partly unconscious but in its end-result conscious intended activity pertaining to his *principium rationis sufficients agendi*. This may, of course, be considered a very special sort of reflex [cf. *K*., 1978].

As regards the macroscopic aspect of our 'idea of causation' in *Hume's* sense, it should be recalled that our sensory perceptions are 'molar', i.e. 'macroscopic'; this self-evident fact was already clearly recognized by *George Berkeley*, who stressed the ('molar') *minima sensibilia*. More recently, *Craik* [1943] stated that our commonest experience of causality is the case where objects obstruct or support one another or in some other way influence each other because of their inability to pass through each other or occupy the same place at the same time. This experience is obviously related to our visual and tactile percepts. But *Craik* justly adds that two gases or solids may occupy the same space as one previously did (at the same pressure in the case of the gases) after chemical combination. Electric and magnetic fields may occupy the same place apparently independently. He could have added that two gases, two fluids, or two dissolved solids may jointly occupy the same space by penetrating each other. Moreover, different percepts of sounds can have identical (vague) spatial relations. Even two different visual perceptual patterns, namely objects in front of one's body, and one's own body with objects behind this latter, may be superposed upon or 'telescoped' into each other, and localized in one and the same region of visual space, if one looks through a glass plate under appropriate lighting conditions. Again, other percepts of consciousness, which are poorly localized and nonconfigurated, such as different emotions, may occupy the same place at the same time.

As regards the 'solidity' and 'impenetrability' of matter, it should also be recalled that atoms, *qua* distribution of 'mass', represent to a considerable extent 'empty space', although being 'impenetrable' under ordinary conditions. Under particular conditions,[69] however, such as the gravitational collapse manifested by 'white dwarfs', 'neutron stars', 'black holes', and the presumable collapse of the universe preceding its rebound as a primordial explosion, the space occupied by apparently 'solid' or 'impenetrable' matter may be greatly reduced.

Craik [1943] concludes that 'macroscopic causation seems to rest on two main principles – the inability of two similar bodies to occupy the same place at the same time, and the transfer and distribution of energy according to the second law of thermodynamics. Microscopic causality appears to consist of certain restrictions imposed by one electron on the possible positions or states of another, and on the transfer of energy by electrons acquiring kinetic energy and losing it. What is the relation between these two concepts of "occupation" and "energy transfer"? Since mass apparently occupies space, and since it is now held that all mass is electrical, it is unlikely that the two concepts can be perfectly unified. Occupation of a certain position in space is not, however, prohibited only by the actual size of the electrons, etc., already occupying that region; these electrons are surrounded by fields, and one electron can occupy a certain position near another only if its energy is high enough. Thus, occupation of space is partly a matter of energy – as we see on a macroscopic scale in the entry of a shell into an armour plate.'

Russell [1948] formulates causal law in its most generalized definition as follows: 'A will cause B if nothing happens to prevent it. Or more simply: A will cause B unless it doesn't.' *Russell* adds here: 'This is a poor sort of a law, and not very useful as a basis for scientific knowledge.' Quite apart from the

---

[69] Cf. the discussion of these phenomena in the preceding section dealing with the cosmology of the physical world.

fact that *Russell* seems not to be aware of his *petitio principii* defining 'causal law' by the undefined term 'cause', one may justly disagree with *Russell's* additional comment, since 'unless it doesn't' has a very significant implication, to wit: if it doesn't, there must be a reason for it, namely the interference by another cause, and this cause as well as its orderly relationship can be found out, at least in principle and within the limits imposed by statistical respectively quantum uncertainties.

There are, however, two important and apparently opposite sources of ambiguity and confusion in our abstract symbolization of experience: objects and events may be given a precision in words which they do not actually possess (hypostatization), while on the other hand words or symbols have an inherent and variable degree of vagueness. Thus, even at best, a certain haziness unavoidably obtains and many not altogether unreasonable arguments must finally remain unconvincing or inconclusive. Strict mathematical formulation eliminates ambiguities as regards certain purely formal or quantitative aspects of events, but with a loss in actuality or relevant validity.

In quantum physics, individual occurrences are not determined by the equations which merely show possibilities. How often each possibility will be realized in a large number of cases can be predicted by statistical rules. Since the initial states are not exactly known, the events appear thus chanced according to the definition of chance given above. This indeterminism includes *Heisenberg's* uncertainty principle which states that there is a theoretical limit to the accuracy with which certain related magnitudes can be simultaneously measured.

A number of physicists have therefore rejected causal interpretation of small-scale events; even the orderliness of macroscopic phenomena has been considered exclusively in terms of statistical regularity.

The logician *Russell* [1948] is inclined to believe that the absence of complete determinism in quantum physics is not due to any incompleteness of the theory but represents a genuine characteristic of small-scale occurrences. To me, this reasoning appears as a negative version of the famous ontologic argument: because in a logical system (quantum mechanics) determinism is excluded, determinism, therefore, cannot exist.

It is true that the statistical character of quantum physics differs fundamentally from that of the kinetic theory of matter. In quantum physics individual laws are entirely discarded and statistical laws are given immediately; there is no room for laws governing the changes in time of the individual object. It is thus impossible to describe positions and velocities of an elementary particle or to predict its path as in classical physics. Such a question has no sense in the theory which determines a highly abstract function, the probability wave. For one elementary particle, the probability wave is, at a given moment, a function of a three-dimensional continuum. For two, three, four, ten or more particles, probability waves become functions in a continuum of six, nine, twelve, thirty and more dimensions. As *Einstein and Infeld* [1938] summarize, there is no place in quantum physics for statements such as: this object is so-and-so, and has this-and-this property. Instead we have statements of this kind: there is such-and-such a probability that the individual object is so-and-so and has this-and-this property.

The indeterminism of quantum physics can still be regarded as indeterminism due to lack of data; it appears irrelevant whether the individual data cannot be ascertained because of physical difficulties as in kinetic theory of matter or in a gambling device, or because the theoretical formulation excludes such data. Intrinsic indeterminism would be a true miracle.

As regards the exclusion of causal data in quantum mechanics, two aspects of the relevant theories should be kept in mind. The first aspect is the required statistical approach, which *eo ipso* excludes causal determinism in favor of probability predictions. The second aspect, particularly manifested in the obsolescent *Bohr theory* of the atom with its quantized orbital levels, is represented by the '*quantum jump*', which precludes any possible description of continuous transitions between 'stationary states'. *Whittaker* [1948] remarks that there are apparently here 'events in the physical world which cannot be represented on the background of space and time'. On the other hand, in contradistinction to *Bohr's* quantized orbits and to *Heisenberg's* matrix mechanics operating with discrete, discontinuous magnitudes, *de Broglie's* and *Schrödinger's* wave mechanics which assume discrete or discontinuous frequencies, do not necessarily preclude a discontinuity consistent with or based on continuity: *ex continuo discontinuum* [cf. *Jaffé*, 1954]. Thus, e.g. a vibrating continuous string with fixation points at both ends can only display stationary waves in the fundamental mode and a series of discrete overtones. Again, the transition of one permissible frequency to the next one can be assumed as instantaneous, but without disruption of the continuous wave motion.

Concerning this topic, *Brancazio* [1975] brings the following comments. 'It is rather ironic that while *Schrödinger's* mathematical theory won great acclaim, the physical meanings that he attached to his findings were generally rejected. In particular, *Schrödinger* believed that he had done away with the idea of discontinuous quantum "jumps" within the atom – an idea that had been particularly disturbing to the more classically oriented physicists. *Schrödinger* visualized the atom as a nucleus surrounded by a three-dimensional wave pattern with fixed vibration frequencies. (The waves are *de Broglie* waves, and the standing wave pattern comprises the electron cloud.) He pictured energy transitions in the atom in terms of changes from one wave pattern to the other, comparable to the way in which the different harmonies of a violin string can be produced by bowing or plucking the string in a different manner. Through this analogy with classical wave phenomena, *Schrödinger* thought that the quantum jump could be discarded.'

'In the fall of 1926, *Schrödinger* was invited to discuss his ideas with *Bohr* and his students. The discussion turned into a marathon debate, which lasted several days. *Schrödinger* was not nearly as energetic or as forceful a debater as *Bohr*, and he gradually gave ground. Eventually, *Schrödinger* had to admit the inadequacy of his model. In his despair (and exhaustion) he shouted at *Bohr*, "If we are going to stick to this damned quantum jumping, then I regret having ever been involved in this thing!" – to which *Bohr* replied, "But the rest of us are thankful that you did, because you have done so much to promote the quantum theory".'

'*Schrödinger* never brought himself to accept the idea of quantum jumps. As time progressed, he drifted further and further from the main lines of thought in quantum mechanics. Yet the *Schrödinger equation* remains as the single most important equation of this theory.'[70]

Be that as it may, I believe, in agreement with the classically oriented physicists, that the substitution of true indeterminism for uncertainty is not justified. Although doubts remain concerning an appropriate evaluation of the quantum jump postulate, neither the limit of observation nor the concepts of a wave particle or of a probability wave appear to be valid arguments for the denial of the principle of sufficient reason in its first application (*principium rationis sufficientis fiendi*).

Concerning the small-scale events *Craik* [1943] states: 'Most quantum physicists regard indeterminism as a characteristic of real phenomena and I (tentatively, because I am unable to follow the mathematical detail of their theories) do not.'[71] Viewed in terms of anatomy of mathematics, quantum theories represent logical systems with certain sets of postulates, and follow the *principium rationis sufficientis cognoscendi* (*et essendi*); if the validity of this principle is denied, then the validity of the theories becomes eo ipso nullified. *The principium rationis sufficientis fiendi*, applicable to individual events, is excluded in the premises. Thus, as mentioned above (p. 93) in quoting *Bertrand Russell*, and regardless of the mathematical details, such theories, showing that significant results can be obtained without the *principium rationis sufficientis fiendi* (causality, determinism), do by no means

---

[70] With respect to quantum mechanics, *Schrödinger* is also quoted by *Hoyle* [1975b] to have said: 'I don't like it, and I am sorry that I ever had anything to do with it.'

[71] *Craik* was perhaps here unduly impressed by the redoubtable mathematical notations of quantum physics and underestimated his own ability. While it is evident that only the mathematically highly competent quantum physicists can properly handle their complex equations, it is nevertheless possible for intelligent outsiders who do not shun some hard work (which is well worth the trouble) to understand the essential meaning, i.e. the gist, of their formulations and the significance of the thereby obtained results.

disprove the actuality of determinism or causality. As *Craik* points out, the physicists 'seem to have a certain curious belief that they have constructed things rather than discovered them'.[72] The quoted author then adds: 'Neither the limit of observation imposed by the disturbing influence of the observing electron or quantum, nor the intangible nature of the conception of a wave-particle justifies us, surely, in imposing on reality the burden of supporting the shortcomings of our own intellects and instruments.'

It is, moreover, of particular significance that *Max Planck*, who originated the quantum concept, and *Albert Einstein*, who was an important contributor to the development of quantum theory, firmly upheld the concept of causality. Likewise, *Schrödinger's* objection to quantum mechanics, of which he himself developed a relevant aspect, was pointed out above.

Planck [1933] stated: '*In dem Weltbilde der Quantenphysik herrscht der Determinismus ebenso streng wie in der klassischen Physik, nur sind die benutzten Symbole andere, und es wird mit anderen Rechenvorschriften operiert.*'

Einstein [1934] expresses the view that 'the scientist is possessed by the sense of universal causation'. He was particularly opposed to the view that 'events in nature are analogous to a game of chance' [1950]. In this respect, however, I am inclined, in apparent contradiction to the latter remark by *Einstein*, to consider many aspects of cosmic as well as of organic evolution, and of other natural events, although causal and strictly determined, comparable to a game of chance with loaded dice, whereby the doubtless obtaining randomness (disorder) becomes controlled by constraining parameters which may or may not remain hidden. It seems evident that events in a gambling device or in the throwing of dice can be considered strictly determined, but that, because we cannot know all the variables, the predictions must be based on the theory of probability.

There is no theoretical reason why the motions of a single die, coin, or gas molecule could not be described precisely in terms of causal interactions. But in the theories of quantum mechanics, as stated above, such sorts of interactions have no logical existence, and the mathematical symbols deal exclusively with 'expectation values' (averages). The axiomatic formulations do not permit the introduction of concealed parameters with the help of which the indeterministic description could be transformed into a deterministic one. Hence, if any future theory should be deterministic, it cannot be a modification of the present quantum theories but must be essentially different [*Born*, 1964]. Physicists concerned with quantum mechanics point out that this could not be done 'without sacrificing a whole treasure of well-established results' [*Born*, 1964].

---

[72] Yet, in a sense, physicists did contrive to 'construct things', namely artificial atoms (elements) apparently not existing in nature (cf. above, p. 18).

Meaningful individual causal events, which are highly significant in everyday life macroscopic perception as well as in classical physics, have no logical existence and are therefore meaningless in quantum theories. 'In quantal physics a pure, indecomposable collection in a mixture has not the character of a causal collection' [*De Broglie*, 1955].

In this respect, the mathematician *Thom* [1971] justly remarks: 'Any mathematician endowed with a modicum of intellectual honesty will recognize that in each of his proofs he is capable of giving a meaning to the symbols he uses. Because of this, his work differs from that of the theoretical physicist who very frequently does not hesitate to put his trust magically in the virtues of blind formalism in the hope (often deceived) that the light at the end of the tunnel will dispel the intervening darkness.' Yet, it remains a fact that 'blind formalism', in some instances, although devoid of an intelligible meaning, has led to some indisputable results (e.g. *Dirac's* antiparticles).

On the other hand, the eminent mathematician *Poincaré*, in his '*Dernières Pensées*' [1913b], stresses that 'science is deterministic; it is so a priori; it postulates determinism because, without it, it could not exist. It is deterministic a posteriori also; if it began by postulating it, as an indispensable condition for its existence, it proves it later by the very fact of existing, and each of its conquests is a victory of determinism'.

What *Poincaré* means here by 'a priori' can be regarded as a so-called 'axiom of order' based on 'intuition' in that author's sense. 'Intuition' is here the capacity to construct 'axioms of order' and relevant mathematical theorems or physical 'laws' based on the exact part of our thoughts. This capacity exists in us before any experience, because, without it, experience would be impossible and would be reduced to brute sensations, unsuitable for any organization; and 'because this intuition is merely the awareness of this faculty' [*Poincaré*, 1913b].

Quite evidently, this faculty is provided by the organization of the Human brain, particularly of its cerebral cortex and can thus, with some degree of justification, be called 'a priori'. Our 'awareness', i.e. our knowledge concerning said faculty and its results, are, nevertheless, based on mature experience, and therefore 'a posteriori', requiring previous sensory input and its subsequent processing by the cerebral mechanisms.

Radioactive disintegration is often cited as a typical example of an undetermined or spontaneous phenomenon. It is impossible to state why and when an individual atom will disintegrate. Yet the process of disintegration is most orderly and the half-life of radioactive substances can be accurately predicted. Many details of nuclear structure, especially concerning so-called binding forces, are poorly known, quite apart from the fact that particular causal events have no logical existence in quantum mechanics. There may be numerous periodicities and cyclic processes crudely comparable to the wheels in a gambling device where one particular combination hits the jackpot. While an observer could not predict this event, it would be possible, in a large series of such devices playing under constant conditions, to predict statistically the number of such events in a given time. However, as stated above, the introduction of relevant deterministic parameters into the formulations of quantum mechanics is logically inconsistent with the mathematical structure of said theories and thus impossible.

It could also be said that among physicists dealing with and thoroughly familiar with quantum theory, *Planck*, *Einstein*, and to some extent also *Schrödinger*, uphold causality identified with determinism, while *Bohr*, *Born*, and particularly *Heisenberg* uphold indeterminism and reject causality (in the classical sense). *Dirac* [1963], one of the most brilliant exponents of quantum mechanics, stands on the sidelines, as it were, with regard to the controversy between determinism (causality) and indeterminism.

Born [1964], however, claims that causality (in his definition) is not identical with determinism, and thereby, in contradiction to *Einstein*, believes that indeterminism does not eliminate causality. In *Born's* definition, causality is the postulate that one physical situation depends on the other, whereby causal research means the discovery of such dependence. This is said to be 'still true in quantum physics, though the objects of observation for which a dependence is claimed are the probabilities of elementary events, not those events themselves'.

'We have the paradoxical situation that observable events obey laws of chance, but that the probability for those events itself spreads according to laws which are in all essential features causal laws' [*Born*, 1964]. To this, one could reply that the observable events are nevertheless determined, but, in the formulations of quantum physics, which significantly differ from the statistical approach in thermodynamics, can only be expressed in mathematical terms excluding any permissible formulation representing the dynamics of single events.

It can be maintained, with *Hume*, that causality involves necessity, that is 'constant union' between cause and effect or, in other words, determinism. Although the rules are certain and infallible, when we apply them, our uncertain and fallible faculties, the inconstancy of our mental powers and the irruption of other causes prevent our complete understanding. By this means, as stated by *Hume* [1748] 'all knowledge degenerates into probability, and this probability is greater or less, according to our experience of the veracity or deceitfulness of our understanding, and according to the simplicity or intricacy of the question'.

In his explicit denial of causality the mathematician *von Neumann* [1932] stresses that, in macroscopic physics, no experiment proves causality. To this it can be answered that causality is indeed, as an aspect of the principle of sufficient reason, an unprovable postulate. Experiments, however, are not designed to prove causality but conversely to corroborate or to demonstrate relationships between physical (in the wider sense) phenomena on the consciously or unconsciously assumed basis of the principle of causality. This is even done by quantum physicists which, although they may deny causality, nevertheless investigate particle tracks and collisions in cloud or bubble chambers. Thus, in present-day particle physics, based on advanced theories of quantum mechanics, the relevant experiments represent strictly causal games of chance which can be likened to a random mechanical play of billiards. A beam of highly accelerated 'particles' is blindly shot at other 'particles', e.g. 'atoms' which, if hit, may become disrupted into their constituent fragments, and the results of these collisions are analyzed in terms of the above-mentioned mathematical concepts.

In contradistinction to *Born*, one could thus maintain that causality is identical with determinism, but in contradiction to *Einstein* also maintain that all games of chance are deterministic (i.e. causal), and that many causal events in the physical world result from random interactions ('chance') constrained by hidden parameters (e.g. 'loaded dice'). Such events, in accordance with expressions used by *Schrödinger*, represent order produced from disorder. Other sorts of events, per contra, represent order produced from order.

Moreover, in agreement with the quantum physicists, one can regard their formulations as fully justified, but with the qualification that they concern aspects of events which, for a diversity of reasons, must be dealt with in the manner of a *Vaihinger* fiction, that is to say *as if* determinism of single events did not obtain. On the basis of this postulate, it becomes necessary to express the orderliness of events in probabilistic terms entirely excluding any introduction of causality (determinism).

Yet, on the other hand, statistical laws and probability can be considered as merely an alternate formulation of the inherent orderliness of events, that is of causality. The whole theory of probability is accordingly founded on causal ideas. *Craik* [1943] states that it is meaningless to lop off the causality and hope to retain the notion of finite probabilities and to associate them with events. He remarks furthermore that he has 'not been trying to prove by this means that causation exists but only to show that any attempt to dispense with it is meaningless'. This brings us back to the statement that 'the principle of sufficient reason cannot be proved since it forms the basis of proof'.

There exists, nevertheless, a practical proof of the principle of sufficient reason, including its application as causality and determinism, as well as any probabilistic approach: on the basis of these concepts it becomes possible to predict future events, and the validity of such predictions can be corroborated by their actual fulfillment. Conversely, the validity of theories may be tested, according to the principle of sufficient reason, by probing whether predictions based on such theories are substantiated. As regards this practical aspect, 'the fairly high probability of certain "chance" or "misleading" (i.e. causally indirect) conjunctions' [*Craik*, 1943] must be kept in mind.

We may now summarize our proposition: a four-dimensional physical world, stripped, as we have assumed, of all qualities of consciousness, represents an orderly manifold of movable magnitudes and magnitudes of motion. This orderliness, conceived as strictly determined, can be expressed either in terms of causal or of statistical laws. Certain events in this manifold occur in patterned groups, representing matter. Orderly relations between these events are formulated as laws of physics and chemistry.

3. Organic Life

We shall next consider the phenomena of life occurring within this orderly manifold. Again assuming to exclude consciousness (psychic phenomena, mind *sensu latiori*) we may describe or define life as a series of events related to various aqueous colloidal systems of proteins, nucleic acids, carbohydrates, lipids and other substances, separated from the environment by a macromolecular boundary membrane. Such systems are designated as protoplasm and, in certain states, display the characteristics of life which can be enumerated in abbreviated form as follows: (1) metabolism (respiration, assimilation, excretion, secretion), (2) growth, (3) reproduction (heredity, transmission of specific characters), (4) irritability (reaction upon stimulus), (5) conductivity (transmission of impulses), (6) contractility (motion). The first three, occurring in plant and animal life, may be said to represent the vegetative functions, the last three, generally more pronounced in animals than in plants, may be designated as animal functions. It is difficult to outline the zone of demarcation between living and non-living matter; viruses perhaps represent a form of life near this vague boundary zone. Concerning phylogenetic speculations it must nevertheless be stressed that the known viruses are parasitic, that is, feed on higher forms of life. It has been suggested that these viruses represent parasitic descendents of very primitive Prokaryota or that on the other hand, they have evolved from prokaryote cell components which became independent. Since 1971, so-called 'viroids' have been identified which consist of a naked one-stranded RNA-helix arranged in a closed ring, and acting as pathogens for certain plants. So far such viroids have not been observed as animal pathogens [cf. e.g. *Frese*, 1978]. It is now, however, suspected that similar naked DNA viroids might occur, some of which could be animal pathogens.

With regard to the evolution of Eukaryote organisms from Prokaryote ones, it has been recently shown that considerable differences obtain between those two organic forms *qua* biochemistry of messenger RNA formation.

These differences are so profound as to suggest that sequential prokaryotic to eukaryotic evolution seems unlikely. The now discovered noncontiguous sequences in eukaryotic DNA that encode messenger RNA may reflect an ancient, rather than a new, distribution of information in DNA, and suggest that Eukaryotes evolved independently of Prokaryotes [*Darnell*, 1978].

The cited author points out that if a sequential evolution did not occur, then it seems not only possible but logical that the basic rules of genome organization might also differ between present-day prokaryotes and eukaryotes. If the molecular basis of eukaryotic gene regulation is to be explained in relation to developmental biology or cancer biology or endocrinology or many other topics, it is at least possible that we cannot rely on bacterial models but must again solve the molecular control mechanisms of eukaryotic genes [*Darnell*, 1978].

Be that as it may, even if present-day Prokaryotes, or at least some of them, such as Bacteria, evolved independently of Eukaryotes, it seems most likely that, in organic evolution, all Eukaryotes passed through a Prokaryote phylogenetic stage. On the other hand, considering the exceedingly long duration of prebiotic and earliest biotic evolution, considerable biochemical changes in various Prokaryote populations might well have occurred, thereby not precluding a branching off from a primitive Prokaryote population, whereby permanent prokaryotes and progressive Prokaryotes evolving into Eukaryotes became separated.

Darnell's [1978] remark concerning the doubtful applicability of bacterial models to molecular control mechanisms of Eukaryote genes (as e.g. implied by the *Jacob and Monod hypothesis*) seems, however, quite justified, and such doubt was also previously expressed by myself [*K.*, 1973a, p. 11, footnote 8].

Motion, which may appear to be spontaneous but can be causally interpreted as responses to external or internal events (stimuli etc.), has been particularly stressed since *Aristotle's* dictum 'ὁβίοϛὲν τῇ κίνησεί ἐοτί'. Even nonmotile living plant cells show protoplasmatic streaming and motion of the organoids. Time-lapse cinemicrophotography demonstrates considerable, often rhythmic or pulsating motions of entire cells or cell components in tissue cultures. The frenzied bubbling of the protoplasm during mitotic division is a spectacular feature of such pictures. Nevertheless, movements, whether obviously caused or apparently spontaneous, whether random or directed, cyclic, rhythmic or pulsating, can hardly be considered a specific manifestation of organic life.

The foregoing definition and enumeration of characteristics has, however, only considered generalized processes, of which many are cyclical or reversible.

There are, however, besides the surface boundary of a whole organism, boundaries of subsystems. In Metazoa and Metaphyta, the organism's sur-

limitations

face boundary becomes complex. Internal boundaries of subsystems are cellular and intracellular biologic membranes, which play an important functional role. Cellular boundaries may be provided by additional surface structures superimposed upon the biologic membranes.

Of particular import, and subsumed under the general concept of metabolism as enumerated above in abbreviated form, are the cyclic processes pertaining to 'intermediary metabolism' whereby the required energy for the 'vital' functions is obtained. Such types of reaction chains which are 'self-perpetuating' as long as the particular individual life is sustained by the metabolism, are, among others, the anaerobic glycolytic pathway (*Embden-Meyerhof pathway*), the pentose pathway (hexose-monophosphate shunt) and the citric acid or monoxycarbolic acid cycle (*Krebs cycle*), which is an aerobic pathway that completes the breakdown of energy-containing fragments remaining from the first two pathways [cf. e.g. *Patton*, 1963].

Thus, in the *Embden-Meyerhof pathway*, adenosine triphosphate (ATP) and adenosine diphosphate (ADP) play an important role. Two ATP molecules are expended and four are gained, having a net gain of two high-energy phosphates trapped in the process. In the pentose pathway, high-energy phosphates are trapped by the so-called pentose shunt reaction. In the *Krebs cycle*, also referred to as the 'metabolic mill', citric acid is produced and proceeds through a series of enzyme-controlled reactions during which there is a net gain of 15 mol of ATP. The cycle ends with production of malic acid, which, converted to oxaloacetic acid, renews the cycle. Carbon dioxide and water are given off, representing the final breakdown of the original carbohydrate.

Still more generally speaking, the biological transformations of energy ('vital interactions', 'vital forces', '*Lebenskraft*' in the 'non-vitalistic', 'mechanistic' sense) display oxidation-reduction potentials with various phases of hydrogen transfer involving complex enzyme activities, including the cytochrome and cytochrome oxydase systems.

In addition to enzyme activities, the actions of vitamins and of hormones represent relevant parameters for numerous vital chemical processes characterizing 'higher' forms of life. Vitamins are diverse organic substances necessary in minute quantities for the nutrition of most metazoan animals and some metaphytic plants. They act especially as precursors of coenzymes in the regulation of metabolic processes, but do not provide energy or serve as building units. They are present in various foods or may be produced within the body. The Human body and that of some other organic beings cannot 'manufacture' all its necessary compounds by digesting fats, carbohydrates and proteins. The additional compounds needed to that effect cannot be built up by the body and must be obtained from the diet.

Hormones are chemical compounds which control the overall functioning of the diverse enzymes. Some hormones are proteins, and others have a chemical structure containing cyclic alcohols (sterols), being thus called steroids.

However, all these above-mentioned important aspects of biology, that is to say of organic life, as far as their details are concerned, have no direct bearing upon the problems here under discussion.

Singh [1961] quotes *J. B. S. Haldane* said to have defined life 'as a self-perpetuating pattern of chemical reactions'. Yet, in accordance with the cited definition, a cyclic nuclear reaction, such as obtaining in the sun and other stars, would then characterize these stars as 'living organisms'. On the other hand, considering 'life' as defined above, the difference between a star and a living organism seems evident. The stellar nuclear reactions proceed from, and rise up, the original mass of the star. The cyclic energy-producing processes of living organisms result from the synthesis, by said organisms, of their own complicated specific material from indifferent or nonspecific compounds of the environment, the boundary between environment and living system being provided by the highly important biologic membrane [cf. *K.*, 1970, 1973a]. These processes, resulting, as it were, into 'order from disorder' are directed by the negentropy encoded in the genome.

The important vital characteristic of reproduction correlated with various degrees of complex ontogenetic development, depending on the particular organic form, results from the behavior of loci in the chromosomes. These loci, originally called 'genes', represent the hereditary factors that are passed from parent to offspring, either by asexual or by sexual reproduction.

A chromosome is essentially a long nucleotide chain consisting of desoxyribonucleic acid (DNA, formerly called 'thymonucleic acid'). These chromosomes are located within the cell nuclei of Eukaryote organisms, being the so-called chromatin material. In Prokaryote organisms the chromatin is not enclosed by a nuclear membrane but appears as a more diffuse agglomeration of chromosome strands forming a 'nucleus equivalent' or 'nucleoid'. There are here, moreover, also 'plasmids', namely ring-like molecules of DNA diffusely distributed in the cytoplasm, and therein replicating autonomously.

Another nucleic acid, namely ribonucleic acid (RNA) is also found in all cells, principally outside the nucleus, but does not play the primary hereditary role.[73]

---

[73] However, in certain viruses and tumor-inducing agents RNA does represent the genetic material. Generally speaking, a nucleotide consists of a pentose (five-carbon sugar), namely desoxyribose or ribose, connected with a phosphate group on one side, and a purine (adenine or guanine) or pyrimidine (cytosine, thymine, uracil) on the other side. Such nucleotides, either of the desoxyribose type, or of the ribose type (but not of both types) are linked together by their phosphate groups (cf. fig. 15). DNA contains desoxyribose, but no ribose and no uracil. RNA contains ribose but no desoxyribose and no thymine.

K. Voit[74] and myself, about 1932, were apparently the first to point out, against strong opposition from a noted expert on cytology, the significance of DNA as the active nuclear substance concerned with the transmission of variety [*K.*, 1932]. On the basis of our studies on DNA in cell nuclei [*K. and Voit*, 1932] we recognized that DNA was the essential component of chromatin respectively chromosomes [cf. *K.*, 1970, pp. 100–109]. About 12 years later, *Avery* et al. [1944] demonstrated the role of DNA in the reproduction of Bacteria, and are now generally credited with the 'discovery' of said component's significance.

After 1950, when studies of nuclear acid structure by means of the X-ray diffraction method were initiated, *Watson and Crick* [1953] elaborated their now well known model of DNA molecule as a pair of DNA polynucleotide chains wound around a common axis, thus forming an interlocking double helix. The pentose phosphate components provide the backbone of the two helical chains; these are linked together by their bases (purines and pyrimidines) which point inward toward the central axis.

Because a purine consists of two rings and a pyrimidine of one, the four bases will fit into the assumed structure of constant width only in certain pairs, such that any pair must include the combination of a long (purine) and of a short (pyrimidine) base. Again, the only pairs fitting into the model are adenine-thymine, and guanine-cytosine (cf. fig. 15). Evidently, in long nucleotide chains of this type, a very large amount of variety comparable to that of a binary notation, can be provided by the alternating, that is, the permutational pattern of the sequences. Depending on the dinucleotide combination (doublets) or trinucleotide (triplets), an initial variety of 4 bits (16) or of 6 bits (64) could be encoded. Thus, while doublets would not suffice, triplets would already provide a redundant code for all those amino acids (about 20) which, by their various combinations and sequences, build up the specific protein molecules. Said triplets became identified as 'codons' whose significance as symbols of the biologic coding system has been elucidated, whereby a decipherment (or 'code-breaking') of the basic genetic code[75] was accomplished through the joint investigations of numerous authors.

The obtaining DNA variety, moreover, is easily transmissible: the two helical chains, if separated and unwinding, can provide molds or templates for

---

[74] *Voit* [1925, 1927] was, moreover, the first to detect and to demonstrate the presence of DNA in Bacteria.

[75] It is evident that this does not amount to a complete 'breaking' of the entire genetic code system but merely to a preliminary general identification of one of its aspects involving relevant symbols. The 'genetic code' as well as the related 'biologic codes' are based on complex systems of 'superencipherments' [cf. *K.*, 1961, pp. 393f.; 1973a, pp. 30–34].

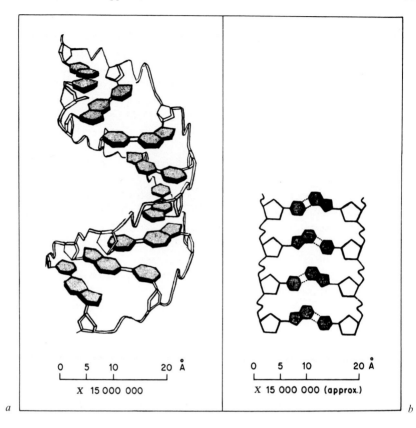

Fig. 15a. Structural model showing a pair of DNA chains wound as a double helix around a central axis [after *Crick*, 1955]. The pentose sugars are the white pentagons, the phosphate groups are represented by the kinks in the outer lines, joining the pentose groups. From each pentose unit there protrudes a base (pyrimidine, single, purine, double) shown as stripped hexagons or pentagons. Each base is linked to an opposing one at the same level by a nitrogen bond. These base-to-base links act as transverse support across the axis of the double helix and hold the chains together. As shown by the scale, the depicted model involves an approximate fictional magnification of 15×10^6, where 1.5 mm corresponds to 1 Å.

Fig. 15b. Simplified and flattened representation of pattern shown and explained in figure 15a [after *Crick*, 1955]. Approximate fictional magnification as in figure 15a.

RNA transcriptions upon DNA templates

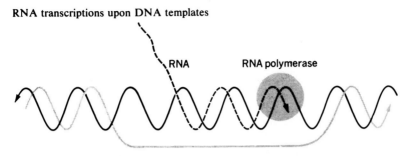

Fig. 16. Diagram purporting to illustrate template effect of DNA (transcription) by means of a semi-conservative duplication mechanism [after *Watson* from *Handler*, 1970]. Attachment of RNA polymerase opens the DNA helix by partial separation without breakage of either strand, and bases of RNA pair complementarily with those on one selected DNA strand whose anti-codons are transcribed into codons of the synthetized RNA strand which, as it grows, is said to 'peel off' by elimination of pyrophosphates.

their complements. Because of the specific pairing of the bases the sequence of the pairs of bases will be exactly duplicated.

The DNA chains, moreover, can also provide templates for RNA chains, that is, build up RNA molecules out of ribonucleotides forming complementary sequences, substituting, in these replicas, uracil for thymine.

The nuclear DNA thereby provides, by transcription, corresponding 'messenger RNA' molecules which move into the cytoplasm and there, with the added action of 'transfer RNA' ('soluble RNA') and through the mediation of ribosome RNA, become essential agents in protein synthesis. In other words, during such synthesis, the amino acid sequence of the polypeptides is assumed to be determined by the interaction of a 'messenger RNA' with 'transfer RNA' specific for a given amino acid. The structure of 'transfer RNA' is considered to represent the significant link.

The matching process between the amino acid, t-RNA, anticodons and the messenger codons, that is to say the translation mechanism, occurs on the ribosomes. These latter attach to messenger RNA molecules at specific 'initiator signals', and the amino acid t-RNA complex, which can register the initiator signal, is bound. This provides a reading frame, and now, as the ribosome moves along the filament of 'messenger RNA', each subsequent triplet codon comes into register, the appropriate amino acid t-RNA is bound, and the amino acid is polymerized onto the growing end of the protein chain, which grows one amino acid at a time. The sequence in which amino acids are polymerized is determined by the order in which messenger codons come into register and their matching by each amino acid t-RNA anticodon. This

Second Position

First Position		Second: U	C	A	G	Third Position
U	U	18	06	19	15	U
	C	18	06	19	15	C
	A	05	06	31	33	A
	G	05	06	32	17	G
C	U	05	08	20	12	U
	C	05	08	20	12	C
	A	05	08	14	12	A
	G	05	08	14	12	G
A	U	04	07	13	06	U
	C	04	07	13	06	C
	A	04	07	11	12	A
	G	16	07	11	12	G
G	U	03	02	09	01	U
	C	03	02	09	01	C
	A	03	02	10	01	A
	G	03	02	10	01	G

Fig. 17. Messenger RNA codons represented by trinucleide triplets specifying a particular amino acid, e.g. UUC indicating *l*-phenylalanine (18). Codons UAA, UAG, and UGA (31, 32, 33) are the so-called 'terminator-triplets' or 'punctuation marks', not yet entirely understood, but presumed to indicate chain terminations. In the relevant literature, UAA is usually referred as 'ochre', and UAG as 'amber'. The numerals from 01 to 20 indicate amino acids 01: glycine (gly); 02: *l*-alanine (ala); 03: *l*-valine (val); 04: *l*-isoleucine (ilu); 05: *l*-leucine (leu); 06: *l*-serine (ser); 07: *l*-threonine (thr); 08: *l*-proline (pro); 09: *l*-aspartic acid (asp); 10: *l*-glutamic acid (glu); 11: *l*-lysine (lys); 12: *l*-arginine (arg); 13: *l*-asparagine (asn); 14: *l*-glutamine (gln); 15: *l*-cysteine (cys); 16: *l*-methionine (met); 17: *l*-tryptophane (try); 18: *l*-phenylalanine (phe); 19: *l*-tyrosine (tyr); 20: *l*-histidine (his); 31, 32, 33: terminators; A: adenine; C: cytosine; G: guanine; U: uracil. C and U are pyrimidines, A and G are purines. [modified and adapted from *Handler*, 1970].

proceeds until a terminator triplet is reached, whereupon the completed protein is released by hydrolytic removal of the t-RNA still fixed to the last amino acid in the chain. Figures 16–18 illustrate the transcription mechanism, the messenger RNA code, and the translation mechanism in accordance with a somewhat more detailed description given by *Handler's* [1970] publication. For further particulars, not relevant in the present context, the reader may be referred to said publication as well as to the *Textbook of Human Genetics* by *Levitan* [1977] and to the comments included in volumes 3/I and 3/II of the present author's *Central Nervous System of Vertebrates* [*K.*, 1970, 1973a].

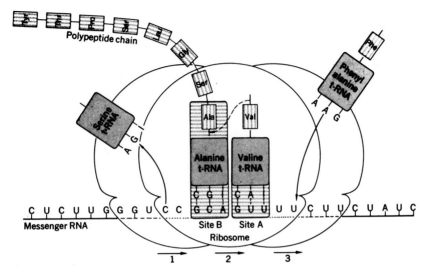

Fig. 18. Diagram purporting to illustrate 'translation' mechanism. Protein synthesis takes place on m-RNA strand 'threaded' through a ribosome. The protein chain grows one amino acid at a time, the sequence of amino acids being determined by the order in which m-RNA codons are matched by each amino acid t-RNA. The ribosome is supposed to move along the m-RNA from left to right. The formation of a specific polypeptide chain proceeds until reaching a terminator triplet, whereupon the completed protein is released by hydrolytic removal of the t-RNA still fixed to the last amino acid in the chain. The first amino acid representing one of the chains in process of synthesis is shown at upper left (Tyr). At the actual site of synthesis the bond between alanine and valine is just about to be effected. At left, the unchanged serin t-RNA is departing, and at right the charged phenylalanine attached to its t-RNA is shown to arrive. I (e.g. in GGI) stands for inosine, a base closely resembling guanine [after *Crick*, 1966, from *Handler*, 1970].

Although the significance of DNA and RNA as well as the basic transcription and translation mechanisms discussed above appear well-substantiated and represent a generally accepted theoretical basis of macromolecular genetics respectively biology, numerous details of the pertinent events and relationships still remain poorly understood and controversial. Among these gaps in the resulting 'models' one could mention the unsettled question concerning the relationship of DNA to proteins, most histones and to other constituents of the chromosomes. Uncertainty obtains also about the number of DNA strands present in each cytologically definable chromosome displays by the various organisms.

As regards the concept of a 'gene', separate terms for units of genetic

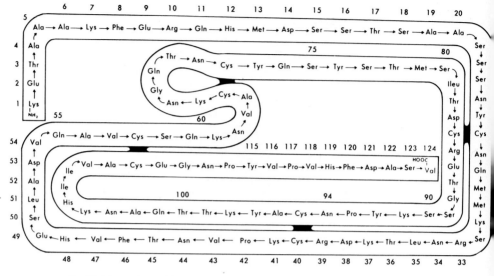

Fig. 19. The amino acid sequence of the enzyme ribonuclease [after *Smyth* et al., from *Handler*, 1970]. The dark patches represent stable cross-bridges formed between amino acids within the same polypeptide chain.

recombination, of mutation and of function have been introduced, named recon, muton, and cistron.

Levitan [1977], however, in agreement with some other authors, points out that these new terms do not replace the gene, 'but only emphasize that operationally we may sometimes perceive only a part of the whole gene'. The recon may thus represent the interchanged portion of an entire gene. The muton (mutable site) would provide a change that gives rise to a new allele. Generally speaking, many genes could be considered equivalent to a single cistron (or unit of gene action). The number of 'genes' in man, estimated some years ago at about 50,000, is now assessed at a few millions. These genes seem to fix permanently certain function rules, which are relatively few in number, but are capable to direct a sequence of further events: the function rules must be fixed, their application flexible, thus providing for 'plasticity' [cf. *Ashby*, 1952]. It seems likely that, in the relevant further events, 'superencipherment' by additional biologic 'codes', superimposed on the variety encoded in the genome proper, plays a substantial role.

It seems that most, possibly all, genes function by acting as indirect patterns for polypeptides which form the organism's proteins, and thereby governing the synthesis of proteins. These latter can be classified as

(1) structural proteins, (2) enzymes, and (3) regulators of gene activity [cf. *Levitan*, 1977].

Enzymes, namely organic catalysts, are of particular significance for the regulation of the metabolic and energy transport mechanisms mentioned further above. These enzymes are either pure proteins or have non-proteins ('coenzymes') attached to them. It is widely assumed that, *qua* genetic action, one gene corresponds to one enzyme.

Recent advanced techniques, such as paper chromatography, electrophoresis and other biochemical procedures have resulted in a 'fingerprinting' of amino acids and in the determination of their sequences. Figure 19 shows, as an example, the amino acid sequences of the enzyme ribonuclease, which is a single polypeptide chain of 124 amino acid residues, containing 8 residues of cystine which are joined by four specific disulfide bonds.

With regard to the highly relevant three-dimensional configuration of complex protein and other organic molecules, the method of X-ray diffraction has yielded significant results. It became evident that the biological properties of proteins are based on their particular three-dimensional structures.

Reverting to the significance of the genes, an important aspect of their activities is their tendency occasionally to change, within certain limits, their structure and composition without thereby losing the capability to duplicate themselves. Such structural changes, which then exert a different biochemical effect, represent mutations,[76] which give rise to characteristic differences in the resulting phenotypes. These variations, maintaining much of the overall pattern, generally differ in certain details.

Yet, either continuous small mutations (micromutations) or perhaps sudden greater changes (macromutations) as postulated by *Goldschmidt*, are of fundamental importance for the origin of new varieties, subspecies, species, as well as additional phylogenetic changes. Constrained by *Darwin's* natural selection and favored by 'adaptation' these changes are presumed to be the essential causes of organic evolution.[77]

Mutations seem to arise 'spontaneously' and can also be induced by external agents (induced mutations). Their exact mechanism still remains unknown at the time of this writing. As regards extrinsic mutagenic agents, it is now customary to distinguish (1) radiations, (2) temperature changes, and (3) chemicals [cf. the tabulation given by *Levitan*, 1977, pp. 746–747].

---

[76] In a wider sense, 'mutations' also include gross chromosomal changes related to the meiotic processes, including chromosome aberrations, but the term mutation is now commonly restricted to changes within a gene or cistron, that is to 'gene mutations'.

[77] Further details on problems of evolution as interpreted by the present author are elaborated in his treatise on *The Central Nervous System of Vertebrates* [*K.*, 1967–1978, e.g. vol. 1, pp. 84–155, vol. 5/II, chapt. XVI, et passim].

Thus, the mechanism of heredity, whose basic features were first shown by *Gregor Mendel* (1822–1884), includes both a persistent and a modifying trend, upon which the constraints obtaining in somatic life are superimposed.

As regards one of the persistent trends, it should be mentioned that, despite the random 'shuffling' obtaining in meiosis, some 'genes' tend to remain linked. My esteemed old friend and former associate in the Department of Anatomy at the whilom Woman's Medical College, *Prof. Max Levitan*, was among the first geneticists to demonstrate that linked genes stay together in evolution far more often than prior genetic theory seemed to suggest.

With respect to the just mentioned 'shuffling' in meiosis, whereby the diploid set of 46 Human chromosomes is reduced to a haploid of 23, there obtains, as it were, a game of chance, in which at least, and discounting 'crossing over', 2^{23} different sets of haploid gamete chromosomes could result, that is to say somewhat more than 8 millions.[78]

Discounting the very numerous still unclarified problems of inheritance and evolution, and referring to the concepts selection and adaptation, the following summary of organic evolution could be given.

Given an overall open system consisting of a set of closed transformations with increasing variety, and with a number of transitory transforms, representing subsets characterized by variety, such that, by a peculiar type of one-many transformations one or two transitory transforms, e.g. one spore or two zygotes, become operands that may result in a number of additional instances of transitory transforms (or subsystems) greater than the original number.

There exist, in this system, very complex parameters providing constraints, such that only certain successions of transforms (trajectories or lines of behavior) are possible, thus limiting the transformations as regards variety, number of instances of similar types representing transforms, and total duration of any subset of transformations representing a line of succession.

A number of transforms become hereby eliminated as operands of transformations which might involve potentially (or presumptively, conceivably) possible additional variety. Because variety of diverse sorts is eliminated from further one-one or one-many transformations, the resulting possible actual variety within the system at any given time period of this succession of events will be less than the conceivably 'possible' variety.

It is evident that the constraints, by reducing variety, thus 'select' the 'permissible' amount of variety. Again, it is evident that the subsystems

---

[78] Cf. the discussion on pages 99–101, chapter XIV, volume 5/II of *K*. [1978]. Through an inadvertent error in arithmetic, however, 2^{23} was erroneously said to be roughly 44 million. It should be 8,388,606 or roughly 8.4 million, which is still a rather large number in the aspect under consideration.

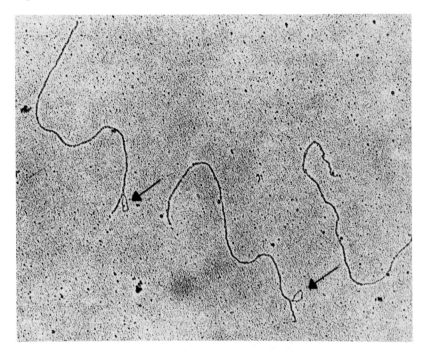

Fig. 20. Electron photomicrograph showing plasmids subsequently to opening of their ring structure through the effect of 'restriction enzymes' [from *Hintsches*, 1977b]. The inserted 'passenger gene' can be recognized as loops indicated by the arrows. Each of the three DNA strands has a length of about 2 μm. The magnification is roughly somewhat over 100,000.

manifesting variety, and persisting under the constraints, that is, 'selected' by the constraints, are thus 'adapted' to the constraints.

'Adaptation' or 'determination' as mentioned above on page 111 with reference to 'functional requirements' accordingly simply means that, if a variety of structural forms does 'randomly' arise, only those compatible with certain functional situations will survive throughout a series of generations.

Reverting once more to the concept of mutations, recent developments since about 1973 have made it possible to experiment in vitro with the preparation of individual genes and with the incorporation of such genes from a donor into the genome of a recipient (recombinant DNA research, 'genetic engineering').

Such experiments are based on the properties of enzymes involved in cleaving and replicating DNA. Thus, the so-called restriction endonucleases have the capability to cut DNA at sequence-specific sites (fig. 20).

The self-explanatory figure 21 illustrates the principle of recombinant

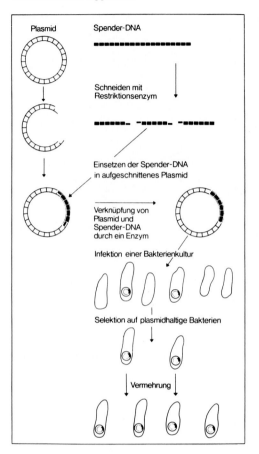

Fig. 21. Diagrams illustrating the procedure of experimental DNA recombination [from *Hintsches*, 1977b].

DNA experiments, as particularly undertaken with prokaryote Bacteria (e.g. *Escherichia coli*). The DNA taken from the donor is commonly called the 'passenger' inserted into a 'vehicle' pertaining to the recipient. The plasmids, which are small, circular DNA molecules capable of self-replication independently of the nucleoid's chromosomes, provide convenient 'vehicles'. Another 'vehicle' is a well-studied bacteriophage lambda. As regards 'passengers' of various provenance, it even became possible to synthetize a wholly artificial gene correcting a mutational defect in the just mentioned bacteriophage [cf. *Maugh*, 1976].

The recombined DNA technology has used a number of different vehicle-host systems, involving unrelated species and including mammalian cells in tissue cultures [cf. e.g., the summary by *Abelson*, 1977].

Because of the danger that new, highly resistant and uncontrollable pathogens might result from 'genetic manipulation', a public debate concerning recombinant DNA research arose and stringent safety guidelines have been discussed and proposed [cf. e.g., *Goodfield*, 1977; *Rogers*, 1977; *Singer*, 1977; *Wade*, 1977; *Abelson*, 1978].

As regards organic life, the definition given above on page 101 and the foregoing discussion of significant vital processes have, however, only considered some generalized aspects. It should, moreover, be kept in mind that an overall definition of life, because of the great extension (*Umfang*) of said term, necessarily involves a rather low degree of intension (*Inhalt*).

Configuration must be included as one of the most important characteristics, in some respects perhaps as the intrinsic feature. Thus life can also be defined as the state of a protoplasmic body which retains its essential form throughout a constant change of matter. *Schopenhauer* [1851] stated this as follows: '*Das Leben läßt sich definieren als der Zustand eines Körpers, darin er, unter beständigem Wechsel der Materie, seine ihm wesentliche (substanzielle) Form allezeit behält. – Wollte man einwenden, daß auch ein Wasserstrudel, oder Wasserfall, seine Form, unter stetem Wechsel der Materie, behält, so wäre zu antworten, daß bei diesen die Form durchaus nicht wesentlich, sondern, allgemeine Naturgesetze befolgend, durch und durch zufällig ist, indem sie von äussern Umständen abhängt, durch deren Veränderung man auch die Form beliebig ändern kann, ohne das Wesentliche anzutasten.*'

Organic form or configuration is, of course, less pronounced in a virus particle or in an Ameba than in higher Metaphyta or Metazoa. Nevertheless, even in the primitive manifestations of life, a definite structure is displayed.

The stream of matter through organic configurations has two aspects. There is an atomic or perhaps better molecular turnover in metabolism which, on the basis of recent studies, seems to be fairly rapid and complete. It has been estimated that in 1 year approximately 98% of the atoms in the human body will be replaced by others.

There is furthermore in many higher Metazoa of comparatively long life duration, especially mammals and man, a turnover of entire formed entities, that is cells. *Labile* or *unstable elements* including blood cells, epidermal epithelium and similar cells are constantly destroyed and replaced during the life of the individual. *Stable elements*, including many glandular epithelia, connective tissue, and neuroglia cells, do not, under normal conditions, manifest extensive changes involving destruction and regeneration, but may have a limited turnover. *Perennial elements*, represented by nerve cells, cardiac musculature and possibly a few other structures, have little or no ability to regenerate. Their life duration can correspond to the entire life span of the individual; however, their material substance may have changed many times through metabolism.

We have thus a flow of energy and matter through an organic configuration. This statement can be reversed and organic form may be understood as 'an enduring order impressed upon a flow of energy' [v. Bonin, 1946]. We might perhaps even go farther and state that life is an evolving, relatively enduring configurational order impressed upon a flow of matter and energy through a protoplasmic matrix which represents an open system, separated from the environment by a boundary.

Morphologic studies of organic forms disclose a remarkable interdependence of structure and function. Structural forms are adapted to or may perhaps even be determined by functional requirements which differ from species to species in correlation with different modes of life. On the other hand, a highly stable fundamental pattern may appear genetically predetermined for large groups of organisms, despite considerable differences in functional demands, and functional requirements are constrained to adapt themselves to a given spatial order.

The concepts of homology and analogy result from a comparison of diverse organic forms, and the distinction between two different sets of principles can be made: one is concerned with change, the other with persistence.

The principle of persistence is manifested by fundamental features preserved throughout all stages of differentiation. Formanalytic studies deal with the abstract aspects of this organic configuration which has topologic and gestalt properties. In this respect the two *Ehrenfels* criteria of wholeness and transposability should be particularly stressed. Since spatial order seems to prevail over temporal events in these relationships, time can be eliminated for practical purposes of analysis. The theoretical formulation thus excludes causality, and the principle of sufficient reason must be applied in its third form, as *principium rationis sufficientis essendi*, that is, as geometric and topologic orderliness. Concepts such as *Grundformteile, Bauplan, Grundbestandteile*, and *Formbestandteile* have been defined [*Haeckel*, 1866, 1898; *Gegenbaur*, 1898; *Jacobshagen*, 1925; *K.*, 1929, 1956]. *Thompson* [1942] has elaborated a method of coordinate transformation.

A morphologic pattern or *Bauplan* represents an elementary topologic space [*K.*, 1967a]. Configurations which, by the topologic procedure of 'mapping', are shown to display identical connectedness within a given *Bauplan* or its *Grundbestandteile*, are *homologous*.[79] Configurations which are not homo-

---

[79] '*Organe, die in einem Bauplan oder dessen Grundformteilen denselben Bestandteil verkörpern, nennen wir, unbekümmert um etwaige Form- und Funktionsunterschiede, homolog*' [*Jacobshagen*, 1925]. Further details on the significance of homology and analogy are elaborated in *K.* [1978, vol. 5/II, chapter XVI].

logous but display certain identical configurational invariants (similarities) or identical or similar functions, are *analogous*.

A hierarchy of orders obtains in various respects; in a very tentative and simplified classification we could, for instance, distinguish internal configuration (structure, texture), which may be repetitive in a randomly, that is nonsignificant fashion, from significant outline or form. *Gegenbaur* distinguished '*Bau*' and '*Struktur*'. A cranial bone, for instance, has a structure of bony (and other) tissue, i.e. a grain, a morphologic form value as an individual configuration, and again another morphologic value as component of a significant higher configuration (*Bauplan*).

It may be possible to classify configuration or pattern in an arbitrarily formulated theoretic scale, such as first, second, and higher (ascending) or lower (descending) order. Further discussion of these still insufficiently clarified relationships must remain outside the scope of this presentation. Geometric or topologic configuration of matter occurs in non-living substances as crystallization. Various kinds of substances have in this respect their natural geometry. There is a definite but as yet insufficiently analyzed relationship between crystallography and the form-analytic study of organisms. *Schrödinger* [1946] suggests that a gene or perhaps a whole chromosome fiber may represent an aperiodic crystal.

Concerning the principles associated with change, that is the active four-dimensional aspect of the physical world in accordance with the *principium rationis sufficientis fiendi*, the morphologist can consider the organism mechanistically in terms of functional anatomy, or historically as a product of organic evolution. Morphology as an evolutionary science 'assumes that certain forces such as natural selection have acted on organisms and – over millions of years – moulded their shape'; *v. Bonin* [1946], whose formulation is quoted here, has defined these relations in terms of 'types and similitudes'.

In ontogeny, we see that organic structures evolve and multiply by reproduction, transmitting their characteristics through a mechanism of heredity. During early and critical ontogenetic stages, Human and other mammalian embryos exhibit morphologic patterns directly comparable with patterns characteristic for Anamnia. Branchial and aortic arches, the urogenital system with its unfolding of pronephros, mesonephros, metanephros and associated ducts, and many regions of the neuraxis as well as other systems display this phenomenon. From a morphological viewpoint, it appears valid to speak of a formal recapitulation of presumably ancestral stages; because of many complicating factors, caution and reserve in the interpretation of these form relationships is imperative. Nevertheless, a satisfactory morphological understanding of adult human organization can be reached only on a broad comparative base including lower vertebrates and key stages of mammalian embryonic development.

Despite a number of errors and exaggerations, *Haeckel's* biogenetic principle, based on the earlier 'law of reduction' ('*Reduktionsgesetz*') formulated by *J. H. Meckel*, appears fundamentally sound and applicable to both vertebrate and invertebrate ontogenesis.

In a publication entitled *Analysis of Development*, compiled by numerous proponents of experimental embryology, *Oppenheimer* [1955] proffers an extreme critique of the biogenetic principle. Needless to say, I completely disagree, not only with her conclusions, but also with the general tenor of her review. Various other authors, particularly also *Medawar*, have likewise expressed views based on a complete misunderstanding not only of said principle but also of basic aspects of morphology.

Considering ontogenetic development we must distinguish quantitative growth processes (*Wachstumsvorgänge*) and qualitative formative processes (*Gestaltungsvorgänge*). Besides this, a structural differentiation of individual cells occurs. Undirected growth would merely lead to an amorphous or at best crudely globular cluster of cells. However, proliferation, migration, grouping and differentiation of cells proceed in compliance with a typical regional pattern which is an expression of negative entropy. Since an orderly arrangement of material units takes place in a three-dimensional organization, a physical agent must be assumed as cause. *Gurwitsch* [1930] has introduced the concept of the biologic field for the factors determining such a pattern. *Weiss* [1939] regards this concept as an abstraction trying to give expression to a set of phenomena observed in living systems; this author also points out that inasmuch as the action of fields produces spatial order, it becomes a postulate that the field factors themselves possess definite order. A three-dimensional organization and heteropolarity of the field must be assumed and the gradual decrease of the field intensity around the imaginary center has led to the concept of field gradients. *Child* [1941] has stressed the significance of physiological gradients which represent spatial patterns in living organisms and are characterized by a gradual progressive differentiation in certain expressions of physiological condition. Morphologic gradients appear during embryonic development and presumably correspond to physiological field gradients. A mitogenetic radiation of the type assumed by *Gurwitsch* [1923] has not been corroborated.

Experimental embryology (developmental mechanics) has tested a number of causal factors and provided some attempts at interpretation. Among external factors studied by experimental methods are mechanical, physicochemical (osmotic pressure, ionic action etc.), biochemical, and radiational effects. Internal factors are related to interactions of embryonic structures; these factors have been investigated by means of isolation, explantation, destruction or excision, transplantation, implantation, fusions, and other methods.

Experimental embryology has, by such means, yielded information concerning polarity, prelocalization, fertilization, cell lineages, ranges of potency, degree of plasticity as shown in regulative development, and determination; the concepts of organizers, induction, competence, and others have been established.

Many fundamental problems still remained unexplained; inductors of various order can be recognized, and even dead tissue is effective under certain conditions. Organizers not only elicit activity in a field but may, to a certain extent, control the emerging field powers. Some factors seem to lie within the responding tissue, and others in the organizer, but on these questions little can be said with any reasonable degree of certainty. Neither the very promising field and gradient concepts nor the various other theories have led to a comprehensive and plausible theory of organic development, growth and regeneration. Nevertheless, we see that a few useful general ideas begin to take shape.

The phenomena of organic life are of overwhelming complexity and it must be admitted that their interpretation in terms of physicochemical concepts has remained unsatisfactory in some respects. Many events cannot be fully explained. The results of experimental embryology nevertheless clearly indicate a succession of orderly, determined (causal) manifestations.

In the second half of the 19th century numerous biologists assumed that chemical laws and physics in its classical Newtonian form might provide a complete explanation of the phenomena of life. The old theory of animal spirits as well as *Bichat's* vital forces and *Magendie's* vital principle were no longer in favor. Since then, vitalism has been revived in various forms. It is claimed that vital processes have a character radically different from purely physicochemical phenomena, and that a qualitatively different concept must be introduced, such as '*élan vital*' (*Bergson*), '*entelechy*' (*Driesch*) and '*telefinalism*'.

It may be reasoned that we can assume vital principles, but certainly not we must. The vitalist's argument is somewhat similar to that of the quantum physicist denying determination or causation. In addition, the concepts of entelechy and telefinalism have definite weaknesses. *Driesch* [1921, 1924] emphasizes a specific principle responsible for wholeness, '*eine besondere ganzmachende Kausalität*' which is not assumed to act in space, but 'into the space', and designates it in *Aristotle's* terminology as *entelechy*. A principle of this type indeed exists as the properties of configuration or gestalt, according to the *principium rationis sufficientis essendi*, but it is by no means a characteristic of life. The orderliness inherent in pattern applies to the entire range of the physical world and cannot be said to represent a vitalistic principle. As concisely stated in a 'symposium' by *Brain* [1950]: 'An atom is a pattern of electrons, a molecule a pattern of atoms. There are patterns of patterns, and so on indefinitely. The most complicated patterns we know are in the brain.'

Telefinalism (*Zielursächlichkeit, Zweckmäßigkeit*) of *G. Wolff* [1933] and of others assumes a purpose which, in turn, must necessarily imply a consciously and intelligently envisaged plan. These views merely represent a thinly disguised modern version of the well-known ancient teleologic or physicoteleologic argument. By definition, we have attempted to eliminate the attributes of consciousness from the postulated physical world and it would be inconsistent to reintroduce such attributes for any single group of events. Phenomena of life require a set of certain conditions which are indispensable or can be said to represent *a conditio sine qua non*. If, and only if, we assume a conscious intention, the events resulting from these conditions can be regarded as purposeful.[80]

Although organic life appears characterized by a number of specific phenomena, I do not see any reason to assume a different set of fundamental principles for any separate group of events in the physical world, whether these events concern living or non-living matter. Numerous new physical 'forces' or rather effects may result from patterned, vectorial and even scalar combination of other physical interactions, and account for a peculiar, but strictly determined situation in which 'existing order displays the power of maintaining itself and producing orderly events' [*Schrödinger*, 1946].

Schopenhauer, a strict determinist, considered himself a vitalist, following *Bichat* and others. Despite numerous weaknesses, which may in part be attributed to the less advanced scientific knowledge at his time, he made many excellent statements on organic life. In an amusing, and perhaps not entirely unjustified vitriolic diatribe directed against *Agassiz*, the following pertinent remark is given, which may be considered devoid of any vitalistic implication: '*Auch er steht noch vor der selben Alternative, daß die organische Welt entweder das Werk reinsten Zufalls sei, der sie, als ein Naturspiel physikalischer und chemischer Kräfte, zusammengewürfelt hätte; oder aber ein am Lichte der Erkenntnis (dieser functio animalis) nach vorhergegangener Überlegung und Berechnung klug verfertigtes Kunstwerk. Eines ist so falsch wie das andere ...*' (Parerg., und Paralip. II, *Zur Philosophie und Wissenschaft der Natur*, § 91).

Schopenhauer's remark, however, requires a very relevant qualification. The concept '*reinster Zufall*', that is to say, 'pure chance', is a rather vague one, as pointed out above (p. 76 et passim) in the section on causality 'Chance' does by no means exclude 'necessity'.[81]

It can be maintained that organic life at its prebiotic stage resulted from

---

[80] The significance of the terms purpose and teleology, as defined by *Rosenblueth* et al. [1943] will be discussed in vol. 2, chapter IV, section 3, page 33.

[81] The publication '*Le hasard et la nécessité*' by *Monod* [1970] can hardly be taken seriously, since this author entirely fails to understand the significance of both chance and necessity as well as the relationship between these two concepts. The late *Jaques Monod* [1910–1976] is a typical

an apparently 'random' interplay of physicochemical processes in accordance with the 'law of large numbers' discussed in the just cited section (p. 78), and comparable to a procedure 'by trial and error'. The interplay of the four basic 'natural forces', however, presumably provided constraining parameters, precluding an 'equiprobability' obtaining in an ordinary game of chance such as, e.g., the throwing of 'normal' dice. The random but nevertheless strictly determined (i.e. necessary) events leading to prebiotic stages and finally to organic life can therefore be likened to a game of chance with loaded dice. In another wording, as formulated by *Schrödinger* [1946], organic life originated in accordance with 'order resulting from disorder'.

The concept of order based on disorder may, *prima facie*, appear as a paradox or as a meaningless platitude [cf. e.g. *K.*, 1961, p. 349]. However, if disorder is conceived as 'randomness' respectively 'chance' (lack of purpose, lack of ascertainable relation or connection), it will be seen that 'chance' nevertheless involves necessity, and that randomness, in accordance with the 'law of large numbers', involves various aspects of orderliness. If 'order based on disorder' is conceived to imply the just mentioned orderliness, then said concept becomes justified and expresses the gist of cosmic and prebiotic evolution. In subsequent organic evolution an additional principle becomes manifested by the negentropy provided through the peculiar properties of nucleic acids. Thus, in organic evolution 'order from (or based on) order' becomes superimposed upon, or combined with 'order from (or based on) disorder'. The concept of 'order based on order' (that is to say feeding on negentropy) was also clearly elaborated by *Schrödinger* [1946].

It should also be recalled that *Ernst Haeckel* was apparently the first author who postulated and defined in the modern sense abiogenesis ('spontaneous generation', archegony), that is to say the origin of prokaryote Biota ('Monera') from prebiotic evolutionary processes.

The origin of life at its prebiotic stage can, moreover, be regarded as resulting from an inevitable 'degeneration', 'disease', or (in the figurative sense, introducing here a logically illicit, i.e. fictional axiologic valuation) 'putrefaction' of 'matter', intrinsically related to the given properties of cyanamide compounds and of the nucleic acid macromolecules.

It is likely that the primordial explosion or 'fireball' resulting in the formation of the present (or any similar previous) universe caused a random (chance) but nevertheless strictly determined distribution of mass and energy

---

example of numerous 'superspecialists' who, because of their particular substantial achievements, have been canonized by the Establishment and subsequently believe that they are thus qualified to express pontifical views on topics beyond their narrow grasp. Other such examples are *Medawar* with respect to his pronouncements on phylogeny and related topics, as well as *Eccles* and diverse quantum physicists elaborating their 'philosophic' views.

with evolving galaxies and stars. This included the formation of organic compounds which, in turn, provided for prebiotic evolution. This latter, nevertheless, required particular conditions which, within the framework of cosmic evolution, seem to be relatively perhaps extremely rare, although in view of the extensive size of the universe, such conditions may obtain in a large number of cases.

This inevitable 'degeneration' of matter is substantiated by the large variety of molecules, including complex organic ones, recently discovered in interstellar space [cf. *Rank* et al., 1971; *Metz*, 1973; *Turner*, 1977]. The list of molecules detected now exceeds 25 and includes H_2O, OH, NH_3, NH_2CHO, CO, H_2CO, CS, SiO, HCN, CH_3CN, HCOOH, CH_3OH, H_2S, and others. Mixtures of such molecules as H_2O, HCN, NH_3, and H_2CO are common starting points for primitive synthesis experiments to examine possible processes that can initiate organic life in accordance with *Haeckel's* 'Carbogen-Theorie' and *Pflüger's* 'Cyan-Theorie' [cf. *K.*, 1970, p. 650]. In such experiments, HC_3N and HNCO are typical important products, which can play a role in further synthesis. Although the interstellar molecules cannot initiate relevant prebiotic processes in the interstellar environment extremely hostile to life, the fact that such molecules can form even in such environment supports the view that they can readily be formed in planetary atmospheres.

The number of stars with planetary systems in our galaxy and in the universe at large might be substantially less than that of stars without such system, but is, nevertheless, now estimated to be quite large.[82]

Again, if our solar system is taken as an example, most planets might be entirely inhospitable to further prebiotic evolution and thus remain sterile. Besides our own planet, only Venus and Mars were believed to be suitable for organic life, but Venus was subsequently shown to be unsuitable,[83] and the experiments performed on Mars by the 1976 Viking robot landing mission remained inconclusive up to the time of this writing. It seemed evident, however, that if organic life does exist on Mars, it would merely occur in a very 'low' state, precluding the evolution of sentient and 'intelligent' forms.

This would agree with the opinion expressed by *McCrea* [1975] who pointed out that the formation of 'true planets' is an exceedingly complicated process, which does not result in 'standard models' but in an extremely large number of possible types. The cited author believes that even if rudimentary

---

[82] *Hoyle* [1975a] assumes 10^{11} stars of sun-like size and presumably with planets, in our galaxy. If this latter contains 10^{12} stars, this would be a ratio of one in ten. Apart from the uncertainty about the presumed numbers, *Hoyle's* estimate is perhaps unduly high. Further comments on this topic will be given further below.

[83] Discounting, of course, a bare possibility that, following cooling and appropriate chemical changes, life might there originate in a very distant future (cf. above, p. 66).

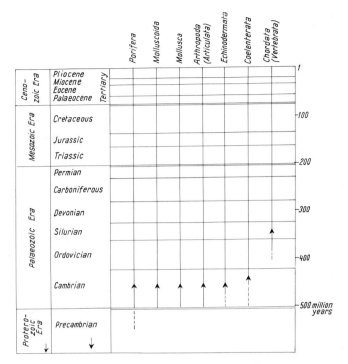

Fig. 22. Rough diagram of Geologic Time Chart including lineal representation of paleontologic records concerning seven major animal phyla [from *K.*, 1967a]. The pleistocene and recent epochs cannot be shown at this scale. Although coelenterates and echinoderms (cf. fig. 23) could be regarded as phyla with very 'primitive' morphologic features, their earliest records are less ancient and distinct than those of some other phyla (e.g. arthropods). This may be due to various circumstances not related to actual ancientness, and not precluding such greater ancientness. Again, in many outlines of this sort, the width of the vertical line or band is drawn in proportion to the known variety or numerousness of the particular phylum in each of the geological periods. Sacrificing detail to conciseness, this procedure was not followed here, particularly since it involves many and considerable uncertainties as regards proper interpretation.

life could originate in numerous regions of the cosmos, the conditions for the origin of Human beings (respectively of comparable intelligent beings) are extremely rare (cf. further below, p. 130).

Reverting to the evolutionary events on our planet as discussed on page 66 in the section on the physical world, one could distinguish prebiotic and subsequent biotic events. Assuming the presence of a hot atmosphere, volatile organic compounds could have been present in vapor or clouds. Sunlight may have induced the synthesis of amino acids, carbohydrates and other complex molecules, which all fell to the surface in rain, providing solutions in ocean or

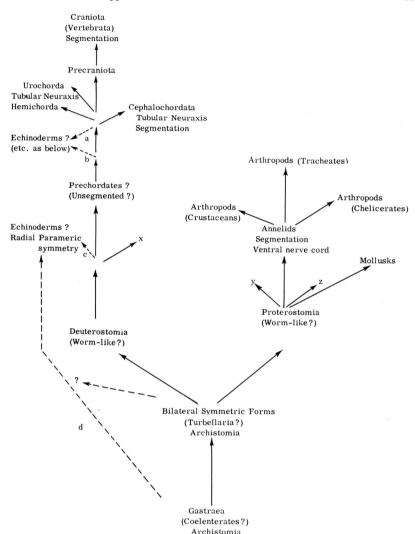

Fig. 23a. Hypothetic main evolutionary relationships in Metazoa, illustrating a possible general derivation of vertebrates from invertebrates [from *K.*, 1967b]. a, b, c, d: 'Logically' permissible different phylogenetic derivations of echinoderms, whose 'origin' is difficult to establish; x: Chaetognatha (and possible additional 'minor' groups as might be demonstrated to be Deuterostomia); y: protostome lophophorate Metazoa; z: other 'minor' groups. Archistomia have only one blastopore (stomodeum). In Proterostomia, the blastopore persists as the adult mouth, the anal opening being secondary. In Deuterostomia, the blastopore becomes the anus the oral opening being secondary.

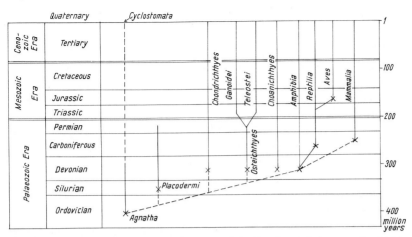

Fig. 23b. Generalized hypothetic genealogic tree of the Vertebrate phylum correlated with Geologic Time Chart [from *K.*, 1967a]. It should be recalled that *Ernst Haeckel* was the first to elaborate this sort of genealogic tree (*Stammbaum*) whose overall concept has remained much the same despite the many new additional data.

lagoons. Subsequent random combinations resulted, until by 'chance' self-replicating systems arose, leading to biotic events.

Assuming on the other hand, a lower early temperature, the prebiotic chemicals might have initially arisen in the ocean or in land-locked pools [cf. e.g. *Hoyle*, 1975b].

It can be presumed that the prebiotic events resulted, about 3 Eons ago, in the origin of Procaryotes (*Haeckel's* Monera) such as early photosynthetic Bacteria and photosynthetic blue-green Algae. It seems likely that the activities of these organisms contributed to, or even produced, the oxygen content of the atmosphere [cf. e.g. *Schwartz and Dayhoff*, 1978]. Other Bacteria produced carbon dioxide and hydrogen, on which, in turn, anaerobic, methan-producing micro organisms, so-called 'methanogens' lived. It is claimed that 'methanogens' represent a third group of Prokaryotes differing from Bacteria [*Maugh*, 1977].

The origin of Prokaryotes was doubtless related to the production of chromosomes by the random interactions involving DNA and RNA. This initiated a new stage in organic evolution, at which 'order based on disorder' became supplemented, but not entirely replaced, by 'order based on order', whereby organic life 'feeds on negative entropy' [*Schrödinger*, 1946].

About 2 Eons ago, Eukaryote Protophyta and Protozoa may have evolved, from which, about 0.6 Eons (i.e. 6×10^8 years) ago, Metaphyta and

Metazoa originated. Figures 22–24 illustrate the presumed course of meta-zoan phylogenetic evolution.[84]

It is also appropriate to keep in mind the exceedingly large number of different Prokaryote and Eukaryote organic forms, including extinct and still extant recent ones. In the present author's *Propaedeutics to Comparative Neurology* [K., 1967a] approximate numerical estimates were given. Altogether, there may be substantially more than 340,000 'different species' of plants (extant and fossil) and more than 1 million of (fossil and extant) 'different species' of animals, both plant and animal species being subsumed under a lesser but still rather large number of genera, families, orders, classes and phyla. The process of phylogenetic evolution displays, as it were, a branching off at random in diverging directions of 'radiating lines' (phyloge-netic radiations, 'phylogenetic trees'). The randomness and the number as well as the extent of the 'radiations' are limited by numerous constraining parameters, such as 'natural selection' etc.

With respect to the phylogenetic evolution of mammals and presumably also numerous submammalian vertebrate and other animal and vegetal or-ganisms, the faunal and floral isolations related to the now generally recog-nized *continental drift* appear to have played an important role.

Although a few previous authors, impressed by the jigsaw-like fitting outlines of African and South American coasts, had suggested a splitting of these continents, *Alfred Wegener* (1880–1930) was the first to propound a systematic theory of '*Verschiebung der Kontinente*' [1915] or continental drift, which became, some years after mid-century, further elaborated by the plate tectonic theory.

It is now assumed, in overall conformity with *Wegener's theory*, that at the transition from Paleozoic to Mesozoic eras (Permian-Triassic periods), about 200 million years ago, our planet's land areas formed a single continent, Pangaea, surrounded by a single ocean, Panthalassa.

---

[84] Comments on further details of organic evolution in accordance with the present author's views are included in volumes 1, 2, 3/II and 5/II of *The Central Nervous System of Vertebrates* [K., 1967, 1973, 1978]. Relevant discussions on organic evolution, e.g. by *Remane*, are contained in the publication 'Evolution' edited by *Scharf* [1975], which also includes, on pages 396–416, a 'Round Table Discussion' on '*Zufall und Notwendigkeit in der Evolution*', in which the zoologist *E. Mayr* participated. This gentleman had the effrontery to proclaim verbatim [p. 410, loc. cit.]: '*Von all den Herren, die hier an diesem Tische sitzen, kann ich wohl sagen, dass ich der einzige bin, der seinen "Führerschein" als Biologe hat. Aber die anderen Herren, die aus der Chemie kommen oder aus der Physik, sie kennen einen Teil der Biologie, aber die Kenntnisse sind etwas mangelhaft.*' Although a modicum of competence in his specialty may be conceded to the quoted *Harvard* pandit, his conduct deserves censure. Despite his self-issued '*Führerschein*' (official 'license'), I have reasons to believe that his vaunted knowledge remains far below his own estimate of it.

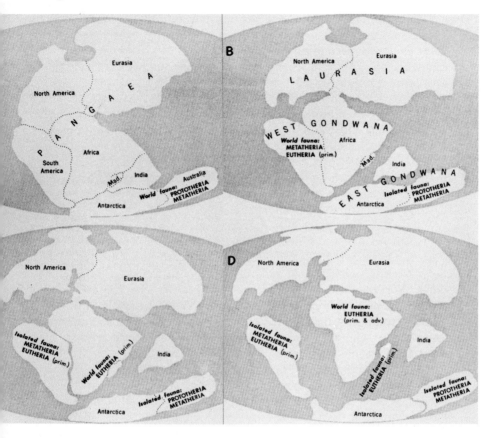

Fig. 24. Hypothetic maps illustrating the break-up of Pangaea [simplified after *Dietz* and *Holden*, from *Fooden*, 1972]. A: At end Palaeozoic (ca. 200 million years ago); B: near end of Triassic (perhaps 165 million years ago); C: at upper Jurassic or lower Cretaceous (perhaps roughly 135 million years ago); D: during Cretaceous period (ca. 135–75 million years ago).

There is, moreover, some evidence that this continent was initially entirely submerged, and that its emergence from a primordial ocean, covering the entire globe, occurred in the Precambrian, about $3-4 \times 10^9$ years ago. This emergence of a continent from beneath the primordial sea may have been a slow process, occupying most of the Precambrian time.

During the Mesozoic era, at the Jurassic-Cretaceous periods, about 135 million years ago, a northern landmass, Laurasia, seems to have split from a southern one, Gondwana, from which, in turn, Antarctica and India split off, with India heading toward Laurasia. Perhaps in the lower Cretaceous, Laurasia split into North America and Eurasia, while South America split off from Gondwana, whose remainder became Africa. During the Cretaceous, Madagascar began to separate from Africa, and Australia-New Guinea may have started to drift away from Antarctica.

In the Paleocene epoch of the Cenozoic era, perhaps 65 million years ago, the North Atlantic and Indian Oceans took shape, the South Atlantic widened, and India was still floating toward Eurasia, which it joined, possibly in the Miocene epoch, some 20 million years ago, thrusting up the Himalaya range. North and South America likewise became joined in the Tertiary period. During this period, concomitantly with collisions of the African and Eurasian continents, the Mediterranean sea repeatedly dried up and became again flooded. One such major flooding within that sequence seems to have occurred in the middle Pliocene, about 5 million years ago.

It is believed that the still shifting crust of the earth represents a mosaic of perhaps about 20 'plates', about 50–150 km thick. These plates, slowly sliding over a hot, semiplastic layer ('asthenosphere') carry the continents and ocean basins with them. Earthquakes and volcanic eruptions occur along some boundaries, 'faults' or 'cracks' between the plates, while other edges slide beneath an opposing plate. Polar wandering is supposed to have taken place in connection with these events, and the present Sahara may have been at the South Pole about 450 million years ago, in the Paleozoic era, at the Cambrian period.

Figures 24A–D illustrate current concepts of the breakup of Pangaea and indicate some of the implications for Mammalian phylogeny. The aboriginal land Mammal faunas in Australia and New Guinea (Prototherians and Metatherians), and Madagascar (Eutherians only) can be considered to represent successively detached samples of the evolving world Mammal fauna as it existed when each of these land masses became faunally isolated from the rest of the world as a result of the progressive fragmentation of Pangaea [*Fooden*, 1972]. Isolation of aboriginal Prototherians and Metatherians in Australia and New Guinea may date, according to the cited author, from the Upper Jurassic-Lower Cretaceous; isolation of aboriginal Metatherians and Eutherians in South America may date from the Middle Cretaceous-Upper

Cretaceous; isolation of aboriginal Eutherians in Madagascar could date from the Paleocene-Eocene.

Reverting now to *Schopenhauer's* diatribe against *Agassiz* quoted above on page 120, it could be stated that the strictly determined and thus inevitable or 'necessary' evolution toward the *'organismische Welt'* may indeed be likened to a cosmic game of chance based on an interplay of physicochemical 'forces', in which, as it were, the dice are loaded in favor of the apparently highly 'improbable' origin of organic life.[85] Subsequently to said origin, 'chance' (i.e. randomness) became further constrained (but not eliminated) by the orderliness (negentropy) encoded in the nuclear acid genome. The entire course of these events including prebiotic evolution and succedent phylogeny can thus be said to display a predestined spatial and temporal pattern manifesting itself along the time coordinate. 'Predestined' means here 'necessary' respectively 'inevitable', and 'chance', means both 'random' and 'purposeless'.

With regard to extraterrestrial life, it is evident that on the basis of the available evidence, merely very vague conjectures are possible. One might, nevertheless, assume that since an identical orderliness of anorganic 'matter' involving subatomic, atomic, molecular, and large-scale events seems to hold in the entire observable universe, an identical biological orderliness should likewise obtain. This would imply a substantial uniformity of prebiotic and prokaryote as well as eukaryote evolution leading to Protista, Protophyta, Protozoa, Metaphyta and Metazoa, invertebrates and vertebrates.

One could thus discount speculations concerning bizarre forms of 'life' based, e.g. on the silicon instead of on the carbon atom. On the other hand, neither the presence of oxygen nor relatively low or high temperatures, nor higher levels of radiation might preclude the origin of anaerobic or otherwise adapted primitive organic systems. Such conditions, however, might preclude the evolution of 'higher' forms. The presence of water, nevertheless, would presumably be a prerequisite for any origin of organic life.

The problem of extraterrestrial life, moreover, is not quite identical with the problem of extraterrestrial intelligence and civilizations. One could maintain that 'intelligence' presupposes sentient (conscious) organic beings endowed with a central nervous system as briefly discussed below in the next section.

---

[85] With respect to the two alternatives mentioned by *Schopenhauer*, namely *'reinster Zufall'* or *'am Lichte der Erkenntnis (dieser functio animalis) nach vorhergegangener Überlegung und Berechnung klug verfertigtes Kunstwerk'*, there is thus a third one, provided by constrained chance (order from disorder), subsequently combined with a relatively stable orderliness (order based on order) nevertheless still subject to disturbance by 'noise', that is to say by random factors, which, however, continue to remain controlled by constraints.

Although a tubular dorsal neuraxis as characteristic for vertebrates may, in this respect, be superior to the ganglionic Invertebrate nervous system,[86] it could, nevertheless, be possible that some extraterrestrial 'intelligence' or 'civilizations' might develop among unknown invertebrate forms.

Again, although vertebrate intelligence and civilization, as developed by Man, has reached a high degree of technology and of knowledge extending to the structure of the entire observable universe, the existence of still 'higher' extraterrestrial civilizations remains a possibility. It should, however, be kept in mind that Human civilization seems already to have passed its 'acme' and can be regarded as beginning to degenerate, having entered its stage of paracme (cataplasia, *Rückbildung*) in *Haeckel's* formulation.

Nothing certain whatsoever can be said about the possible number, in the universe, of planets (1) with organic life, (2) with sentient organic beings, and (3) with 'civilizations' developed by 'intelligent life'.

If there are 10^9 galaxies and 10^{11} planetary systems in an average galaxy, perhaps 10^{20} planetary systems might exist. Arbitrarily assuming one such system in 1,000 to have developed organic life on one or two of its planets, an order of magnitude corresponding to 10^{17} obtains. If, again, the ratio of $1:1,000$ for sentient beings with a central nervous system holds, we obtain 10^{14}. Assuming the same ratio for 'intelligent life' with civilizations, the number would be in the order of 10^{11} (hundred billion). Even with this very large number, the odds for extraterrestrial civilizations are about $1:10^9$. Yet, one might also assume a much smaller number of planetary systems and much higher odds against 'intelligent life', such as e.g. $1:10^{12}$. Even this would give an order of magnitude corresponding to 10^8 (hundred million).

Thus, while not only 'intelligent life' but also organic life in general might be regarded as extremely 'improbable' or rare phenomena in the cosmos,[87] these phenomena would, because of the large numbers involved, nevertheless manifest themselves in very numerous instances.

Again, assuming, in our galaxy, an undefined large number (e.g. 10^6 to 10^8) of other planetary systems on which life may have arisen, and given the emergence of 'intelligence', for how long on the average can we expect such an intelligence to persist? [cf. *Hoyle*, 1975b].

Denoting the average duration of intelligent life by L, one can hardly

---

[86] Cf. *K.* [1978, vol. 5/II, p. 396] with reference to views expressed by *Elliott* [1969].

[87] As regards the inevitable occurrence of organic life in our present universe, it should also be kept in mind that, in some of the possible universes resulting from the succeeding primordial fireballs the composition of the cosmic material would preclude the formation of carbon and of molecules necessary for life (cf. also above, p. 66), in the section on the physical world). Thus, in the cycles of expansion and collapse, a 'reprocessed' universe might not manifest the required conditions for life to form. Accordingly, we may now merely sample a particular form of cosmos

expect that L will be at all comparable to the total age, say T, of our galaxy. With L less than T the number of planetary systems with intelligent beings existing at the same time, and therefore theoretically able to communicate with each other, must be less than the assumed total of one million favorable cases by the ratio L/T.[88] Only a fraction of the cases might overlap with each other, or there might be no effective overlap at all, and interstellar communication would not be possible.[89]

Yet a search for 'extraterrestrial intelligence' or 'extraterrestrial civilizations', including perfunctory attempts at interstellar communication is now seriously considered by competent authors and organizations [cf. *Hoyle*, 1975b; *Kuiper and Morris*, 1977; *Sagan* et al., 1977].

The American spacecraft Pioneer 10, launched March 3, 1972, took a 21-month-long flight to the vicinity of Jupiter in order to provide data on this planet, and then continued on a course toward interstellar space beyond our solar system. Assuming the bare possibility that the craft might be intercepted by an intragalactic civilization, it contained a graphic message engraved on an aluminium plate giving information on the craft's origin as well as a few data concerning Human beings and scientific thought. It was assumed that the message could be deciphered by intelligent beings of an advanced civilization.

Again, a project 'Cyclops', consisting of an array of 1,500 radio antennas, has been suggested which could transmit and receive coded interstellar information, restricted, however, to our galaxy. A preliminary attempt was made to transmit a message in binary code toward the great cluster in the constellation Hercules from the radio telescope at the Arecibo observatory in Puerto Rico.

Given the great distances, the limited speed c of electromagnetic radiation, and the thinly scattered stars, the odds against a positive result are evidently considerable. In addition, there would necessarily be an interval of very many, perhaps a few thousand years between transmission of a message and reception of a response.

Still more difficult would be the problem of interstellar space travel, even if spacecrafts with nuclear power could be accelerated to speeds significantly approaching c. On the basis of contemporary astronomical, physical and mathematical knowledge as well as technology, the possibility of Human

---

from a whole ensemble of them, many of which would pass unobserved by intelligent sentient beings. Thus our existence would still be an accident, but one that must inevitably occur in a universe which reconstitutes itself in different forms, again and again. In this perspective, *Spengler's* [1927] reference to the '*Zufall Kultur*', the '*Zufall Mensch*' and the '*Zufall Leben*' appear fully justified, particularly also with respect to the denotation implying 'lack of a purpose'.

[88] *Mutatis mutandis*, similar considerations apply to the universe in toto.

[89] To this must be added the limitations imposed by the limit c for radio communication and still more for space travel extending beyond the solar system as again pointed out further below.

interstellar travel over distances of a few light years appears at least highly improbable in the foreseeable future and, for the still greater interstellar and intergalactic distances, such travel, involving at present insuperable problems, seems to be practically impossible.

In recent years, the problem of unidentified flying objects (UFO) has generated speculations that our Earth is observed by spacecrafts (e.g. 'flying saucers') from extraterrestrial advanced civilizations. Most 'UFO' reports can be explained as optic illusions, mistaken identity of conventional flying contraptions, (e.g. meteorologic balloons), natural phenomena and hoaxes. The few 'unexplained' cases might represent still poorly understood meteorologic respectively psychologic phenomena. The widespread 'UFO' craze can be evaluated as a symptom of the evident present-day generalized psychopathic degeneration and thus be discounted, quite apart from the improbability that intelligent extraterrestrial visitors would not have made serious attempts at únequivocal communication

As an aside, it is perhaps appropriate to mention three speculations on this topic, which are of some historical interest.

Among the grandiose cosmic phantasmagories of Mahâyâna Buddhism the famed shorter *Amitâbha Sûtra* (*Bussetsu Amida Kyô*, Sino-Japan; *Budhabâsita Amitâbha Sûtra* or *Sukhâvati-vyûha*, Sanskr.), dating back to approximately between 50 BC and 50 AD, purports to be a sermon on the 'Pure Land' (*Jôdo*, Sino-Japan; *Sukhâvatî*, Sanskr.) given by the historical Buddha *Shakyamuni* at *Shrâvasti*. In this Sûtra, addressed to *Sâriputra*, one of *Shakyamuni's* main disciples, the following passage can be found:

'*Sâriputra*, just as I now praise the inconceivable excellences of *Amitâbha* Buddha, there are also in the Eastern region Buddha *Aksobhya*, Buddha *Meruprabhâsa*, Buddha *Manjugosa* and other Buddhas as numerous as the grains of sand in the River Ganges. Each of these Buddhas proclaims the Law with such eloquence that his teachings spread throughout three thousand great Chiliocosms.' This is repeated five times with the names of additional Buddhas, for the other three cardinal directions (South, West, North) as well as Nadir and Zenith.

In Western literature, subsequently to *Giordano Bruno's* interpretation of the 'fixed stars' as distant suns, the concept of extraterrestrial inhabited worlds pertaining to other solar systems was elaborated by diverse authors. It will here be sufficient merely to quote *Voltaire* and *Schopenhauer*.

In *Voltaire's* tale '*Memnon*' [1747], a spirit, denizen of the world of Sirius, is made to state: '*dans les cent mille millions de mondes qui sont dispersés dans l'étendue, tout se suit par degrés. On a moins de sagesse et de plaisir dans le second que dans le premier, moins dans le troisième que dans le second, et ainsi du reste jusqu'au dernier, où tout le monde est fou.*' '*J'ai bien peur, dit Memnon, que notre petit globe terraqué ne soit précisément les Petites Maisons de l'univers dont vous me faites l'honneur de me parler'. 'Pas tout à fait, dit l'esprit; mais il en approche.'*

In his tale *'Micromégas' Voltaire* [1752] introduces an interstellar traveller from *'une de ces planètes qui tournent autour de l'étoile nommée Sirius'.* Together with an inhabitant of Saturn, he visits Earth. In a discussion with Earthlings, one of a group of terrestrian philosophers, *'plus franc que les autres'*, comments on the status of his globe: *'si l'on en excepte un petit nombre d'habitants fort peu considérés, tout le reste est un assemblage de fous, de méchants, et de malheureux.'*

Schopenhauer begins the first chapter of the second volume of his main work (*Welt als Wille und Vorstellung*, 1844) with the statement: *'Im unendlichen Raum zahllose leuchtende Kugeln, um jede von welchen etwa ein Dutzend kleinerer, beleuchteter sich wälzt, die inwendig heiss, mit erstarrter kalter Rinde überzogen sind, auf der ein Schimmelüberzug lebende und erkennende Wesen erzeugt hat; – dies ist die empirische Wahrheit, das Reale, die Welt. Jedoch ist es für ein denkendes Wesen eine missliche Lage, auf einer jener zahllosen im grenzenlosen Raum frei schwebenden Kugeln zu stehen, ohne zu wissen woher noch wohin, und nur Eines zu seyn von unzählbaren ähnlichen Wesen, die sich drängen, treiben, quälen, rastlos und schnell entstehend und vergehend, in anfangs- und endloser Zeit'* ... *'– Da hat nun endlich die Philosophie der neueren Zeit, zumal durch Berkeley und Kant, sich darauf besonnen, daß Jenes alles doch nur ein Gehirnphänomen und mit so grossen, vielen und verschiedenen subjektiven Bedingungen behaftet sei, dass die gewähnte absolute Realität desselben verschwindet und für eine ganz andere Weltordnung Raum lässt, die das jenem Phänomen zum Grunde liegende wäre, d.h. sich dazu verhielte wie zur blossen Erscheinung das Ding an sich selbst.'*

4. The Nervous System

Animal organic life above a certain level of organization is characterized by a nervous system acting as a correlating and integrating communication and control mechanism, based on the diverse functional characteristics of nervous tissue.

The relevant functional characteristic is customarily designated as conductivity (cf. above, p. 101 with regard to the definition of organic life). This term refers to the transmission, through a given path or channel, of an electrochemical disturbance, called 'impulse' and representing a 'signal', encoding variety.

Nervous tissue, again, consists of conducting elements, namely nerve cells with their elongated processes ('nerve fibers'). Several sorts of supporting elements may be closely related to the nerve cells and their branching extensions.

The relevant biological activities of nerve cells involve here (1) irritability, that is to say the property to be excited (disturbed) by a stimulus, and (2) the propagation of the disturbance. This latter, again, may then result in an end-effect, such as motion, or secretion; electric discharges (by some fishes), or emission of light (bioluminescence of some fishes and some invertebrates).

Such activities imply receptors, for the stimuli, conductors of the 'impulse', and effectors. In *Sherrington's* [1906, 1947] words the manifestations of behavior 'in which there follows on an initiating reaction an end-effect reached through the mediation of a conductor, itself incapable either of the end-effect, or, under natural conditions, of the inception of the reaction, are reflexes'.

The cited author also emphasized the integrative aspect of nervous function: in the higher Metazoa, it is mainly[90] nervous reaction which integrates the organism, that is 'welds it together from its components, and constitutes from a mere collection of organs an animal individual'.

Such integration, combining different nerve impulses so that they combine or 'cooperate' toward a common, significantly describable effect includes 'coordination' and requires, in addition to the conduction of impulses ('signals') their processing by a nervous network characterized by 'circuits' and their 'switches'. These latter are devices for making, breaking or changing the connections within the circuits.

In the nervous system, the surfaces, or membranes of separation between two connected conducting elements provide the required switches. These latter, if transmitting the impulse in one direction only, are designated as synapses (*Sherrington*), being thus 'polarized', and play a most important role in highly differentiated central nervous systems. Another type of nexus, particularly in very primitive nerve nets, may be 'unpolarized' or 'asynaptic', transmitting impulses in either direction. Again, there seem to obtain facultatively polarized connections which may be called 'protosynaptic'.

Synapses may either be excitatory, that is, transmitting the impulse from one conducting unit (neuron) to the next one, or inhibitory, that is preventing the connected conducting unit from responding or 'reacting' to neural signals.

Reverting to the concept of receptors, conductors and effectors, the receptors may be represented by diverse 'sense organs', 'adapted to' (that is to say with a low threshold of excitation for) particular stimuli,[91] or by free

---

[90] Some integration can also result from the biochemical effect of substances (e.g. hormones) distributed by body fluids, and from the effects of blood or fluid circulations in general.

[91] My senior Breslau colleague *H. Winterstein* was wont to stress the distinction between '*Reizung*' ('stimulation') and the different aspects of '*Erregung*' ('excitation'). Stimulation is said to represent the local energy or force (interaction) changes produced at the 'reception locus', and excitation subsumes the physicochemical changes triggered by the stimulation ('*die durch die Reizung ausgelösten physikalisch-chemischen Vorgänge*'). It may be taken as well substantiated that excitation involves an 'expenditure of energy'.

endings of receptory ('sensory') nerve fibers. Accordingly, with regard to the stimuli, one may distinguish mechanical receptors, chemoreceptors, and receptors to radiation. Effectors are represented by muscles, glands, and more rarely, as mentioned above, electric organs and luminescent (photogenic) organs.

The connections between a nervous system and the elements of a sense organ or of an effector also represent particular types of synapses.

The essential features of a nervous system involve thus input and output of signals through afferent respectively efferent nerve fibers and, particularly in centralized, well-differentiated nervous systems, the 'processing' of these signals by so-called 'centers', whose details of circuitry may be only partly elucidated on the basis of the available data. Some 'centers' then represent 'black boxes' in engineering terminology. Black box designates here some system with input and output, manifesting determinate or, at least, statistically definable behavior. Said system, however, is either unspecified or not open to inspection, such that its internal working arrangement remains unknown. Yet, upon a describable sort of input, a describable sort of output can be expected.

Again, in terms of engineering, as discussed above in connection with causality, synapses are transducers, namely devices which convert one form of condition, of event, of force, respectively of energy into another, such as, in artificial devices, electrical energy in sound energy or vice versa. Thus, a transducer may convert pressure, temperature, acceleration, mass, time, distance, radiation, and a multiplicity of other events into electric signals. The use of such a device makes possible the conversion of any physical, chemical or biological phenomenon into a mechanical, optical or electrical signal for transmission, recording or actuation. More generally speaking, transducers convert variety of one type into variety of another type, such that the energy of the transform, namely of the signal emitted by the transducer is not provided by the 'detected' energy, but derived from a local source, as in a so-called servomechanism.[92]

As regards neurobiology, sensory receptors, synapses and nerve endings on effectors must be rated as transducers. Although sensory receptor endings,

---

[92] A servomechanism in the terminology of the engineer [cf. e.g. *MacColl*, 1945] has the characteristic of imposing upon the output signal y(t) the same functional form as the input signal x(t), subject to the restriction that the energy associated with y(t) shall be derived from a local source and shall not be furnished by the input signal. In other words, a load at high power level is made to follow the fluctuations of a control operating at low power level. Since the energy of a muscular contraction is not directly furnished by the nervous impulse acting as a stimulus at the neuromuscular junction, muscular activity controlled by nervous action thus corresponds to the engineer's concept of a servomechanism. Some analogies *qua* synapses likewise obtain. Additional comments can be found in section 3, volume 1 of *K.* [1967a].

responding e.g. to stretch or to radiation etc., differ in certain respects from synapses which transmit a neural signal, namely a 'nerve impulse', from one nerve cell to another nerve cell, or from a nerve cell to an effector (e.g. muscular or glandular element); all above-mentioned three sorts of endings, converting a variety or a signal into another variety or signal, quite evidently represent transducers and can be conceived as three different categories of synapses.

Another important aspect of particular 'processing centers' is the storage and retrieval of information. Such storage involves changes and the subsequent effects of these changes that may or may not become manifest in the further activities of the system. *Semon* [1904, 1909, 1920], adapting previous ideas propounded by *Hering* [1870, 1905], introduced and elaborated the concept of mneme, and coined the term engram for the relevant information stored by living structures, particularly by the nervous system. Engraphy refers thus to the storage process, engram denotes the stored variety, and ecphory the retrieval of the engram.

Semon's formulation of the principle of engraphy is, moreover, very similar to present-day concepts of the conditioned reflex, based upon the work of *Pavlov* [1927]. In oversimplified manner, *Pavlov's* principle can be expressed as follows: given a reflex resulting in a response C to a stimulus B, and given that the animal was simultaneously and frequently subjected to the stimulus A, not normally resulting in the response C, the stimulus A may then cause the response C in the absence of B. In this respect, not only simultaneity but antecedence in the overlapping sequence of two stimuli has been stressed. Thus, with a repetition of such combinations of stimuli, an 'engraphic' change in the nervous network has occurred, whereby, e.g. the antecedent stimulus may elicit the same response as the second stimulus.

'Instrumental' or 'operant conditioning' as subsequently elaborated by diverse schools of behaviorists, makes use of favorable and unfavorable input, respectively attraction ('reward') and avoidance ('punishment') situation, as e.g. in maze run training or other sorts of training.

Skinner [1938, 1969] devised a box with a small lever near the bottom and a trough located near that lever. A hungry rat, placed into that box may accidentally depress the lever in the course of random explorations. The lever is wired to a food container in such a way that a pellet of food is delivered into the trough when the lever becomes depressed. The rat soon learns to press the lever in order to obtain more food.

The learnt response is here instrumental in providing food as a 'reward'. In the original *Pavlovian conditioning* the learnt response (e.g. salivation) is not instrumental in producing the presence of food. Thus, in contradistinction to '*classical*' *Pavlovian conditioning*, which deals primarily with responses by the autonomic nervous system, '*instrumental conditioning*' deals with responses by the 'somatic' nervous system, mainly involving what could be called 'voluntary' activities. However, since *Pavlov* elaborated the basic features of 'conditioning', I believe the differences in technique are not sufficiently relevant to preclude the inclusion of 'operant' or 'instrumental' conditioning under the general concept of *Pavlovian* conditioning. Much the same could be said about the type of response called 'imprinting' obtained in newly hatched birds exposed to a moving 'model' during a critical period subsequent to hatching, and developing a more or less long lasting 'preference' for, or 'attachment' to the 'model' initially followed. This may be considered a special case of 'conditioning'.

Again, a further adaptation of the so-called '*Skinner-box*' with its lever or pedal resulted in the experiments with self-stimulation through an electrode implanted into particular regions of an animal's brain, and activated by pressure on the pedal. These experiments, devised by *Olds*, *Delgado*, and others, are briefly discussed further below on page 147, section 7 of chapter IV in volume 2.

Using the terminology of his 'operant conditioning' ('adversive reinforcers', 'positive reinforcers' etc.) *Skinner* [1972] made a rather naive attempt to show how an improvement of the deficiencies of Human society could result from 'controls' based upon the principles which he derived from his experiments (cf. vol. 2, chapter IV, section 11, p. 317).

All these and related behavioral activities appear, in an overall abstract or theoretical formulation, reducible to manifold combinations and permutations of rather few and elementary circuit activities, such as storage (engraphy, ecphory), stimulation (excitation, activation), inhibition, and sequence programming. There are, of course, numerous complicating parameters (*Zustandsbedingungen*) related to the phylogenetic and ontogenetic stage of development and varying of fluctuating physiologic states of the nervous system depending on multitudinous factors.

The distribution of stimuli, excitation, impulses respectively encoded signals in an organism with nervous system is evidently determined by the extrinsic and intrinsic connections of the conducting elements, and by the fluctuating, but presumably determinate functional states of receptors, conductors, switches and effectors. Distribution of excitation etc. is thus with the just mentioned functional qualifications a correlate of structural arrangement which, in turn, can be considered an innate, genetically determined characteristic, pertaining, in addition to the individual, to such fictional or abstract collective entities as subspecies, species, genus, and so forth.

The manner in which the organism reacts to the environment is an effect of the distribution of excitation, being thereby a correlate of the organism's action system. This latter, as the product of an inherited structure, is thus not only determinate but to some extent invariable or stereotype.

Yet, Metazoa with a nervous system may manifest, in addition to this invariable innate behavior common to all individuals of a given subspecies, species etc., a variable, individually acquired type of behavioral reaction which adapts itself to particular environmental conditions and is based on processed individual experiences resulting in the storage of variety as discussed above.

The activities of the nervous system may thus be roughly classified into two types [*K.*, 1927; *Ashby*, 1952], namely into stereotype, inborn behavior, and into 'learned' or 'acquired' adaptive behavior. Both types of behavior can be regarded as strictly determinate although not accurately predictable, but to a variable degree uncertain. This uncertainty of the nervous system results (a) from the 'unreliability' of its elements exposed to numerous disturbances, and (b) from a multitude of unascertainable parameters. While not accurately ascertainable nervous activity, nevertheless, remains statistically predictable within particular ranges of 'probability'. Seen from still another viewpoint, 'spontaneous' activity of the nervous system can initiate, within an organism, significant behavioral manifestations not directly 'triggered' by external events, but by 'intrinsic' events whose causal factors are physicochemical processes involving nerve cells and neuronal circuits. Such behavior is then, in the aspect under consideration, apparently unrelated to specific environmental input or states. Furthermore, insofar as behavior is correlated with environmental states, such 'intrinsic' or 'spontaneously initiated' neural activities can be presumed to represent an important aspect of exploratory behavior, which may be considered a manifestation of 'higher' neural functions. Together with 'adaptive' behavior, spontaneous or input-related 'exploratory' activities can also be interpreted as directed, that is, may appear as if 'goal seeking'. Moreover, some such sorts of behavior are customarily subsumed under the abstraction 'intelligence'.

Reverting to the concepts of input and output, a fictional and diagrammatic simple reflex arc, which would mediate, by means of a synaptic mechanism, a response to a stimulus, is directly comparable to the type of mechanism designated as open cycle or non-reset, input actuated control. Subsequent input (i.e. stimuli) remain here independent of the result of the operation, that is, of the effect of the response, or, in other words, remain unaffected by the output. It is rather doubtful whether simple mechanisms of this type play a very significant or, at least preponderating role in nervous activities.

Of greater import for the behavior of organisms controlled by a nervous system is the closed cycle, reset (error actuated), or feedback control system in the terminology of the engineer. The control is here actuated by a quantity which is in turn affected (either decreased or increased) by the result of the control operation, that is, of the output. The feedback can be either positive or negative.[93]

In biological terminology, we may simply state that the organism affects the environment and that the environment affects the organism: such a system can be said to have feedback [*Ashby*, 1952].

The concept of feedback in nervous and neuromuscular activities is relatively old. A striking example was demonstrated by *Breuer* in 1868 and designated as '*Selbststeuerung der Athmung durch den Nervus vagus*'. Inspiratory inflation of the lung inhibits further inspiration through stimulation of afferent vagus nerve fibers and contributes to initiate expiration. Expiratory collapse of the lung has the opposite effect, presumable through another set of nerve endings and of afferent vagus fibers. This double system of negative and positive feedback operates through the respiratory centers[94] which activate or inhibit motor nerve cells stimulating the respiratory muscles. These, in turn, through their action affect inflation and deflation of the lung, thus closing the feedback loop, that is, providing the 'closed cycle' cited above. It will be noted that the 'channel' effecting the closure is non-nervous, consisting of physiologic and physical events in thorax and lung. Other examples of feedback obtain in the reciprocal innervation of flexor and extensor muscles as described by *Sherrington* [1906, 1947].

Purely nervous closed cycles (closed circuits), wherein an 'impulse', by means of a nerve fiber, is carried back to the nerve cell in which the event originated, were apparently first pointed out by the present author [*K.*, 1927] on the basis of the neuron theory, and were subsequently discussed by many others. The psychologist *James* [1890], however, had already postulated closed neural circuits, but did not take into account the type of nexus between nerve cells as now generally assumed and based on the neuron theory established by *Forel* [1887] and *His* [1886], supplemented by *Sherrington's* concept of the synapse.

Again, attempts at a rigorous definition of feedback (*Selbststeuerung, Reafferenzprinzip, Rückkoppelung, Regelung, geschlossene Regelkreise*) lead to various semantic and logical difficulties when the interconnections between the parts of a system become complex. *Ashby* [1958] justly points out that when there are only two parts joined so that one affects the other, the

---

[93] The centrifugal governor controlling the speed of a steam engine, and invented by *James Watt* about 1790, is a typical and frequently cited example of (primarily) negative feedback. The generator principle (*Dynamoprinzip*) of *W. von Siemens* (1816–1892), embodied in the construction of electric generators, generating current by a self-reexciting loop, is an example of positive feedback.

[94] These 'centers' correspond to the 'processing' 'black boxes' referred to above, and contain terminal arborizations of nerve fibers (neuropil) with excitatory and inhibitory synapses.

properties of the feedback give important and useful information about the properties of the whole. But when even as few as four parts are so joined, then 20 circuits can be traced through them; and knowing the properties of all the 20 circuits does not give complete information about the system. Such complex systems cannot be treated as an interlaced set of more or less independent feedback circuits, but only as a whole. *Ashby* adds here that 'complex systems, richly cross-connected internally, have complex behaviours'. These behaviors can be directed, that is as if 'goal-seeking', in complex patterns.

The 'ethologist' *Lorenz* [1975] has summarized his views on the phylogenetic evolution of behavior. He is, nevertheless, compelled to admit that the concepts elaborated by 'ethologists' on the evolution of animal behavior are quite vague. The cited author assumes a complex and hierarchically integrated interplay of three 'elements' as enumerated further below. He fails, however, to indicate precise factors leading to said phylogenetic evolution and properly to distinguish phylogenetic and ontogenetic events. He claims, moreover, to define 'homologies' of behavior ('*homologe Verhaltensweisen*') but has evidently not understood the relevant distinction between morphologic homology and analogy.[95] His 'homologies' represent, in many if not most cases, mere analogies.

The three 'elements' pointed out by *Lorenz* [1975] as significant for the evolution of behavior in higher Metazoa with a central nervous system include (1) the genetically determined prefunctional neuronal mechanisms whose innate tendency toward 'triggering' ['*angeborener Auslösungsmechanismus*', AAM, *Lorenz*, 1975] depends, in turn, on (2) receptor adaptation and 'filtering' within the synaptic channels. With this is combined (3) the so-called 'appetitive behavior'[96] ['*Appetenzverhalten*', *Lorenz*, 1975]. The interplay of these factors is said to result in 'consummatory action'.

Receptor adaptation and 'filtering' as conceived by *Lorenz* correspond of course to the concept of 'analyzers' or 'analysors' elaborated by *Pavlov* and his school. These 'analyzers' are said to represent specialized components of the nervous system which control the reactions of the organism to changing external conditions. 'Analyzers' comprise a receptor together with its central connections, by means of which 'sensitivity to stimulations' is differentiated. The 'analyzer' concept has been extended to the connections with effectors. Thus the *Pavlovian* neurobiologist *Sarkisov* [1966] enumerates motor, cu-

---

[95] The confusion resulting from said lack of understanding is conspicuously displayed in a lecture delivered by *Lorenz* [1974] upon the occasion of his canonization at Stockholm.

[96] This 'appetitive behavior' evidently corresponds, at least in a relevant part, to what I have designated above [p. 138; cf. also *K.*, 1967, p. 18] as intrinsic neural activities leading to 'exploratory behavior'.

taneous, optic, auditory, vestibular, olfactory, taste and interoceptive[97] 'anal-yzers'. The Russian textbook of the cited author, available in the 1966 English translation, is of interest since it expounds the orthodox Soviet views based on the 'dialectical-materialistic approach' and on the *Marxist-Leninist* ideology, besides containing an extensive bibliography of Russian publications em-bodying recent Soviet neurobiological research activities. It should be under-stood that the foregoing very brief and summary account is merely meant to point out the overall significance of a nervous system as seen from an un-prejudiced, purely empirical 'materialistic' approach, differing thereby from the 'Marxist' one.

The multitudinous details involved in the transmission of the nerve 'impulse', namely the changes of electric potential, the velocities of conduc-tion, the significance of transmitter substances, and the roles of neuro-secretion and its output upon 'target cells', moreover the significance of neurohormones, etc., are here entirely irrelevant with regard to the abstract point of view adopted in said account meant as providing a first approxima-tion to an understanding[98] of the manner in which the mechanisms of a nervous system perform, that is to say of the common features of a nervous system. In the vernacular this may be expressed as 'what an organism's nervous system is all about'.

---

[97] The term 'interoceptive' is based on *Sherrington's* [1906, 1947] classification of stimuli respectively input. Exteroceptive stimuli occurring in the organisms environment affect the external body surface, interoceptive stimuli arise within, and affect the internal surface such as the digestive canal. Proprioceptive stimuli arise 'within the depth' of the organism and effect e.g. muscle and tendon receptors. *Sherrington* also used the term 'receptive fields', consisting of the proprioceptive field, the exteroceptive field, and the interoceptive field. The vestibular system is commonly included into the proprioceptive field. Cf. also the discussion in *K.* [1973, vol. 3/II, chapt. VII].

[98] A publication by *Eccles* [1977], entitled *The Understanding of the Brain*, insofar as it deals with the empirical data (chapters 1–5) is typical for the extremely narrow, excessively myopic viewpoint of a canonized superspecialist. It brings a poorly organized jumble of partly even controversial details, whereby the forest cannot be seen by restricting the vision not even to the trees but to the leaves. Said author's publication should properly be entitled 'How Not to Understand the Brain'. As regards its 'philosophical' chapter 6, one may quote *Schopenhauer's* quip [vol IV, p. 119]: '*Philosophen aus der Apotheke und dem Clinico, Leute, die nichts gelernt haben, als was zu ihrem Gewerbe gehört und nun ganz unschuldig und ehrsam, als sollte Kant erst geboren werden, Ihre Alte-Weiber-Spekulation vortragen, über "Leib und Seele", nebst deren Verhältnis zu einander disputieren, ja (credite posteri!) den Sitz besagter Seele im Gehirn nach-weisen. Ihrer Vermessenheit gebührt die Zurechtweisung, dass man etwas gelernt haben muss, um mitreden zu dürfen, und sie klüger thäten, sich nicht unangenehmen Anspielungen auf Pfla-sterschmieren und Katechismus auszusetzen.*' In the case of *Eccles*, one could say: '*Anspielungen auf Microelectroden-Nadelstechen und Katechismus*'. As regards said author's 'philosophy' he merely absorbed the peculiar lucubration of the neoprimitive professional 'philosopher' ('*Fachphilosoph*') *Popper*.

Further comments concerning the important neuroregulators (neuro-transmitters and neuromodulators) will be found in volume 2, chapter IV, section 4 (Parameters).

Figure 25 depicts in terms of engineering the overall functional aspects of a central nervous system, illustrating the concepts of open cycle and of feedback mechanisms, as well as of processing centers representing 'black boxes'.

As regards the Vertebrate respectively the Human central nervous system or neuraxis, it will here be sufficient, for the orientation of readers who are not biologists or physicians, to mention said system's main subdivisions, as illustrated by figures 26 and 27.

The entire Vertebrate neuraxis arises, in ontogenetic development, as the wall-differentiation of an embryonic neural tube which, with certain transformations essentially retains its original lumen in modified form (as 'central canal' or 'ventricles', containing fluid).

Two main subdivisions are the spinal cord in the vertebral canal, and the brain in the cranial cavity. The brain consists of five main parts, namely (1) the telencephalon (endbrain, cerebral hemispheres) with cerebral cortex and basal ganglia[99], (2) the diencephalon (betweenbrain) which connects the endbrain with (3) the midbrain (mesencephalon). Caudalward the rhombencephalon[100] consists of (4) the dorsal cerebellum (metencephalon) and (5) the ventral (basal) medulla oblongata, which, as 'myelencephalon' is continuous with the spinal cord. Midbrain and medulla oblongata, this latter with a rostrobasal addition called pons, pertaining to the cerebellar system (metencephalon) and characteristic for Mammals, represent (without the cerebellum) the so-called brain stem.

Peripheral input and output connections are provided by cranial (cerebral) and spinal nerves as diagrammatically indicated in figure 27. Spinal and

---

[99] The term 'ganglion' generally refers to a swelling in peripheral nerves, containing nerve cells with or without their synapses. In some instances (as e.g. basal ganglia) it designates, however, an assembly of nerve cells with their synaptic connections, located within the central neuraxis. It then corresponds to some sort of 'processing center'. Such central ganglia and other assemblies of nerve cells with synapses and with terminal arborizations of nerve fibers are also called a 'griseum' or 'grisea' because of their gray appearance in fresh and unprocessed preparations. Other designations for central ganglia are 'nucleus' respectively 'nuclei' or descriptive terms such as e.g. 'corpus striatum' for some basal ganglia. It should be added that the terms 'white' and 'gray substance' refer to the presence or absence of a lipid myelin sheath surrounding nerve fibers. The significance of myelin for the impulse conduction shall be discussed in section 4 of chapter IV, volume 2. It will here be sufficient to state that nerve fiber terminal arborizations with synapses (neuropil) are devoid of myelin sheaths, and thus pertain to the 'gray substance'.

[100] Rhombencephalon refers to that brain portion's ventricle, whose floor is the 'rhomboid fossa'.

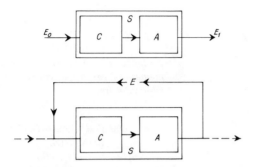

Fig. 25. Diagrams illustrating the neuraxis as conceived in terms of open cycle control mechanisms (above) and of control mechanisms with feedback (below). The systems with their subsystems are represented as 'black boxes' whose internal arrangements remain undefined. A: Actuating part of system, providing output; C: part of system, processing input and providing control; E: environment; E_0: state of environment acting an open circle mechanism; E_1: state of environment resulting from open system control mechanism; S: system as distinguished from environment [from *K.*, 1967a, 1978].

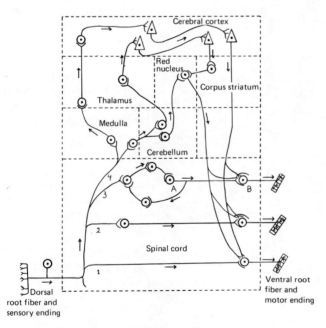

Fig. 26. Diagram illustrating essential arrangements of the Mammalian neuraxis. A closed circuit is indicated in spinal cord [after *Bayliss*, modified by *Ranson*, from *K.*, 1967a, 1978].

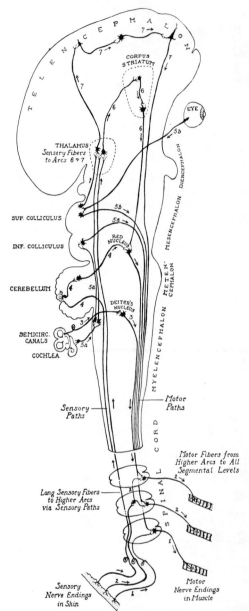

ARC 7
VOLUNTARY AND INHIBITORY CONTROL
Choice of response based on memory of past experiences. (Via pyramidal tract.)

ARC 6
AUTOMATIC ASSOCIATED CONTROL
of complex muscular actions. (Via striato-rubro-spinal tract.)

ARC 5
a. AUDITORY REFLEXES
e.g. Automatic response to sudden noise.
b. VISUAL REFLEXES
e.g. Automatic response to blinding flash of light.
(Both via tecto-spinal tract).

ARC 4
SYNERGIC CONTROL
Automatic coördinating control of muscular actions. (Via rubrospinal tract.)

ARC 3
EQUILIBRATORY CONTROL
Automatic balancing reactions. (Via vestibulo-spinal tract.)

ARC 2
INTERSEGMENTAL REFLEX
Impulse carried by association neurones to neighboring segments causing coördinated response of muscles in several segments.

ARC 1
INTRASEGMENTAL REFLEX
Response limited to segment stimulated.

Fig. 27. Schematic drawing showing main communication channels in the Mammalian neuraxis and including a functional classification of so-called 'arcs' [after *Patten*, from *K.*, 1978].

most cranial nerves display a metameric arrangement, that is to say a serial sequence of homologous configurations along the longitudinal extension of the neuraxis.

As regards processing centers or so-called grisea, one can thus distinguish segmental and suprasegmental[101] mechanisms. The most important suprasegmental griseum for 'higher' neural functions in Man and Mammals is the cerebral cortex, while the grisea indispensable for the immediate maintenance of the body's life are located in the medulla oblongata.

Figure 26 illustrates, in schematic and oversimplified fashion, synaptic connections in the diverse subdivisions of a Mammalian central nervous system. The diagram includes a 'closed circuit' within the spinal cord, as well as one peripheral input channel and three peripheral output channels with receptor respectively effector transducers.

The likewise diagrammatic figure 27 depicts the approximate outline of a Mammalian neuraxis with its subdivisions and includes a classification of so-called reflex 'arcs' from an overall functional viewpoint.

Turning now to a few relevant data of comparative anatomy from which, by judicious extrapolation and interpolation, presumptive phylogenetic inferences can be drawn, a very primitive nervous system can be found in Coelenterates. These forms are characterized by a more or less diffuse network of nerve cells (conductors) connected with receptors (sensory cells) and effectors (muscle cells) as shown in figures 28–31. Some condensations into 'nerve rings' (fig. 31) may obtain.

The nerve cells may be joined by 'syncytial' fusion and thus display asynaptic connections. In other instances they seem connected by apposition, with unpolarized, asynaptic connections or, in some instances, by protosynaptic, facultatively synaptic connections. Figure 28, in particular, indicates an early sort of differentiation into receptor, conductor, and effector.

Within the multitudinous phyla or groups of Invertebrate Metazoa (cf. fig. 23) a commonly obtaining configuration of the central nervous system displays a solid[102] brain ganglion dorsally to the rostral end of the gut (alimentary canal). This brain ganglion is directly continuous, through a 'ring' surrounding the gut, with a double or single (fused) longitudinal cord located ventrally to the gut and displaying, in annelids and arthropods segmental, metameric ganglia. Brain and ganglia are provided with nerves. If two cords

---

[101] Suprasegmental grisea are e.g. the cerebral cortex, the basal ganglia, the roof of the mesencephalon (particularly its so-called optic tectum in the 'superior colliculus' of mammals), the cerebellar cortex, and the so-called reticular formation below the ventricular space of the brain stem.

[102] 'Solid' means here: without an internal cavity, in contradistinction to the vertebrate tubular neuraxis with its lumen.

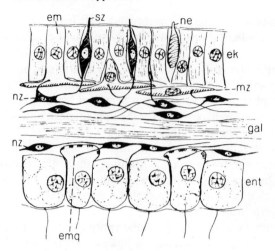

Fig. 28. Diagram of primitive nerve system as displayed in some Coelenterates [combined after *Plate*, other authors, and personal observations, from *K.*, 1927, 1967b]. ek: Ectoderm; em: epithelioid muscle cell; emq: cross-section through epithelioid muscle cell; ent: entoderm; gal: mesenchyme; mz: muscle cell; ne: nettle cell; nz: nerve cell; sz: sensory cell (receptor).

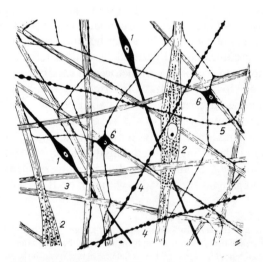

Fig. 29. Ectodermal nerve plexus of the coelenterate Scyphozoan Rhizostoma [after *Bozler and Beccari*, from *K.*, 1967b]. 1: Small bipolar cell; 2: large bipolar cell; 3, 4: various nerve fibers; 5: nerve fiber ending by apposition (contact); 6: multipolar cell.

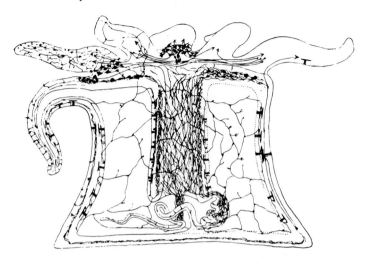

Fig. 30. General arrangement of the nerve net in a coelenterate Actinia [after *Wolff*, from *K.*, 1967b].

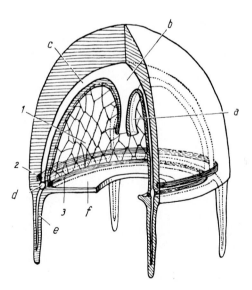

Fig. 31. Nerve net in a coelenterate Hydromedusa, including nerve rings [after *Bütschli and Beccari* from *K.*, 1967b]. 1: Subumbrellar nerve ring; 2: external nerve ring; 3: internal nerve ring; a: manubrium; b: stomach; c: radial canal; d: circular canal; e: tentacle; f: velum.

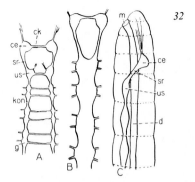

32 *33*

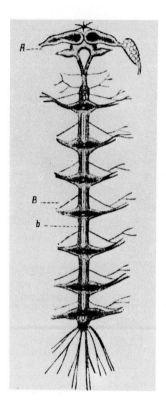

Fig. 32. Semi-schematic drawing illustrating the general configuration of the central nervous system in annelid worms [from *K.*, 1927]. A: Rope-ladder pattern in Sabella (Polychaete), modified after *B. Haller*; B: Earthworm (*Lumbricus terrestris*); C: Topographic relationship of ventral nerve cord and of brain to gut in Lumbricus; ce: cerebral ganglion ('brain'); ck: cerebral commissure; d: gut; g: ganglion of ventral nerve cord (interconnected by transverse connections with antimeric one in A); kon: longitudinal connective; sr: pharyngeal ring; us: subesophageal ganglion. In B and C the two ventral longitudinal cords with their segmental ganglia are fused in the midline. The stumps of some of the peripheral nerves are shown in A and B.

Fig. 33. Rope-ladder central nervous system of the isopod crustacean *Porcello scaber* ('Wood-louse', 'Sowbug'). A: 'Brain'; B: ventral cord; b: unpaired median accessory connective [after *Leydig and R. Hertwig*, from *K.*, 1967b].

are present, they are commonly interconnected across the midline by transverse connections and display a 'rope-ladder' pattern ('*Strickleiternervensystem*'). The gut thus passes through the 'pharyngeal ring' of the central nervous system (cf. fig. 32 and 33). The most 'intelligent' Invertebrates with segmental bodies are insects such as bees and ants, whose brain, shown in figure 34, contains intricate processing centers, such as the corpora pedunculata ('mushroom bodies', *Pilzkörper*) and others, which mediate the complex behavioral activities of these 'intelligent' animals.[103]

The central nervous system of the unsegmented, but bilaterally symmetrical mollusks, presumably derived from unsegmented worms in phylogenesis, likewise displays solid ganglia and nerve cords. The Cephalopods, such

---

[103] The behavior of ants was particularly studied by *Forel* [1910, 1921–23], and that of bees by *v. Frisch* [1950, 1953: cf. also the short summaries in *K.*, 1967b, vol. 2].

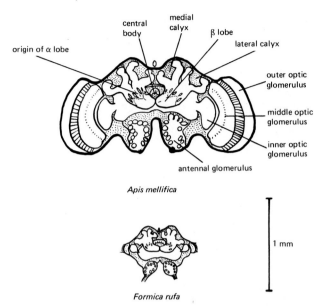

Apis mellifica

Formica rufa

Fig. 34. Semi-schematic drawings comparing the brain of a Bee with that of an Ant [after *Vowles*, from *K.*, 1967b].

as the Decapod Sepia (squid) and the Octopod Octopus possess a highly differentiated central nervous system (cf. fig. 35 and 36). The rostral gut (esophagus) runs through the cerebral mass made up of fused ganglia, and diverse smaller peripheral ganglia are present. As regards 'intelligence' the Cephalopods compete with ants and bees as the most 'intelligent' Invertebrates.[104] *Young* [1964, 1971] made very detailed studies on their nervous system. Said author's treatise '*A Model of the Brain*' [1964] is mainly based on the investigation of the Cephalopod nervous system, particularly in Octopus, but also in Sepia, by *Young* and his collaborators, and was followed by a comprehensive monograph on the nervous system in *Octopus vulgaris* [1971].

The Vertebrate central nervous system is characterized by its tubular origin and configuration and by its location dorsally to the gut, from which it is separated by cranial base and by axial skeleton. The brain becomes enclosed in a cranial cavity, and the spinal cord in a vertebral canal.

---

[104] The psychologist *Piéron* [1911], who undertook pioneering studies on the memory functions of the cephalopods comments as follows '*Le niveau mental auquel arrivent les Céphalopodes est relativement très élevé, et le Poulpe (Octopus vulgaris), en particulier, semble supérieur à un grand nombre de vertébrés, en particulier à des poissons ou des batraciens, et peut-être même des reptiles.*'

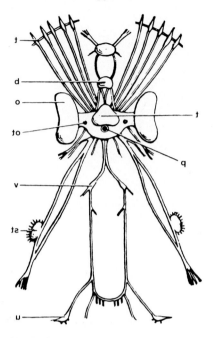

Fig. 35. Simplified drawing of the nervous system in the cephalopod Sepia [after *Ihering and Selenka-Goldschmidt*, from *K*., 1967b]. b: Superior buccal ganglion; o: optic ganglion; ot: optic gland; p: pharynx; st: stellate ganglion; t (upper): tentacle ganglia; t (lower, mislabelled for c): cerebral ganglion; u: branchial ganglion; v: visceral ganglion.

Among Invertebrates only some Chordates, from which Vertebrates are assumed to have evolved (cf. fig. 23), display a tubular central nervous system dorsally to the supporting notochord (chorda dorsalis), which represents the 'precursor' of the vertebrate column.

Elliott (1969) considers the Vertebrate phylogenetic ascent, culminating in the Human brain and in the emergence of 'superior intelligence', as intrinsically resulting from the development of a neural tube, whose potentialities, in his opinion, are superior to those inherent in an invertebrate ganglionated central nervous system. Be that as it may, the course of higher Metazoan evolution on the surface of our planet at least appears to corroborate *Elliott's* surmise.

It seems evident that, as far as 'successful' and 'superior' 'intelligent behavior' is concerned, the Human brain has here attained the highest stage of development which, however, is not correlated with the greatest size respectively volume. In this regard, the brains of Elephants and of Cetacea surpass that of Man. Said animals, moreover, display a relatively high degree of

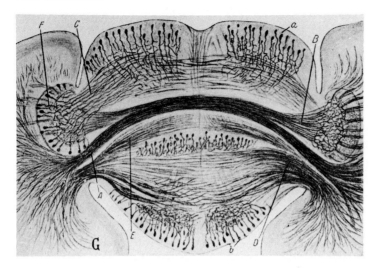

Fig. 36. Horizontal section through cerebral ganglion of the cephalopod Sepia [after *Cajal*, from *K.*, 1967a]. A: Crossed optic pathway; B: end of crossed pathway in peduncular ganglion; C, D: optic connections; E: middle optic pathway; F: peduncular ganglion; a: posterior part of cerebral ganglion with nerve cell bodies; b: anterior part of cerebral ganglion.

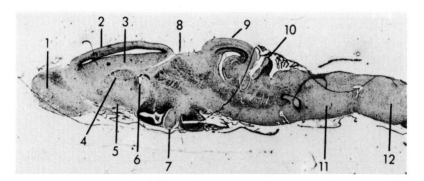

Fig. 37. Sagittal section (cell stain) through brain and rostral spinal cord of the amphibian frog [from *K.*, 1978]. 1: Olfactory bulb; 2–5: grisea of telencephalon; 6: interventricular foramen; 7: optic chiasma and supraoptic commissures; 8: diencephalon; 9: mesencephalon; 10: cerebellum; 11: medulla oblongata; 12: spinal cord.

'intelligence' (cf. e.g. *Lilly* [1963, 1975] and *Lilly and Miller* [1961] in dolphins).

Supplementing the preceding brief account of the main structural, configurational and functional features of a Vertebrate central nervous system (fig. 26, 27), it will be sufficient, in this context, to show a very simple Vertebrate neuraxis, represented by that of an Amphibian Frog, which represents a paradigma illustrating the manifestations of the fundamental morphologic pattern characteristic for the neuraxis of all Vertebrates (fig. 37), in comparison with the neuraxis of Man (fig. 38; this figure should be compared with figure 27). Again, for comparison with head and brain of an Insect (fig. 39), a section through head and brain of Man is depicted in figure 40.

In concluding this generalized account of the nervous system in Metazoans with particular emphasis on that of Vertebrates including Man, the following comments are perhaps appropriate.

It is evident that, in the Vertebrate series, the neuraxis displays a remarkable conservatism as regards the topologic features of its configuration, that is to say of its morphologic pattern as well as of its main communication channels and of its peripheral nerves.

Although specific progressive differentiations have taken place in phylogeny, no additional 'new' topologically fundamental component has been added to the basic *bauplan* of telencephalon, diencephalon, mesencephalon, cerebellum, oblongata and spinal cord characteristic for all Vertebrates, nor to thereto pertaining basic griseal neighborhoods (*Grundbestandteile*). All progressive differentiations have resulted from one-many transformations of the given topologic neighborhoods pertaining to fundamental longitudinal zonal systems. A few special cases of differentiation also involve secondary many-one transformations.

This orderliness is doubtless encoded in the genome and results from physicochemical interactions during ontogenesis. The genome, in turn, is causally related to the organism's phylogenetic evolution, and no purpose is here implied.

Yet, despite the obtaining genetically predetermined orderliness of configuration and of communication channels, involving specific functionally relevant fiber connections, the multiplicity of the factors resulting in morphogenesis subjects this latter to numerous internal and external disturbances. Considering the end-effect displayed by the approximately stable adult organisms, one is indeed justified to speak of a 'superb architecture' combined with inevitable 'slipshod workmanship'. Although the configuration, structures and *modus operandi* of the nervous system may be conceived as resulting from 'predetermined order', the actual end-results remain, to a large extent, probabilistic. The just mentioned obtaining orderliness or 'stability', however, becomes favored by significant factors of redundancy.

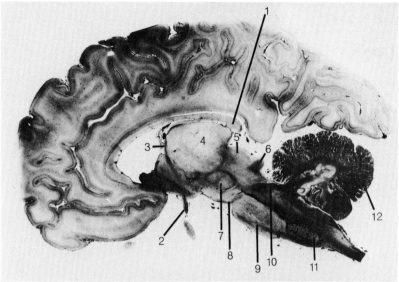

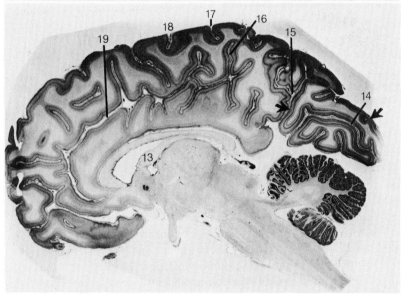

Fig. 38. Two sagittal sections through a Human brain (newborn), showing some of the medullated fiber tracts (a) and processed with the Nissl stain for cells (b) [from *K.*, 1978]. 1: Corpus callosum; 2: optic nerve; 3: medullated stria of thalamus; 4: thalamus (diencephalon); 5, 6: superior and inferior colliculus of mesencephalon; 7, 8: grisea of mesencephalon; 9: pons; 10: a cerebellar pathway; 12: cerebellum; 13: fornix (a tele-diencephalic communication channel); 14: fissura calcarina (the two arrows in b indicate boundaries of an optic projection cortex – area striata); 15: fissura parieto-occipitalis; 16: ramus marginalis of sulcus cinguli; 17: sulcus centralis; 18: sulcus praecentralis; 19: sulcus cinguli.

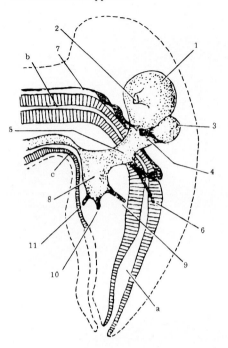

Fig. 39. Drawing showing relationships of brain and head in an insect (the cockroach Periplaneta) as seen in lateral view for comparison with figure 40 [after *Beccari*, from *K.*, 1967a]. 1: Protocerebrum; 2: optic peduncle; 3: deuterocerebrum; 4: antennal nerve; 5: tritocerebrum; 6: labral nerve; 7: stomatogastric nerve; 8: subesophageal ganglion; 9: mandibular nerve; 10, 11: nerves of first and second maxilla; a: buccal cavity; b: esophagus; c: duct of salivary gland.

The interplay of relatively 'precise' genetic coding and 'chance' factors allows for an overall 'specific' organization of the central nervous system in terms of neuronal interconnections combined with features pertaining to a 'random network'.

The concept of 'random networks' has been challenged by *Eccles* [1977] in three of his so-called 'general statements' making the following claims.

'(1) At no stage in the development are the neurons of the brain connected together as a random network. (2) Only in a few special regions has there been evidence of an excess of unused and unwanted neurons which rapidly die. Elsewhere it can be assumed that there is no redundancy. No doubt there appears to be a redundancy in the enormous populations of neurons in many parts of the brain, but we may assume that this appearance derives from our deficient understanding of the modes of operation. (3) The organization of the brain is highly specific, not merely in terms of the number and location of

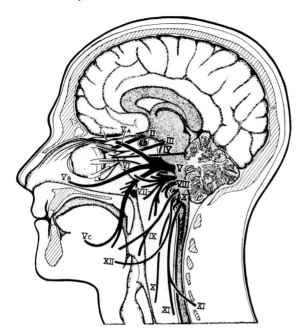

Fig. 40. Drawing of midsagittal section through Human head, showing brain *in situ*, and indicating overall arrangement of cranial nerves I to XII [after *Neal and Rand*, from *K.*, 1978]. VA, B, C: ophthalmic, maxillary and mandibular branches of Vth nerve (trigeminus).

synaptic knobs upon different parts of the same cell' ... 'and the precise distribution of synaptic knobs arising from that cell.'

It must be admitted that, as already stated above, there obtains indeed a high degree of orderliness in configuration and structure of the nervous system, involving even instances of constant cell numbers. Such numerical cell constancy, combined with constancy of their interconnections, that is to say of their circuitry, occurs in diverse Invertebrates as well as Vertebrates. In the former some such instances of numerical cell constancy may even apply to the entire nervous system, while, in the latter, said constancy remains restricted to a few cell types and circuit systems (cf. volume 2, chapter IV, section 6).

Nevertheless, despite the obtaining degree of orderliness, each one of the dogmatic 'general statements' by *Eccles* [1977] quoted above remains highly questionable. *Burns* [1968] has rather convincingly shown, on the basis of experimental evidence, that the Mammalian central nervous system, especially the cerebral cortex, displays many of the properties that can be theoretically predicted for the activity or behavior of random networks. *Eccles'* denial of redundancy and overemphasis on 'specificity' is belied by the results of many severely destructive lesions which are followed by restitution of function despite irrevocable loss of the allegedly 'specific' elements and connections (cf. volume 2, chapter IV, section 6, page 95). An 'excess' of 'unused and un-wanted' undifferentiated elements which do not 'rapidly die' is clearly in-dicated by the subependymal cell plate displayed by diverse regions of many Mammalian brains.

The cerebellum is indeed characterized by a specific peculiar monoto-nously 'grid-like' parallel and orthogonal arrangement of its cortical fiber system, and by peculiarities of its synaptic structures. But even there, random and redundant network features persist, which are, moreover, evidenced by the results of experiments with some lesion and even complete extirpation of that 'expendable' brain subdivision, as discussed in chapter X, volume 4 of *The Central Nervous System of Vertebrates* [*K.*, 1975]. It seems likely that the views expressed in the quoted 'statements' of *Eccles* may have been subcon-sciously suggested by that author's particular interpretation of, and concern with, the peculiar organization and functional aspects of the cerebellum. Although based on partially valid interpretation or on what could be called 'half truths', said 'statements' by *Eccles* evidently represent an instance of misleading 'reductionism' characterized by the viewpoint of 'nothing but' (cf. volume 2, chapter IV, section 2, page 9).

Ashby [1952] has plausibly shown that the ability of the nervous system to produce adaptive behavior can be explained on a purely mechanistic basis. This system contains many variables that behave as step functions and as part functions; despite the above-mentioned orderliness of its genetic determina-tion, it seems to be assembled largely at random, so that its details are determined not individually but statistically. *Ashby* demonstrates a funda-mental tendency for systems of this type to arrange their internal pattern to action that, in relation to their environment, they become stable. The prin-ciples of stability and ultrastability can be formulated in mathematical terms; with a mechanical model embodying these principles and designated as home-ostat, *Ashby* is able, at least in a rudimentary way, to imitate vital behavior of ultrastable type.

Logical operations, symbolization and memory functions can likewise be conceived in strictly mechanistic forms. *Craik* [1943] pointed out that the brain must contrive to model external events by using a symbolism com-parable to that by which a calculating machine represents the pattern of a given information. Computing machines handling information and perform-ing such operations as calculation, conclusion and selection, are commonly designated as mechanical brains. The binary system and the statistical concept

of information as negative entropy[105] have proved to be of particular significance in this connection. In analyzing automatic relay and switching circuits,
Shannon [1938] demonstrated that the algebra applying to such circuits is
none other than the algebra of logic or *Boolean* algebra. *McCulloch and Pitts*
[1943] have used this approach in constructing theoretical models of nerve
nets.

As regards memory, we must distinguish short-term memory, intermediate memory, and long-term memory[106] as required in the storing of
experience and learning and for the retrieval of such stored variety
(information).

The shortest memory, required in the execution of complex reflex patterns
involving time intervals of some duration, may be mediated by some arrangements of the self-reexciting closed circuits, that is to say on the basis of a
feedback mechanism which I pointed out in 1927 following earlier and less
clearly defined concepts proposed by *James* and by *Cajal*. Other sorts of
relatively short-term memory effects may correspond to the so-called habitu-
ation and sensitization displayed by ganglia of diverse Invertebrates.
'Memory' is doubtless a complex, multifactorial property of the nervous
system and seems also to include a poorly understood 'intermediate memory'.
The engrams of long-term memory may be represented in the cerebral cortex
by spatially extensive configurations of affected synapses with specifically
lowered resistance [*K.*, 1927, and subsequent other autors]. Engrams would
thus be properties of the network rather than of the cellular units, although the
individual neurons may play an important biochemical role. Conversely, one
and the same neuron, through various synaptic connections, may represent a
link or element in a large number of entirely different engrams. So long as the
essential pattern of a given combination is allowed to remain, a substantial
number of nerve cells and fibers pertaining to such a pattern may be destroyed
without affecting its significant code value – thus a given configuration shot
through with sieve-like holes may still kepp its recognizable features. This,
again, represents evidence for redundancy as well as for 'random network'
structural aspects.

There is, moreover, as regards the storage and retrieval (ecphory) of an
engram, an interesting general analogy with the principle of holography,
discovered by *Gabor* [1972] about 1948. Holography is a new and ingenious

---

[105] Entropy ('disorder', 'randomness', 'probability') and negentropy ('order'), if the relevant variety is numerically ascertainable, can be expressed in terms of logarithms. The binary
system (0, 1) is here particularly convenient for the expression in 'bits', which are the logarithms to
the base 2. 'Bit' is here derived from 'binary digit'. Cf. *K.*, [1961, §68, pp. 354–358].

[106] Further details on memory respectively 'storage', or 'engraphy' are discussed in volume
2, chapter IV, section 6. Cf. also *K.* [1978, vol. 5/II, chapter XV, section 6].

method for recording a three-dimensional image of a scene. It records not only the light waves issuing from the scene, but a second set of waves called the reference beam. The two sets of waves interfere with each other, and this interference pattern is recorded. Holography acts as a complicated diffraction device, causing a beam of coherent laser light to be diffracted in such a manner as to 'reconstruct' a three-dimensional image of the original scene. In other words, holography is an interferometric wavefront reconstruction.

With regard to the diffuse localization of the engram, whose ecphory is not prevented by cortical damage nor by removal of substantial cortical mass, the following similarity with the hologram is of interest. If the latter is cut in half, each half produces the entire image and this is also the case with pieces obtained by further tearing apart. However, when the pieces become very small, the image becomes more and more fuzzy, until from the smallest pieces only a blur is obtained. Again, a large hole punched in the middle of a hologram will hardly affect the produced image. That these properties of the hologram are similar to those of the distributed memory storage in the brain was clearly recognized and pointed out by *Gabor*.

Burns [1968], who stressed the 'random network' of neuronal connections conceived neuronal events spreading through the cortex as a 'wavefront of excitation'. One could thus, in very general and tentative terms, consider 'engraphy' as resulting from the interference of an input wave with a 'reference beam' provided by a 'modulating circuit', the 'reconstruction' (ecphory) being subsequently effected by another 'modulating neural wave'.

The basic similarity of structural and functional principles obtaining in all forms of organic life to those applying to artificial mechanical contrivances, stressed by many authors, and especially by *Kapp* [1877], appears thus well founded. In this respect and as regards the nervous system, a conspicuous analogy of neuronal circuits and certain electrical circuits in electronic devices may be said to have been conclusively demonstrated. *Wiener* [1948] therefore justly emphasizes the essential unity of the set of problems concerning communication, control and statistical mechanics in both machines and organisms. However, in a paper 'on comparing the brain with machines' *MacKay* [1954] states that the question 'how far does the brain resemble existing mechanisms, such as electronic computing machines?' is 'of trivial interest' and dismisses it with the true but in my opinion irrelevant remark that electronic computers are not designed to resemble the brain. I believe that, far from being trivial, the obvious resemblance despite numerous considerable difference is of deep significance since it points to the comprehensive uniformity in the orderliness of events, regardless whether these events are related to organic or to anorganic systems. There are numerous relevant publications concerning the similarities in the overall working principles applying to the performance of computers and related artificial devices *and* to the functions of the brain. It will here suffice to mention the publications by *E. C. Berkeley* [1949, 1959], *Craik* [1943], George [1962], *Kuhlenbeck* [1965a, 1966], *Küpfmüller* [1958], *v. Neumann* [1958], *Steinbuch* [1961], *Turing* [1936, 1937, 1950], and *Wiener* [1948]. This latter author re-introduced the old term 'cybernetics' for control in the animal and the machine.

Notwithstanding many lacunae in factual knowledge and despite the inherent deceptiveness of verbal precision which obstructs the generalization and analysis of the complex problems involved, the materialistic approach appears as a consistent, logical and promising attempt to explain organic life, including animal behavior controlled by a nervous system.

5. Limitations of Materialism: Consciousness

In accordance with *Ashby's* formulation, the nervous system, and living matter in general may be assumed to be identical with all other matter. No use of any specific vital principle needs to be made and all teleological explanations are eliminated. It may be assumed throughout that a machine or an animal behaves in a certain way at a certain moment because its physical and chemical nature at that moment allows no other action. It may be further assumed that the nervous system, living matter and the matter of the environment are all strictly determinate; thus, if on two occasions they are brought to the same state, the same behavior may be expected to follow.

We are, nevertheless, faced with the fundamental fact that the phenomena of consciousness exist and that these phenomena seem to be related in an orderly fashion with certain activities of the nervous system. If the materialistic approach leads to a valid and complete concept of reality, then it should at least be conceivable to explain consciousness on the basis of this concept, or in other words to derive consciousness from the orderliness of the physical world. This, however, is not possible and if such an attempt is forced, then *the entire materialistic concept collapses like a house of cards.*

Materialism is any hypothesis assuming, within a space-time structure, the existence of an objective physical world independent of any conscious perception. If we adhere to this postulate we suppose that a physical or physicochemical process starts from an 'object', affects a sense organ, changes into another physicochemical process, causes yet another such process in an afferent nerve, and finally, through a series of synaptic junctions, reaches certain centers of the brain. All these processes occur with definite velocities along definite distances, in other words as moving magnitudes and magnitudes of motion. Within the brain centers, an additional series of similar processes takes its course as the effect of this causal chain, partly in form of immediate nervous discharges (akin to kinetic energy), partly in form of mnemic changes, that is presumably as enduring modification of synaptic patterns (akin to potential energy). All these effects, which manifest themselves in the behavior of the organism, follow the law of mass-energy conservation. Simultaneously with some of these processes, phenomena of consciousness occur; we are aware of, or see, a red flower, smell a fragrance, feel the softness and shape of a leaf. Yet, no further change in a definite time and along a definite distance can be traced from any of the physicochemical processes to the sensation red or to any other of the modalities of awareness. Neither can the laws of gestalt or configuration be invoked for an explanation of awareness. The properties of configuration merely make it possible, as *Craik* has shown, to conceive the nervous system as a calculating machine capable of modelling or paralleling external events and to suggest that this process of paralleling or symbolization is the basic feature of abstracting invariants, similar to thought, as must be readily admitted, except, however, for the fundamental phenomenon of consciousness. No mathematically or logically conceivable property of configuration has accounted for the miracle that a small-scale space-time model of physical events provided by a pattern of nervous discharges 'transforms' itself into awareness and appears as the phantasmagory, in a private space-time manifold, of a brightly colored flower garden in the midst of a panoramic landscape, accompanied by a variety of sounds and sensations, and a stream of internal feelings.

It is here appropriate to bring a relevant statement made by *Bertrand Russell* as quoted by *Jeans* [1943]: 'So long as we adhere to the conventional notions of mind and matter, we are condemned to a view of perception which is miraculous. We suppose that a physical process starts from a visible object, travels to the eye, there changes into another physical process, causes yet another physical process in the optic nerve, and finally produces some effects in the brain, simultaneously with which we see the object from which the process started, the seeing being something "mental", totally different in character from the physical processes, which precede and accompany it. This view is so queer that metaphysicians have invented all sorts of theories designed to substitute something less incredible ...'

What *Russell* means here by 'conventional notions of mind and matter' should, however, more accurately be worded as follows: so long as we are confronted by the actual, given 'fact' (i.e. existence of experience) of consciousness ('mind' *sensu latiori*) and the conventional notion of 'matter' (physicalisms, i.e. mass and energy), we are condemned ... etc.

Yet, 'miraculous' or 'incredible', this view of 'perception', respectively of consciousness (mind *sensu latiori*) is absolutely inevitable, if we adopt the unavoidable practical postulate of a physical world, which is well-substantiated by the data of natural sciences (physics, chemistry, astronomy, geology, biology), and of mathematics.

It is quite evident that the conscious experience of seeing, and consciousness ('mind') in general, are totally different in character from the assumed physical processes upon which consciousness is empirically shown to depend, and that, *prima facie*, despite being 'incredible', said 'miraculous' view of 'perception' appears to hold, i.e. to be valid. It evidently implies a dualism, namely that between transitory phenomena of consciousness, and persistent events in physical space-time, occurring independently of consciousness.

In order to understand the here relevant significance of consciousness, it becomes necessary to define the meaning of 'reality', which, in the aspect under consideration, has two denotations. *Reality in the first sense* refers to 'existence', 'occurrence' or persistence of events when they are not perceived, that is to say when they do not represent contents of a private perceptual space-time system (i.e. of a consciousness-manifold).

Reality in the second sense, *per contra* refers to 'events' or 'things' correlated with other 'events' or 'things' in a way which experience (or the application of the principle of sufficient reason) has led us to expect.[107]

Since it is logically impossible to derive consciousness from material or physical processes, the materialist must either deny consciousness, or assume the just mentioned inevitable dualistic viewpoint. Behaviorism adopts the policy of the proverbial albeit apocryphal ostrich; while a dogmatic behaviorist is indeed sufficiently obstinate to deny consciousness, the methodological behaviorist chooses to ignore it. The following droll statement to this effect was found in *Ranson's Anatomy of the Nervous System* up to the 8th edition [1947]: 'The behavioristic school of psychology has pretty well undermined the old idea of consciousness.'

In view of the actually obtaining experience, the denial of reality is evidently ludicrous and displays the 'schizophrenic' trends of the Human mind.

With regard to the obvious dualism which the materialist who does not deny consciousness must acknowledge, if he is honest and logical, he may either be an atomistic hylozoist (better: hylopsychist) or conceive matter and mind in more generalized and vague terms, such as 'epiphenomenalism', or postulate a psychophysical parallelism. However, for purposes of a purely practical approach, the fiction of a psychophysical parallelism, about which more will be said below, may be regarded as the least objectionable formulation.

Hylozoism or better hylopsychism conceives 'matter' as endowed with 'spiritual' properties, whatever these undefined 'properties' are supposed to

---

[107] This distinction of reality in both senses was made by *Schopenhauer* and was also given, without reference to that previous author, by *Bertrand Russell*.

be. A prominent exponent of hylopsychism was *Ernst Haeckel* (1834–1919) who not only postulated a '*Zellseele*' but souls of atoms. These 'souls', however, were supposed to be unconscious.[108] Since 'mind' *sensu latiori* respectively 'psychic phenomena' ('soul'), and consciousness should be considered synonymous, the concept of an 'unconscious soul' is evidently a *contradictio in adjecto*, as *Wundt, Kretschmer*, and many others have repeatedly pointed out. Likewise '*unbewusste Vorstellung*', if by '*Vorstellung*' perception is meant, represents such *contradictio*, comparable to a pain which is not pain, respectively to unconscious consciousness. The recently propounded concept of 'panpsychism' corresponds, in this respect, exactly to *Haeckel's* hylozoism, by claiming that the complexes of relations which we call 'matter' are of 'psychical nature', being 'protophenomena', whatever this may mean. The 'conscious processes' correspond to biochemical and biophysical processes, such that the molecules, atoms, and elementary particles áre 'protopsychical' in character. This view is also called 'panpsychistic identism'.[109]

It seems, however, obvious that the experienced state of consciousness significantly differs from the likewise obtaining state of unconsciousness, substantiated by the interruption of consciousness in narcosis, cerebral anemia, severe trauma, dreamless sleep etc.; it is then hardly logical to designate the 'persisting' events as 'psychical', even if labelled 'protophenomena' or 'panpsychistic'.

As regards the origin of true 'psychic' events, which *Haeckel* calls '*bewusste Empfindung*',[110] this author conceived it '*als die höchste psychische Funktion*', arising '*durch Spiegelung der (scilicet: unbewussten) Empfindungen in einem Central-Theile des Nervensystems*'. We may well wonder how such

---

[108] *Haeckel* assumed '*unbewusste Empfindungen*' and stated [1898, p. 91] '*dass auch schon den Atomen die einfachste Form der Empfindung und des Willens innewohnt – oder besser gefasst: der Fühlung (Aesthesia) und der Strebung (Tropesis) –, also eine universale "Seele" von primitivster Art (noch ohne Bewusstsein)*'.

[109] *Sherrington* [1951] justly remarked 'it is not safe even to suppose that mind is universally present in animal life. Most life is, I imagine, mindless. . . .' 'It would seem that though there is matter which exists apart from mind, we know of no instance where mind exists apart from matter; that is, if we define "mind" as we agreed to do.' The alluded definition of 'mind' refers to thoughts, memories, feelings, reasoning and so on.

Sherrington, although not explicitly, appears to have implicitly equated 'mind' with 'consciousness'. *Sherrington* [1951] moreover stated: 'That the brain derives its mind additively from a cumulative mental property of the individual cells composing it, has therefore no support from any facts of its cell structure.' The cited comments by *Sherrington* provide an appropriate reply to the naive hylozoistic or panpsychistic views.

[110] An evident pleonasm, namely conscious consciousness. *Haeckel* calls this '*die höchste psychische Funktion*' while I would simply call it 'the psychic function'. Yet, *Haeckel* rightly states that it must be related to a developed central nervous system.

'*Spiegelung*' ('reflection', in the optic sense) could possibly take place, and we have here an instance of typical pseudosolution of an unsolvable problem by a mere word.

Among comparable pseudosolutions there is the so-called 'psychoneural identity hypothesis' claiming in the face of evidence that both sets of events (biological neuronal and mental, i.e. conscious) are 'identical'.[111]

Reverting to *Haeckel's* '*Spiegelung*' it is of interest that a recent (*Marxist*) neurobiologist [*Sarkisov*, 1966, p. 245] states: 'Consciousness is recognized by the relationship of the processes taking place in the neurons of the brain to the objects reflected in the brain and the phenomena of social activity.' The cited author nevertheless admits that 'however deeply science penetrates into the structural and functional properties of the brain, it cannot reduce consciousness to these'. Yet, he believes that 'further advance in neurology will provide fresh material for *Marxist-Leninist* philosophy, and above all for the fundamental gnosiologic problem – the primary nature of matter and the secondary nature of consciousness'. He emphasizes the official Soviet doctrine that 'in the age of the rapid development of science, the treatment of the philosophical problems of contemporary science on the basis of *dialectical materialism*, as the only scientific method of cognition, has become even more realistic'.

Discounting the *Marxist* dogma of 'dialectic materialism'[112] which would be evaluated as a meaningless cliché, the philosophical approach to the problem of 'brain and consciousness' requires epistemological considerations

---

[111] *Sherrington* [1951] justly remarked that it is 'difficult to bring mind into the class of physical things', or, in other words, that mental events 'seem to lie beyond any physiology of the brain'.

'When I turn my gaze skyward I see the flattened dome of sky and the sun's brilliant disc and a hundred other visible things underneath it. What are the steps which bring this about? A pencil of light from the sun enters the eye and is focussed there on the retina. It gives rise to a change, which in turn travels to the nerve layer at the top of the brain. The whole chain of these events, from the sun to the top of my brain, is physical. Each step is an electrical reaction. But now there succeeds a change wholly unlike any which led up to it, and wholly inexplicable by us. A visual scene presents itself to the mind; I *see* the dome of sky and the sun in it, and a hundred other visual things beside. In fact, I perceive a picture of the world around me. When this visual scene appears, I ought, I suppose, to feel startled, but I am too accustomed to feel even surprised.' Cf. above, page 160, my own remarks and those by *Bertrand Russell*. Although tediously repetitious, the emphasis on the problem at issue seems necessary because its nature and implications are generally ignored.

[112] 'Dialectic materialism' was taken by *Marx* and *Engels* from the logic of *Hegel's* philosophical system. This latter started with the concept '*Sein*' (being, existence), equivalent, because of its emptiness, to its negation, '*das Nichts*' (nothing). The 'oscillation' between the two then becomes '*das reine Werden*' (pure becoming). This is said to be the dialectic method, whereby the negation of a given concept (thesis), its '*Gegenteil*' (opposite, antithesis) leads to a progressive third one (synthesis).   Continued on p. 164

which, in 'modern', i.e. *Post-Cartesian* Western philosophy, may appropriately begin with the argumentation propounded by *Locke* [1689].

This author stated: 'That the size, figure and motion of one body should cause a change in the size, figure and motion of another body, is not beyond our conception; the separation of the parts of one body upon the intrusion of one with another; and the change from rest to motion upon impulses; these and the like, seem to us to have some connexion one with another. And if we know these *primary qualities* of bodies, we might have reason to hope we might be able to know a great deal more of these operations of them one upon another: but our minds not being able to discover connexions betwixt these primary qualities of bodies and the *sensations* that are produced in us by them, we can never be able to establish certain and undoubted rules of the consequence or coexistence of any *secondary qualities*, though we could discover the size, figure or motion of these invisible parts which immediately produce them. We are so far from knowing what figure, size or motion of particles produce a yellow colour, a sweet taste, or a sharp sound, that we can by no means conceive how size, figure or motion of any particles can possibly produce in us the idea of any colour, taste, or sound whatsoever; there is no conceivable connexion betwixt the one and the other.'

To this must, however, be added that, in terms of a physical world, that is to say, of materialism, it is now possible to establish 'what figure, size, or motion of parts produce a yellow color or a sharp sound'. But this, as *Locke* justly remarked, does not provide any conceivable connexion between his primary and his secondary qualities.

The distinction between said two sorts of qualities was pointed out above on page 5 in section 1 of the present chapter II. It will here suffice to recall that the 'primary qualities' of extension, figure, motion, rest, and number represent the experienced aspects of space and time, and are thus, no less than 'solidity' and the so-called 'secondary qualities', essential attributes of consciousness.

Marx and *Engels* likewise teach that all thinking consists of a thesis opposed by an antithesis; after some struggle, they are combined in a synthesis.

Born [1951] illustrates this as follows with a *Marxist* claim concerning physics: '*Newton's* thesis that light consists of particles was opposed by *Huygens'* antithesis that it consists of waves, until both were united in the synthesis of quantum mechanics.' *Born* then adds: 'This is all very well and indisputable, though a little trivial.' One might, however, ask: 'Is it really indisputable?' For practical purposes, light is still dealt with either in terms of photons, or in terms of waves, or in detailed terms of several different systems of quantum mechanics. Where is here the final synthesis? It should, moreover, be added that the relationship of 'thesis', 'antithesis' and 'synthesis', insofar as it contains a modicum of validity, was already elaborated in the *Confucian* treatise *The Doctrine of the Mean* (*Chung-yung*), about 2400 years ago. Some further comments on 'dialectic materialism' will be given in volume 2, chapter IV, section 11, page 312 of the present treatise.

This was first recognized by *Berkeley* [1710, 1713, 1946] who convincingly argued that all 'primary qualities' are likewise only percepts in consciousness, whose existence consists in being perceived.[113]

In *Berkeley's* words: 'Some Truths there are so near and obvious to the mind that a man need only open his eyes to see them. Such I take this important to be, to wit, that all the chair of heaven and furniture of the earth, in a word all those bodies which compose the mighty frame of the world, have not any substance without a mind, that their being (*esse*) is to be perceived or known; that consequently so long as they are not actually perceived by me, or do not exist, in my mind or that of any created spirit, they must either have no existence at all, or else subsist in the mind of some eternal spirit: it being perfectly unintelligible and involving all the absurdity of abstraction, to attribute to any single part of them an existence independent of a spirit.'

Hume [1739–1740, 1748] likewise recognized the cogency of *Berkeley's* argumentation denying the intrinsic difference between secondary and primary qualities. He stated:

'Tis universally allowed by modern enquirers, that all the sensible qualities of objects, such as hard, soft, hot, cold, white, black, etc., are merely secondary and exist not in the objects themselves, but are perceptions of the mind, without any external archetype or model which they represent. If this be allowed, with regard to secondary qualities, it must also follow with regard to the supposed primary qualities of extension and solidity; nor can the latter be any more entitled to that denomination than the former. The idea of extension is entirely aquired from the senses of sight and feeling; and if all the qualities, perceived by the senses, be in the mind not in the object, the same conclusion must reach the idea of extension, which is wholly dependent on the sensible ideas or the ideas of secondary qualities.'

Hume, moreover, also recognized the weakness or *non sequitur* in *Berkeley's* important argumentation, namely that things (or events) not perceived in consciousness must have no existence at all, or else subsist in the mind of some eternal spirit. Quite evidently, since the so-called primary qualities, in essence, merely represent the attributes of space and time, there is a third possibility, namely that an *unknown 'orderliness x'*, *devoid of space and time*, represents reality in the first sense and becomes manifested in consciousness. Because our thinking consists of extrasensory percepts within a private

---

[113] *Berkeley* uses the wording 'ideas existing in the mind', 'ideas' thus representing percepts, and 'mind' being synonymous with consciousness. *Berkeley* stated: 'Their *esse* is *percipi*; nor is it possible they should have any existence, out of the mind or thinking which perceives them.' 'In truth, the object and the sensation are the same thing, and cannot therefore be abstracted from each other.' It should, however, be mentioned that *Leibniz* (1646–1710), although in a much less rigorous manner, had also considered space to be a 'mental' attribute (*ens mentale, ens ideale*).

perceptual space-time system, our thoughts are obviously bound to the symbolism of space-time, and the nature of reality in the first sense remains intrinsically unintelligible.[114]

With regard to this problem, *Hume* remarked: 'Thus the first philosophical objection to the evidence of sense or to the opinion of external existence is this, that such an opinion, if rested on natural instinct, is contrary to reason, and if referred to reason, is contrary to instinct, and carries no rational evidence with it, to convince an impartial enquirer. The second objection goes farther, and represents this opinion as contrary to reason: at least, if it be a principle of reason, that all sensible qualities are in the mind, not in the object. Bereave matter of all its intelligible qualities, you in a manner annihilate it, and leave only a certain unknown, inexplicable something, as the cause of our perceptions; a notice so imperfect, that no sceptic will think it worth while to contend against it.'[115]

It seems evident that, in accordance with the valid aspect of *Berkeley's* argumentation and with the quoted comments by *Hume*, the *space-time of science is absolutely swept away*, and the 'external world of physics' has no existence, except in our thoughts.

It is, moreover, obvious that *Hume's* 'inexplicable something' represents what *Kant* [1781] subsequently designated as '*Ding an sich*' (thing in itself); and that *Hume*, although not explicitly, but very definitely implicitly, anticipated *Kant* with respect to the inevitable conclusion that space and time are merely the given 'forms' or 'formal aspects' of consciousness.[116] *Kant* thus clearly emphasized the distinction between *phenomena* (consciousness, perception) and *reality in the first sense*. His claim, however, that space and time

[handwritten margin note: Without external objects our thoughts would be of nothing AND without experienced sensations in our personal mind - objects do not exist (for us).]

---

[114] An amusing example of an unintelligible relationship is elaborated in the amiable romance '*Flatland*' [1952, reprint] by *E. A. Abbott* (1828–1926), in which two-dimensional sentient beings are unable to conceive the possibility of a three-dimensional world. Somewhat similarly, our spatio-temporal mind is unable to conceive, in intelligent terms, a reality devoid of space-time attributes.

[115] *Hume* furthermore comments as follows on the views of *Berkeley*, whom he greatly admired: 'and indeed most of the writings of that very ingenious author form the best lessons of scepticism, which are to be found either among the ancient or modern philosophers, *Bayle* not excepted. He professes, however, in his Title page (and undoubtedly with great truth) to have composed his book against the sceptics as well as the atheists and free-thinkers. But that all his arguments, though otherwise intended, are, in reality, merely sceptical, appears from this, that they admit of no answer and produce no conviction. Their only effect is to cause that momentary amazement and irresolution and confusion, which is the result of scepticism.'

[116] Since, in *Schopenhauer's* formulation of the principle of sufficient reason, which I have adopted with minor modifications, a 'cause' implies dynamic 'material' interaction in a given space-time system, and thereby implies 'continuity', I prefer here to say that our consciousness is *dependent upon* the unknown 'orderliness x' (*Hume's* 'inexplicable something', *Kant's* '*Ding an sich*') but *not* that this latter, in *Hume's* words, is the '*cause*' of our perceptions.

are given as '*Erkenntnis a priori*' ('knowledge a priori'), cannot be upheld. It seems evident that our 'knowledge' of space (location, configuration) and time (succession) results from the mature thinking analysis of our conscious experiences, and therefore requires these antecedent space-time experiences.[117]

Kant, moreover, convincingly showed that our knowledge remains restricted to phenomena, and cannot extend to so-called 'metaphysics'. This means that our knowledge cannot extend to a 'transcendent' existence beyond our conscious experience.

Schopenhauer, who considered himself a disciple of *Kant*, although he elaborated a detailed and partly justified critique of *Kant's* philosophy, attempted to work out a coherent and universal philosophical system which, despite numerous errors and considerable weaknesses, can be evaluated as most remarkable. His lucid style and his trenchant dealings with the deepest problems of existence are highly stimulating, and compel the critical reader, to clarify his own definitions and to closely scrutinize his own views.

In the present context reference to only four relevant concepts of *Schopenhauer's* system will be sufficient.

(1) *Schopenhauer correctly recognized that our world of consciousness is a brain phenomenon.* However, since the brain itself is a brain phenomenon, we have here the '*brain paradox*', which shall be separately considered in section 6 of the present chapter.

(2) Instead of 'consciousness', *Schopenhauer* uses the term '*Vorstellung*' (representation) with regard to the phenomenal world. '*Vorstellung*', according to said author, implies *ein vorstellendes (erkennendes) Subjekt und ein vorgestelltes (erkanntes) Objekt*, that is to say a perceiving subject and a perceived object. However, the terms '*Vorstellung*', '*Subjekt*', and '*Objekt*' involve considerable weaknesses as well as ambiguities and shall be critically examined further below in a classification of the given aspects of consciousness.

(3) In contradistinction to *Hume* and *Kant*, *Schopenhauer* believed that the 'inexplicable something', respectively the '*Ding an sich*', or the 'orderliness x' could be recognized as, or identified with, 'will'.[118] *Schopenhauer's* conclusion or assertion is quite unconvincing. 'Will' is not only an exceedingly vague and ambiguous term, but, no matter how defined or conceived, it remains definitely a phenomenon of consciousness, that is to say, in *Schopenhauer's* own phraseology, a '*Vorstellung*'.

---

[117] A more detailed discussion of the meaning of '*a priori*' can be found in §47, pages 186–194 of the present author's treatise *Mind and Matter* [K., 1961].

[118] *Schopenhauer* stated [vol. 5, p. 102], '*Ding an sich bedeutet das unabhängig von unserer Wahrnehmung Vorhandene, also das eigentlich Seiende. Dies war dem Democritos die geformte Materie: das selbe war es im Grunde noch dem Locke: Kanten war es = x; mir Wille.*'

(4) In his doctoral thesis of 1813, submitted to the University of Jena, *Schopenhauer* elaborated a very substantial and highly important essay on the principle of sufficient reason, of which he prepared an expanded edition in 1847. Strangely enough, this treatise was subsequently ignored, to the detriment of their argumentations, by many of the later authors dealing with the relevant topics pertaining to that principle of which my own interpretation will be elaborated further below, in the final section 7 of the present chapter.

Reverting now to the definition of consciousness as outlined above on page 2 of the short introducing chapter I, it seems appropriate, in accordance with the sceptical outlook of *David Hume*[119] to point out the different manifestations of consciousness, or, in other words, to delineate the phenomenology of the private perceptual space-time manifold experienced as 'consciousness', which constitutes the one and only one given actuality.

Such private perceptual space-time system, designated as a *consciousness-manifold*, is manifested by its contents, which may be called percepts (*Hume's* 'perceptions'), and thus represents a *plenum*. 'Pure consciousness', that is to say consciousness without contents, is non-existent, except as an abstraction manifested by a conscious thought. All percepts are *localized* and occur in time, i.e. 'here and now'. *Sensory percepts*, pertaining to the conventional five senses and additional modalities as e.g. dealt with in section 1, chapter VII, vol. 3/II of the author's *Central Nervous System of Vertebrates* [*K.*, 1973] can be distinguished from *extrasensory percepts*,[120] represented by thoughts and

---

[119] *Hume* justly emphasized the obvious fact that nothing is ever actually present in the mind (consciousness) 'but its perceptions or impressions and ideas, and that external objects become known to us only by those perceptions'. ... 'to hate, to love, to think, to see, all this is nothing but to perceive'. 'Now, since nothing is ever present to the mind but perceptions, and since all ideas are derived from something antecedently present to the mind, it follows that it is impossible for us so much as to conceive or form an idea of anything specifically different from ideas and impressions. Let us fix our attention out of ourselves as much as possible; let us chase our imagination to the heavens, or to the utmost limits of the universe; we never really advance a step beyond ourselves, nor can we conceive any kind of existence but those perceptions, which have appeared in that narrow compass. This is the universe of the imagination, nor have we any idea but what is there produced.'

[120] I have purposely chosen the term 'extrasensory' instead of 'non-sensory' in order to express my rejection of so-called 'parapsychology', and ESP, and 'mental telepathy'. Insofar as they may not be outright fraudulent, the phenomena of ESP represent, in my opinion, merely unusual coincidences with respect to thoughts. Their emphasized contradiction to mathematical probability concepts merely shows that these latter, although theoretically impeccable, do not correspond to some aspects of actuality. In other words, one should heed a relevant remark of *Einstein*: 'As far as the laws of mathematics refer to reality, they are not certain; and as far as they are certain, they do not refer to reality.' What *Einstein* means here by 'reality' is evidently 'actuality' in the present author's terminology. The uncertainty pointed out by *Einstein* is related to the problem of '*boundary conditions*' or '*boundary value*' referring to the restricted validity of impeccable mathematical formulations when applied to actual events, which generally involve constraining hidden parameters [cf. *K.*, 1973, pp. 40–41].

certain aspects of emotion (affectivity). This distinction corresponds to *Hume's* classification of 'perceptions' into 'impressions' (sensory) and 'ideas' (extrasensory).

Only two sorts of Human vivid sensory percepts, namely optic ones and some body sensations (e.g. tactile and proprioceptive percepts) are in addition to being well localized, also *spatially configurated* (i.e. implying limiting surfaces with outlines and shapes). Acoustic percepts may be vivid, but are less distinctly localized, and, at least in Man, are shapeless, that is, lack spatial configuration.

It should be added, however, that some optic sensory percepts may be shapeless, although spatially extended (e.g. in a diffuse fog, or in complete darkness as a black field of vision). Tactile sensations with closed eyes in still or flowing air or water nevertheless retain the spatial configurational aspect of the body or of a limiting surface.

Olfactory and gustatory modalities may be vivid but are quite vaguely localized with emphasis on nasal cavity respectively tongue, and also lack spatial configuration. Vagueness of localization also occurs with regard to the manifestations of referred pain, which are familiar to the clinician.

Extrasensory percepts, namely, non-eidetic memory images, abstractions, thoughts[121] as well as emotions and vague feelings are poorly localized and likewise without spatial configuration. Extrasensory percepts frequently, but not always, may display a low degree of vividity. Nevertheless, all extrasensory percepts are localized, thoughts, e.g. being generally referred to a region corresponding to the interior of the body, dorsally to the visual space. Not infrequently, sensory and extrasensory percepts may be closely linked together by superposition. If accompanied by vague body sensations, extrasensory percepts may be localized in chest or abdomen. Thus, as e.g. implied by the *James-Lange theory*, the hypothesis of a localization of 'mind' in heart or diaphragm (*phrenes*), as expressed by some views of antiquity, had at least a modicum of justification. However, as justly stressed by authors such as *Flechsig* [1896] and *Forel* [1922], we do not localize our thoughts in our feet or externally to the body.

There is, moreover, a third type of percepts, which could be called *pseudosensory percepts*, being intermediate between the sensory and the extrasensory ones. Such pseudosensory percepts, occurring in dreams or as hallucinations, may display, even quite vividly, the aspects of sensory modalities, without however being mediated by corresponding sense organs. It can be assumed that said pseudosensory events are triggered by activated engraphic complexes pertaining to previously experienced actual sensory events.

---

[121] A detailed definition and discussion of 'thought' is given in the author's contribution to the *Helen Adolf Festschrift* [K., 1968].

As regards localization, however, *Hume's* failure to realize that all percepts whatsoever are localized should be pointed out. *Hume* erroneously claimed that 'an object may exist, and yet be nowhere', and asserted 'that this is not only possible, but that the greatest part of beings do and must exist after this manner. An object may be said to be nowhere when its parts are not so situated with respect to each other, as to form any figure or quantity; nor the whole with respect to other bodies so as to answer to our notions of contiguity and distance. Now this is evidently the case with all our perceptions and objects, except those of the sight and feeling. A moral reflection cannot be placed to the right or left of a passion; nor can a smell or sound be either of a circular or square figure. These objects and perceptions, so far from requiring any particular place, are absolutely incompatible with it, and even the imagination cannot attribute to them.' He also stated: 'What is extended must have a particular figure, as square, round, triangular, none of which will agree to a desire or indeed to any impression or idea.'

It is evident that *Hume* failed to distinguish *location* (or localization) from *spatial configuration*. A moral reflection and a passion most certainly require a localization or particular place (and time: here and now), namely the region of perceptual space-time represented by head and perhaps chest (heart) as well as abdomen ('gut') of the individual experiencing reflection and passion. Since, however, there obtains no spatial configuration, there will evidently be no relationship of right and left between the two, and since no impenetrability obtains, the two percepts will simultaneously occupy either identical or overlapping regions of space (extending from head to chest or abdomen). Yet, a moral reflection may be 'placed' above (in the head) a passion 'localized' in, or extending into chest (heart) and gut.

The diverse sounds of the several instruments in an orchestra experienced as sounds localized outside the body, are simultaneously located, by interpretation, in one and the same ill-defined region of space, but nevertheless can be 'distinguished' from each other.

Even different spatially configured visual perceptual patterns may, by 'interpenetration' occupy either identical or overlapping regions of space, namely objects in front of one's body together with objects behind one's body, being superimposed upon, or 'telescoped' into, each other, and localized in one and the same region of space, if one looks through a glass plate under appropriate catoptric and dioptric lighting conditions.

The consciousness manifold, as manifested by normal adult Human beings, tends to display two distinctive groups or neighborhoods, namely the *'external world'* and the *'internal world'* or *self sensu latiori*. The latter is represented by the perceptual body containing the sensory and motor, or respectively efferent, nerve endings related to the likewise included brain which generates that consciousness (or, of which said consciousness is a dependent variable). The zones of consciousness corresponding to 'internal' and 'external' world complexes have, however, ill-defined boundaries and overlap with wide, fluctuating border zones [*Kretschmer*, 1926]. The body complex, experienced as 'ego' or 'self', and the 'external world' manifest interaction, such that the latter acts upon the former, and vice versa. Some activities of the body are experienced as involuntary and others as voluntary, namely accompanied by a percept designated as 'will' (conation), which can be subsumed under the phenomena of affectivity. It is absolutely impossible to define the experience 'will', except by its relationship, just as it is absolutely impossible to define the sensation 'red'. Both pertain to what *Poincaré* [1909] appropriately called '*qualités pures*', which are intransmissible by words and utterly incommunicable, except for their relationships [cf. *K.*, 1961, p. 241]. '*Will*', moreover, is an exceedingly vague and ambiguous term with a variety of diverse connotations and denotations.

The distinctly localized and spatially configurated sensory optic, tactile (in the wider sense) and proprioceptive percepts, as well as the indistinctly localized and not spatially configurated acoustic, olfactory and visceral percepts are localized externally to the brain. This latter, enclosed in the perceivable head, is likewise perceived *qua* weight through proprioception.[122]

Although all conscious percepts (a tautology) seem to depend upon the function of the perceptual (i.e. perceived) brain, consciousness is thus not localized within this latter, but said brain, contrariwise, becomes localized within the space-time system of the consciousness manifold.

With respect to the above-mentioned obtaining aspects of localization it seems obvious that *Kant's* and *Schopenhauer's* concepts of space as the form '*des äusseren Sinnes*' (of the external 'sense') and of time as the form '*des inneren Sinnes*' (of the internal 'sense') are quite erroneous and based on the following two misconceptions.

(1) Both authors, like *Hume*, wrongly restrict localization to spatial configuration. (2) They also draw, within the consciousness manifold, an arbitrary and unjustified 'boundary' between 'external' and 'internal' 'world', apparently corresponding to the body's surface. Actually, the entire consciousness manifold is experienced as a continuous plenum, consisting of open neighborhoods in the topologic sense.

With respect to the above-mentioned (cf. p. 167) potentially misleading distinction of a perceiving subject and a perceived object, said distinction is merely a rather awkward formulation of the given fact that all consciousness contents ('objects') represent components of an integrated consciousness

---

[122] There is, in the aspect here under consideration, little difference between perceiving, with closed eyes, a dead Human brain held in one's hand, and perceiving one's own living brain enclosed in the head.

manifold ('subject'), namely of a transitory private perceptual space-time system. This latter may be conceived as the transitory 'self', or 'I', in the wider sense, although, in the narrower sense, the 'self', 'I', or *'ego'* is usually restricted to one's body or even to an imaginary 'central point' of the consciousness manifold. The illusion of substantial 'self' shall again be discussed in section 2 of chapter III. Since the phenomenon of consciousness does not involve a perceiving subject and perceived objects as imagined by *Schopenhauer* and others, the percepts and the perceiver are here one and the same phenomenon.[123] The percepts are as they are and not otherwise.

The concept of a perceiving subject is, moreover, closely related to the notion of a 'soul', 'spirit' or 'thinking substance', defined by *Berkeley* [1713] as that 'indivisible, unextended thing, which thinks, acts, and perceives'. Yet that outstanding philosopher had almost reached the proper formulation. We may evidently state that the (private) consciousness manifold, namely mind *sensu completo*, is that indivisible (gestalt-like), extended, four-dimensional whole consisting of thoughts, volitions (emotions), and sensory percepts.

This transitory consciousness manifold can be designated as the 'self' or the *'subject'* in the widest sense, and one may thus, without contradiction, reintroduce the eliminated concept of a 'substantial self' in the guise of an auxiliary fictional construction. That manifold, moreover, might be likened, in some of the aspects under consideration, to *Giordano Bruno's* conception of a *monad*, later adopted, with some modifications, by *Leibniz*.

The fact that a percept must be perceived by a perceiver, i.e. by a mind, or that a perceived object requires a perceiving subject, merely means that, in order to be actualized, a percept must be the content of a consciousness manifold, that is, to occur as intrinsic component of a private perceptual space-time system related to its perceptual brain. *Berkeley* justly stated that 'in truth the object and the sensation are the same thing'. He nevertheless, presumably because of his ecclesiastical status, could not draw the inevitable conclusion and felt compelled to retain the concept of substantial soul, spirit, mind or 'myself', which perceived the perception.

The percepts (or perceptions) represent, however, irreducible given phenomena (*Urphänomene*) which constitute a private consciousness manifold whose sustained 'identity', despite disruptions by periods of unconsciousness, is, as experience evinces, correlated with an awake perceptual brain, pertaining to a given perceptual body. Said percepts, all of which

---

[123] *Schopenhauer* [vol. 5, p. 284] was, in my opinion, mistaken by attributing this identity to the *'erkenntnislosen Urzustand'*, *'ein Zustand, wo der Gegensatz von Subjekt und Objekt wegfällt, weil hier das zu Erkennende mit dem Erkennenden selbst wirklich und unmittelbar Eins seyn würde'*. This identity, in fact, is the characteristic of consciousness [cf. *K.*, 1978, p. 353, fn. 165, referring to a recent author's inability of understanding this important point].

together represent a transitory self *sensu latiori* with a relatively persistent vague self *sensu strictiori*, based on aspects of memory, are as they are and not otherwise. To quote a pithy remark, which the earthy late President *Harry S. Truman* was wont to use in a different context: '*the buck stops here*'. Anything going beyond this 'given' is an extrapolation into the unknown, but remaining within that consciousness manifold as a thought percept in terms of said manifold's spatio-temporal symbolism. This 'unknown' remains, therefore, intrinsically unknowable, thus justifying the statement: *ignorabimus*.

As regards *Berkeley's* extrapolation, the following statement of this author is of interest: 'But whatever power I may have over my own thoughts, I find the ideas actually perceived by sense have not a like dependence on my will. When in broad daylight I open my eyes, it is not in my power to choose whether I shall see or no, or to determine what particular objects shall present themselves to my view, and so likewise as to the hearing and other senses, the ideas imprinted on them are not creatures of my will. There is therefore some other will or spirit that produces them.'

Hume [1738], however, quite correctly recognized that it is not the involuntariness of sensory percepts which suggests their relationship to 'reality' and 'continuous existence', but rather their coherence and constancy despite considerable interruptions of perception.

My own extrapolation, as discussed further above, postulates the unknown orderliness x, which, in some respects, is comparable to *Kant's 'Ding an sich'*. The term 'thing', however, does not seem very appropriate. Neither *Berkeley* nor *Kant*, moreover, sufficiently considered the significance of the perceptual brain.

With respect to 'reality', *Berkeley* designated the 'ideas imprinted on the senses by the author of nature' as the 'real things', and those excited in the imagination as the images or ideas 'of things'. Both 'real things' and ideas of our own framing, imaginations or chimeras 'equally exist in the mind, and in that sense are like ideas'.

In *Berkeley's* 'Third Dialogue between *Hylas* and *Philonous*', *Hylas* asks: 'What think you therefore of retaining the name matter, and applying it to sensible things.' In the guise of *Philonous*, *Berkeley* replies: 'With all my heart: retain the word matter, and apply it to the objects of sense, if you please, provided you do not attribute them to any subsistence distinct from their being perceived. I shall never quarrel with you for an expression.' *Berkeley*, however, then again repeats his strong denial of matter or material substance as concepts 'introduced by philosophers' and used by them to imply a 'sort of independency, or a subsistence distinct from their being perceived'.

Before *Kant*, so-called 'rational psychology' conceived the 'soul', i.e. consciousness, as some sort of 'thing' or 'substance' with the attributes of 'immateriality', 'incorruptibility' and 'immortality'.

This concept was convincingly demolished by *Kant*. *Schopenhauer* likewise justly argued that an individual consciousness, in fact consciousness at all, cannot be attributed to an 'immaterial being', since empirical data clearly suggest that consciousness, as a brain phenomenon, requires the orderliness which, in consciousness, is represented by a perceptual brain pertaining to a perceptual organic body. Much the same can be said about the concept of an 'immaterial' but nevertheless personal 'supreme being' or 'God' with Human 'mental' attributes. The alleged proofs for the existence of such being (ontological argument, cosmologic argument, physico-theological argument) were likewise convincingly demolished by *Kant*.

It will be seen that the structural definition of consciousness, as given and adopted in the present section, conforms to the guidelines set up by *Hume* [1750]:

'Accurate and just reasoning is the only catholic remedy, fitted for all persons and all dispositions; and is alone able to subvert that abstruse philosophy and metaphysical jargon, which, being mixed up with popular superstition, renders it in a manner impenetrable to careless reasoners, and gives it the air of science and wisdom.'

'Besides this advantage of rejecting, after deliberate inquiry the most uncertain and disagreeable part of learning, there are many positive advantages, which result from an accurate scrutiny, into the powers and faculties of human nature. It is remarkable concerning the operations of the mind, that, though most intimately present to us, yet, wherever they become the object of reflection, they seem involved in obscurity; nor can the eye readily find those lines and boundaries, which discriminate and distinguish them.'

'It becomes, therefore, no inconsiderable part of science barely to know the different operations of the mind, to separate them from each other, to class them under their proper heads, and to correct all that seeming disorder, in which they lie involved, when made the object of reflexion and inquiry.'

'And if we can go no further than this mental geography, or delineation of the distinct parts and powers of the mind, it is at least a satisfaction to go so far; and the more obvious this science appears (and it is by no means obvious) the more contemptible still must the ignorance of it be esteemed, in all pretenders to learning and philosophy.'

An example of disclosing a complete misunderstanding of the 'nature' of consciousness is e.g. displayed by a short note which a writer published on pages 184–185 of the *Schopenhauer Jahrbuch* 59, 1978. Said writer, who likewise failed to grasp the meaning of the brain paradox, made the following statement: '*Der Ausdruck "Bewusstsein", ein sprachtechnisches Reifikationsprodukt, bezieht sich nach unserer Auffassung auf die Gegebenheitsweise von Analogprozessen, mittels welcher erlebnishaftes Geschehen einschließlich seiner materiellen und energetischen Aspekte auf der höchsten Schicht des Zentralnervensystems repräsentiert ist.'*

Discounting the meaningless verbiage of '*Gegebenheitsbeweise von Analogprozessen*' etc., which, at most, is an awkward way of stating that consciousness can be conceived as depending on cerebral processes; it will suffice to point out the faulty reasoning involved in conceiving consciousness as a '*sprachtechnisches Reifikationsprodukt*'.

'Reifikation' or 'hypostatization' represents, as justly emphasized by *Whitehead*, the fallacy of misplaced concreteness. Yet, consciousness, of which sensory percepts are one of the most essential features, is thereby characterized by the most substantial concreteness. What could be more concrete than the percept of a rock, of a tree, of a given animal, of another Human being or of one's own body? There are, of course, in the consciousness manifold, less vivid sensory or extrasensory percepts, which, however, in the aspect under consideration, must likewise be regarded as concrete instances.

This was fully understood by *Kretschmer* [1926], who, using the term soul (*Seele*) for consciousness, clearly stated: '*Seele nennen wir das unmittelbare Erleben. Seele ist alles Empfundene, Wahrgenommene, Vorgestellte, Gewollte. Seele ist also z.B. ein Baum, ein Ton, die Sonne, sofern ich sie als Wahrenehmung Baum, als Vorstellung Sonne betrachte. Seele ist die Welt als Erlebnis.*'

It seems evident that *Kretschmer's* 'world of experience' represents consciousness, namely a private perceptual space-time manifold. In this respect, it should be recalled that *Schopenhauer*, already long before *H. Minkowski*, repeatedly stresses the union of space and time into a joint respectively common space-time system. He postulated [Werke, vol. 3, p. 44] '*Vereinigung des Raumes und der Zeit zur Gesamtvorstellung der empirischen Realität*' and also stated '*sogar ist eine innige Vereinigung beider die Bedingung der Realität*'. Reality is here, of course, taken in the second sense.

Concerning the space and time of physics, *Minkowski* [1908] elaborated, in mathematical terms, the four-dimensional space-time concept which proved to be of fundamental importance for *Einstein's* theories of relativity. In his lecture at the Congress of natural scientists and physicians, *Minkowski* stated: 'The views of space and time which I wish to lay before you have sprung from the soil of experimental physics, and therein lies their strength. They are radical. Henceforth, space by itself, and time by itself, are doomed to fade away into mere shadows, and only a kind of union of the two will preserve an independent reality' [*Lorentz* et al., n.d., p. 75].

It might be added that, without any reference to *Schopenhauer, Alexander* [1920, 1966] elaborated on a 'philosophical' and 'metaphysical' space-time concept. Since, however, *Alexander* not only completely failed to understand the relevant arguments proposed by *Berkeley, Hume*, and *Kant*, but also failed to recognize the difference between experienced private space-time and postulated public conceptual space-time system, such e.g. as the space-time of physics, *Alexander's* confused 'metaphysical' treatise can hardly be taken seriously.

Summarizing the relevant conclusions following from the preceding discussion, the inevitably resulting *dualism* becomes obvious, namely the dichotomy or 'cut' between actually given consciousness and that unknowable and unintelligible 'something' (orderliness x) which 'exists' independently of consciousness, or in other words, when there is no consciousness.

The frequently assumed dualism between 'mind' and 'matter', on the other hand, is an illusion resulting from faulty reasoning. Rigorous critical analysis clearly demonstrates that 'mind' *sensu strictiori* (extrasensory percepts) and 'matter' (sensory percepts) are both mere aspects of consciousness.

The term *'monism'* is evidently poorly chosen. At most, it applies to the 'identity' of 'mind' and 'matter'. But this, moreover, involves a *'pluralism'* insofar as innumerable different and disjoint private perceptual space-time systems ('consciousness manifolds') obtain.

Using the term 'substance'[124] *Spinoza* attempted to establish said just mentioned 'monism' in *Pars II, Propositio VII* of his *Ethica, ordine geometrica demonstrata*, by formulating the well known dictum: *'substantia cogitans et substantia extensa una eademque est substantia, quae iam sub hoc, iam sub illo attributo comprehenditur'*.

Retaining for consciousness the term 'substantia' and in full agreement with *Berkeley's, Hume's*, and my own view, *Spinoza's* statement should (and can easily) be modified as follows: *Substantia extensa et substantia cogitans duo attributa sunt unae eiusdemque substantiae, quae conscientia nominatur.*

Reverting now to the materialistic viewpoint it seems evident that the materialist ignores the fundamental fact of his own consciousness. The semantic universe of discourse pertaining to physics and chemistry is based on the concept of orderly events, assuming transformations, respectively interactions, of mass and energy in a public four-dimensional space-time system. These events, as public data, can be registered by the sensory endings (transducers) of the nervous system or by instruments, which, again, can be 'read' by the senses of an observer. Although phenomena of consciousness are experienced by the awake observer, this latter cannot, by means of his senses detect consciousness phenomena extraneous to his own, nor can such phenomena be registered by instruments. Moreover, consciousness has no logical

---

[124] The somewhat ambiguous term 'substance' refers to 'quid est', that is to say denotes the οὐσια, *natura, substantia*, by 'virtue' of which a 'thing' (or 'something') has its determinate 'nature', making it 'what it is' as distinguished from 'something else'. The limitations of Human language are here obvious [cf. also *K.*, 1968].

existence in the universe of discourse pertaining to physics and chemistry. Much the same could be said about most aspects of biology, concerned with the study of organic life, insofar as life represents a physical and biochemical phenomenon displayed by 'matter' (i.e. mass and energy) under particular conditions.

Ashby [1952] in his *Design for a Brain*, although recognizing consciousness as 'the most fundamental fact of all', justly ignores this phenomenon in dealing with his topic: 'Vivid though consciousness may be to its possessor, there is as yet no method known by which he can demonstrate his experience to another. And until such method, or its equivalent, is found, the facts of consciousness cannot be used in scientific method.'

This view, as here applied to brain function, corresponds, of course, to *Watson's* [1925, 1929] concept of *behaviorism*. This author, while originally not denying that consciousness exists, attempted to deal with behavior exclusively in terms of physiological and neurological states which can be recorded by an external observer or by instruments. In this respect, consciousness is indeed neither definable nor a usable concept. Thus, 'psychology as science of consciousness has no community of data' [*Watson*, 1929].

Quite evidently, a presumably conscious living Human or Animal being cannot 'demonstrate' its state of consciousness to an observer. This latter, or for that matter a suitable instrument, can only register the observed being's physical behavior (including e.g. verbal communication) from which that being's consciousness can merely be inferred *per analogiam*. Such unverifiable inference, although in many cases quite 'certain' or rather convincing, is not an actual observation. No conceivable method for such observation can be described in terms of exact sciences, its only equivalent (cf. above *Ashby's* remark) being an inference from observable behavior. Thus, from the viewpoint of 'objective science', methodological behaviorism seems fully justified. Yet, because of the inevitable conclusion that the so-called inner world of thoughts and feelings as well as the so-called external world of material objects are private manifestations of consciousness, it seems evident that the public world of physics and natural sciences becomes a mere fiction. Nevertheless, it appears that only on the basis of this fiction a rational explanation of the experienced phenomena becomes possible. The *fiction* of an orderly 'world', independent of consciousness, and represented by a public physical space-time system, must therefore be considered an indispensable *postulate of practical reason*.

As alreay stated in the present author's old '*Vorlesungen*': '*Sowohl die Gedanken und Gefühle, also die innere Welt, geistige oder Geisteswelt des gewöhnlichen Sprachgebrauches wie die körperlich in Raum und Zeit ausgebreitete äussere (materielle) Welt sind Bewusstseinszustände (Vorstellung, Erscheinung). Das naturwissenschaftliche Weltbild mit seiner unabhängig von einem vorstellenden Bewußtsein vorhandenen objektiven, räumlichen, zeitlichen, kausalen Welt ist eine Fiktion. Aber nur mit Hilfe dieser Fiktion ist ein Verständnis der Erscheinungsreihen möglich'* [*K.*, 1927, p. 2].

Riese [1954] remarks that 'the history of medicine lists no physician daring enough to adopt the idealistic thesis that man's brain is but an idea, if not an illusion', It is evident that my esteemed colleague was not aquainted with my views [*K.*, 1927, 1957, 1961, and other publications], which unequivocally conceived the perceptual brain as an 'idea' in *Berkeley's* sense. There exists, in my interpretation, no physical brain, except as an operatively valid fiction, since the unknowable orderliness x must be assumed devoid of spatio-temporal relationships.

The indeed *real* (*in the second sense*) perceptual brain represents merely, translated into the space-time symbolism of our consciousness, relevant aspects of said independent orderliness. Much the same can be said about the concept of molecules, atoms, particles, quanta, or about the four main sorts of physical interactions (gravity, electromagnetism, weak and strong interactions etc. pertaining to particles).

It should also be emphasized that the idealistic viewpoint, properly understood, does not conflict with the contemporary theories of cosmogony which assume the universe as arisen from the primordial explosion of a superdense mass perhaps about more or less 10^{10} years ago.[125] Within an either early or subsequent later given time the present types of atoms were formed and, in a hierarchy of condensations, galaxies resulted, some stars of which may include planetary systems. In this expanding universe with its populations of galaxies and diverse types of evolving and dying stars, organic life seems to be a rather rare phenomenon. Yet such life can reasonably be assumed as having evolved or still evolving in fairly numerous, widely scattered regions of the universe. Quite evidently, organic life originated much later than the preceding cosmic events, and again consciousness, presumed to be correlated with activities of a nervous system, arose much later than the origin of organic life.

Regardless of unsettled details, these theories appear rather plausible, and pose the problem of their proper formulation in the terminology of the idealistic viewpoint, since it must be presumed that the occurrence of consciousness, in which only spatio-temporal 'material events' become manifested, was preceded by the necessary 'material' evolutionary events. These latter, assumed to be unconscious, were thus not manifested in a conscious-

---

[125] Despite various uncertainties as regards the 'time' of this origin and the sequence in which the present atoms heavier than H and He were formed, the theory of 'primordial fireball' seems well supported and can be assumed to imply a preceding collapse, that is a 'pulsating' or 'oscillating' universe as discussed in section 1.

ness of their own, which would presuppose an adequate nervous system, nor in that of conscious beings, since these did not yet exist. Thus, these 'preceding' states were not spatio-temporal events, but merely unknowable aspects of the unknowable orderliness x. However, if translated into the spatio-temporal symbolism of an intelligent conscious being endowed with reason, these aspects can be conceived as having occurred in the manner postulated by the theories.[126] More naively expressed, if a conscious observer, possessor of a perceptual brain comparable to that of an intelligent Human being, could have been there during these presumed 'periods', said events would have appeared to him as so occurring.

The above-mentioned postulate of practical reason corresponds, of course, to the important concept of operationally valid fictions as elaborated by *Vaihinger* [1913] in his *'Philosophie des Als Ob'*. This author asked the question: *'Wie kommt es, dass wir mit bewusst falschen Vorstellungen doch Richtiges erreichen?'* He then expounded a formulation according to which the fundamental concepts and principles of natural science, mathematics, philosophy, ethics, law, and religions are pure fictions which, although lacking 'objective truth', are operationally valid, that is to say, useful [cf. *K.*, 1961, §72, p. 407f] 'instruments of action'. *Vaihinger* had a deep insight into *Kant's* philosophy and justly interpreted that author's postulates of practical reason as fictions which, depending on the given circumstances or particular aspects under consideration, may be accepted as being useful. *Schopenhauer*, in his critique of *Kant's* philosophy, failed sufficiently to realize this relevant point.

From the viewpoint of the operationally valid fiction postulating the public spatio-temporal world of physicalisms (i.e. mass and energy) respectively natural sciences, including biology, and thereby the existence of a physical nervous system characterized by physiologic neuronal circuit events, it becomes necessary to formulate, in relevant terms, the postulated (fictional) physical events and their correlation with the given actuality of consciousness.

In my own attempts at correlating fictional physical, or behavioristically conceived brain events, with the phenomenon of consciousness, I found it appropriate, adapting and modifying concepts elaborated by *Ziehen*,[127] to

---

[126] Cf. *Schopenhauer* [editio *Grisebach*, vol. 5, *'Zur Philosophie und Wissenschaft der Natur'*, pp. 154–155), and also further below, chapter III, section 6, page 227; chapter IV, section 2, volume 2, page 24. In other words, and from the viewpoint of *Vaihinger's* fictionalism, it is 'as if' the cosmogonic events had taken place or occurred at the postulated periods in a public physical space-time system.

[127] *Ziehen's* formulations shall be critically discussed in section 8 of chapter III. There are also some similarities between R-events and the so-called R-values of *Avenarius* [1888], whose 'system C' is somewhat comparable to N-events, the P-events, again being very roughly comparable to 'E-values' and 'characters' in the terminology of the cited author. Cf. also the comments on *Avenarius* further below on page 183.

distinguish all physicochemical events as R-events (reduced events, roughly corresponding to *Locke's* primary qualities), and all events encoded as *signals* by the nervous system as N-events. In other words, R-events become, at the receptor endings, transduced into N-events, and N-events, in turn, become at the effector level, again transduced into R-events. Roughly speaking, one could also say that all events externally to the nervous system are R-events, and that N-events are all neural signal activities. This, however, requires the qualification that the nervous system itself consists of biological R-events, upon which the N-events are imposed, or which 'carry' the N-events as 'signals' encoding information (variety, negentropy, theoretically expressible in bits[128]). Some, but by no means all N-events[129] appear correlated with consciousness, that is, with P-events ('parallel events'), and such 'physical' N-events may be designated as Np-events. It seems likely that, at least in the Human brain, Np-events represent essentially cortical or corticothalamic events.[130]

Again, in observing another Human (or comparable Animal) being, possessor of an awake, functioning brain, which is located in the private space-time of the conscious observer, this latter cannot observe, nor register by instruments, the corresponding conscious percepts 'produced' by the brain of the observed, and presumably likewise located outside to said brain. It follows that the observer's perceptual space is not identical with the assumed perceptual space of the observed. The different perceptual spaces, respectively space-time systems (or manifolds) are thus strictly '*private*', while the fictional postulated physical space-time system can be conceived as 'public'.

Thus, except for the consciousness of the observer, consciousness (i.e. other consciousness) is always merely an inference from behavior. This inference is experienced as 'certain' for Man and related Mammals, but becomes more and more 'uncertain' as one 'descends' the taxonomic or phylogenetic series. Yet, some sort of consciousness could be reasonably inferred to occur in all organic forms endowed with a central nervous system. One might question its possible occurrence in forms with a diffuse, netlike nervous system

---

[128] It should be recalled that 'bits' merely represent the logarithm to the base 2.

[129] Complex N-events not correlated with consciousness represent that which is misleading but generally called 'unconscious mind', a term involving *a contradictio in adjecto* ('unconscious consciousness'). Such N-events, in a more suitable terminology, should be called 'unconscious cerebration'. This was clearly understood by *Schopenhauer* who compared such unconscious activity with the performance of a mechanical calculator ('*Rechenmaschine*'). This important topic will again be considered in section 3 of chapter IV, volume 2.

[130] This does not exclude the possibility or probability that, particularly in 'lower mammals', in Anamnia and invertebrates, Np-events may occur in other central nervous grisea respectively 'centers'.

such e.g. obtaining in Coelenterates, and, moreover, presume that Animal forms without nervous system (e.g. Porifera and Protozoa) as well as all plants are unconscious (cf. the thoughtful comments by *Sherrington* quoted above in footnote 109). The evident fact that other-consciousness is neither observable nor registrable by instruments, fully justifies methodological behaviorism for a wide domain of natural sciences, but does not justify dogmatic behaviorism, that is to say the encroachment of behaviorism into domains of natural sciences as well as of other realms or 'spheres' concerned with relevant aspects of consciousness (e.g. *qualités pures* of *Poincaré*).

Reverting to the materialistic approach its quandary evidently results from the intrinsic fallacy of its basic premises. Abstracting the so-called secondary qualities, a four-dimensional physical world based on the primary qualities was postulated and it was assumed that this world could be regarded as stripped of all attributes of consciousne, that is of mind *sensu latiori*. Yet, the primary qualities are merely abstract notions of perceptual space-time relationships, and perceptual space-time, in turn, represents the 'matrix' of consciousness, while the secondary qualities must be considered modalities of this matrix. Thus, the postulated physical world is based on the very essence of consciousness. In other words: if consciousness is excluded, then space-time relationships are likewise eliminated. Since, viewed from this standpoint, the concepts of physics are defined and wielded upon a background of irrationality, the resulting paradoxes and the failures in attempting to establish a logical unassailable general basis for physics are not surprising. In conjunction with the increasing amount of new observations, modern physics has steadily moved toward extreme abstractness; the particles have become 'dematerialized' and converted into 'events'; energy and space-time, on the other hand, assume a more 'material' aspect. Thus properties formerly ascribed to 'forces' and 'matter' can be interpreted as characteristics of space which assumes, as it were, the status of a 'stuff': fields are properties of space, which, in turn, may manifest a 'curvature' or may, figuratively speaking, become deformed or 'full of hills' (*Bertrand Russell*) in the vicinity of 'matter', i.e. 'mass'. 'Bodies' follow geodesies around such 'hills'. One is here reminded of the remark, attributed to *J. B. S. Haldane*, that the physical universe 'is not only queerer than we suppose, but queerer than we can suppose'.

The materialistic approach would require an explanation of consciousness as a modification of matter or as a transformation or still better as a causal result of material (physicochemical) processes. If we were to understand how consciousness arises, we should at least be able to have knowledge of something which is not consciousness but becomes consciousness. However, all knowledge and all abstractions, including matter, are merely modalities of consciousness. Therefore it is impossible to solve the problem of consciousness; this problem must thus be relegated with that of squaring the circle with straight-edge and compasses, or that of constructing a working mechanical perpetuum mobile. *Schopenhauer* [1818, 1859] summarizes the frustration of the materialistic attempt as follows: '*Wären wir nun dem Materialismus, mit anschaulichen Vorstellungen, bis dahin gefolgt; so würden wir, auf seinem Gipfel mit ihm angelangt, eine plötzliche Anwandlung des unauslöschlichen Lachens der Olympier spüren, indem wir, wie aus einem Traume erwachend, mit einem Male inne würden, daß sein letztes, so mühsam herbeigeführtes Resultat, das Erkennen, schon beim allerersten Ausgangspunkt, der bloßen Materie, als unumgängliche Bedingung vorausgesetzt war, und wir mit ihm zwar die Materie zu denken uns eingebildet, in der That aber nichts Anderes als das die Materie vorstellende Subjekt, das sie sehende Auge, die sie fühlende Hand, den sie erkennenden Verstand gedacht hätten. So enthüllte sich unerwartet die enorme petitio principii; denn plötzlich zeigte sich das letzte Glied als den Anhaltspunkt, an welchem schon das erste hing, die Kette als Kreis; und der Materialist gliche dem Freiherrn von Münchhausen, der zu Pferde im Wasser schwimmend, mit den Beinen das Pferd, sich selbst aber an seinem nach Vorne übergeschlagenen Zopf in die Höhe zieht.*'

Seen from the materialistic viewpoint, the general problem of localization presents itself as one of the most puzzling aspects of the relationship between brain and consciousness. Disregarding the moot question of special localization restricted to certain regions of the cerebrum, it can be asserted that the neural activities indispensable for the arising of a state of consciousness occur within the brain. As regards external events, these cerebral processes represent, coded in a space-time pattern of neural discharges, with various sorts of modulation and intensity-frequency translations, a complex and highly distorted transposition. Optic, tactile, auditory, gustatory and olfactory consciousness modalities, however, become localized outside the brain and to a great extent also outside the body, displaying the phantasmagory of the material world, not unlike the phenomenon of a phantom limb. Such modalities may even arise as pseudosensory percepts without their adequate sensory stimuli, as in hallucinations, dreams, electrical stimulation of cortex or in the case of the just cited phantom limb.

The most spectacular puzzle of external localization is provided by the visual percepts, although, because of its familiar, commonplace occurrence, it is generally taken for granted and not questioned as an incomprehensible 'miracle' (cf. fig. 29 on p. 211 of vol. 2).

Yet, the classical Greeks, who were somewhat familiar with the anatomy of the eye, but where unable to understand its function, attempted to explain the phenomenon of vision [cf. *Polyak*, 1957]. *Demokritos* and *Epikur* believed that all objects continuously send forth images of themselves into the surrounding air. Reaching the eye, these images 'caused objects to be perceived'.[131] An opposite 'emanation theory' was proposed by *Pythagoras* and accepted by *Euclid* as well as others. According to this view, 'visual rays', emerging from the eye, spread out in the form of a cone. When these rays touched the object, the visual act was consummated in a manner similar to a blind person finding his way about with the help of a walking stick [*Polyak*, 1957]. *Plato* combined both theories of impression and of emanation by assuming that the rays of 'inner lights', issuing from the pupil, united with the rays of 'outer light' originating from a source of light, such as the sun, and reflected by the observed objects.

This hypothesis, particularly elaborated in *Plato's Timaeus* (p. 100–102, *Loeb* edition), attempted to explain why, if some sort of 'light' flowed outward from the light-bearing eyes (φωσφόρα συνετεκτήναντο ὄμματα), objects could not be seen in the dark (when the kindred fire vanishes into night: ἀπελθόντος δὲ εἰς νύκτα τοῦ συγγενοῦς πυρός).

Knowledge of light refraction was lacking during the classical period, although *Euclid, Archimedes* and others had already an understanding of catoptrics (reflection). However, some elementary empirical data of dioptrics related to the property of lenses became available for practical use.

In more recent times, the general problem of externalization has been discussed by many authors; paraphrasing the formulation of *Condillac*, it may be worded as follows: If one admits that sensations are 'caused' by or 'correspond' to neural processes, how does it come about that they appear as objects independent of, and external to the brain? The assumed outward projection of inner 'representation' was also termed 'introjection' by *Avenarius* [1888] who rejected the theory and attempted to substitute his own theory of 'pure experience' which, discounting its artificial ad hoc categories, excessive complexity and verbal acrobatics, includes some fundamental principles of the idealistic approach.

If the materialistic concept of a physical space-time is maintained, an alternative to externalization would be the awkward supposition of a small-scale perceptual space-time manifold, 'located' within the brain and modelled after the large-scale physical space-time of the universe. The world system of a conscious being could thus be likened to a minuscule encapsulated box containing a perceptual space-time model which reproduces to a certain degree features of a gigantic surrounding and pervading physical space-time system. This bizarre notion involves formidable topologic difficulties and would still not help to indicate how consciousness, that is to say a perceptual space-time manifold, could be derived from the entirely different encoded signals of the neural processes, In this respect the following pertinent if

---

[131] *Aristotle* assumed, in this respect, an 'immaterial mediator' by means of which viewed objects affected the eyes.

temperamental comment by *Schopenhauer* [1847, 1851] might well be quoted: '*Man muß von allen Göttern verlassen seyn, um zu wähnen, daß die anschauliche Welt da draußen, wie sie den Raum in seinen drei Dimensionen füllt, im unerbittlich strengen Gange der Zeit sich fortbewegt, bei jedem Schritte durch das ausnahmslose Gesetz der Kausalität geregelt wird*' ... '*daß eine solche Welt da draußen wirklich ganz objektiv-real und ohne unser Zuthun vorhanden wäre, dann aber, durch die bloße Sinnesempfindung, in unseren Kopf hineingelangte, woselbst sie nun, wie da draußen, noch einmal dastände*'.

'*Daß der unendliche Raum unabhängig von uns, also absolut objektiv und an sich selbst vorhanden wäre, und ein bloßes Abbild desselben, als eines Unendlichen durch die Augen in unsern Kopf gelangte, ist der absurdeste aller Gedanken, aber in einem gewissen Sinne der fruchtbarste; weil, wer der Absurdität desselben deutlich inne wird, eben damit das bloße Erscheinungsdasein dieser Welt unmittelbar erkennt, indem er sie als ein bloßes Gehirnphänomen auffaßt, ...*'

It is, of course, possible to avoid some of these difficulties by assuming that the four dimensions of perceptual space-time are not the four dimensions of fictional physical space-time; this supposition, accordingly, implies that phenomena of consciousness involve four public and four private dimensions. The problem of externalization would thus become meaningless, although substituted by the somewhat awkward problem of spatial and temporal correlation between two intrinsically different space-time systems, which have no dimension in common. The possibilities of this formulation will be surveyed in vol. 2 in the discussion of postulational psychophysical parallelism.

If, on the other hand, we assume that the only actual space-time is perceptual, and thus that apart from consciousness space-time does not exist, then we may state, without prejudice to the central role assumed by the brain, that consciousness is not localized in the brain, but that the body including the brain and the external world become localized in consciousness [*K.*, 1927]. This viewpoint, denying the existence of the physical world postulated by materialists, is reached through the idealistic approach, which, following a discussion of the brain paradox (section 6) and of the principle of sufficient reason (section 7) shall then be separately considered in chapter III.

6. The Brain Paradox

The term '*paradox*' is somewhat ambiguous. *De Morgan* (1806–1871), a pioneer in the development of modern logic gave the following definition in his *Budget of Paradoxes* [1954]: 'A paradox is something which is apart from general opinion, either in subject-matter, method, or conclusion.' He also quotes an older definition stating that 'a paradox is a thing which seemeth strange and absurd, and is contrary to common opinion'. We may designate this as a *paradox in the first sense*.

More recent writers [e.g. *Kempner*, 1959] define a true paradox as a chain of flawless reasoning which leads to a result known to be impossible and not true. In medieval scholastics such paradoxes were called *insolubilia*. *Hoyle* [1975a] more correctly stated that a true paradox arises when two different but *seemingly* correct arguments lead to contradictory conclusions. We may designate this as a *paradox in the second sense*. *Hoyle's* inclusion of '*seemingly*' is important, since all logical paradoxes may be solved by pertinent logical analysis, although there obtains no agreement among logicians (e.g. *Russell, Zermelo, Burali-Forti* and others) as to a generalized theory dealing with the flaws in the arguments leading to paradoxes in the second sense.

With regard to the well-known mathematical paradoxes of infinity, as e.g. discussed in §22, p. 89f. of the present author's monograph *Mind and Matter* [*K.*, 1961], the flaws in their argumentation have been concisely pointed out by *Poincaré* [1913a]: there is no actual (given complete or total) infinity. The *Cantorians, Bertrand Russell*, and others have forgotten this, and they have fallen into contradictions. *Russell's* definition of infinity: 'a collection of terms is infinite when it contains as parts other collections, which have just as many terms' includes the obvious flaw of using the concept 'as many terms', since 'as many', which is applicable to a totality of undefined finite numbers, remains entirely meaningless with respect to a sequence intrinsically lacking 'totality'.

A paradox in the first sense is the well-known so-called 'clock paradox' inferred from *Einstein's* relativity theories. We have here the clock time (a) of a non-accelerated particle, with the radiation supplying the 'ticks' of the clock, i.e. the units of time measurement. However, the proper time (b) of an accelerated particle differs from the time (a) in accordance with *Einstein's* theories. While this may seem strange or unexpected, it appears to be an experimentally verified fact.

Among logical paradoxes in the second sense we have e.g. that of *Epimenides*, that of *Jourdain*, and the '*barber paradox*'. *Epimenides* the Cretan stated that all Cretans are liars, absolutely incapable of telling the truth. Is he thereby lying or telling the truth? It is evident that, if, *per impossibile*, heretofore all Cretans should have been absolute liars, than *Epimenides* would become the first Cretan telling a partial truth[132] in accordance with a three-valued logic assuming truth, partial truth (half-truth) and falsity.

In the paradox of *Jourdain*, a card shows on one side the statement: 'On the other side of this card is written a true statement.' On turning the card is found the inscription: 'On the other side of this card is written a false

---

[132] Namely that all Cretans except *Epimenides* are absolute liars.

statement.' Thus, if the statement on the front is true, that on the back of the card is true and that on the front becomes false, but if the statement on the front is false, the statement on the back must be false and hence the statement on the front must be true. Both statements, on front and back, by themselves, display no logical flaw.

Discounting the writing on both sides of a card as a mere shenanigan used in order to generate confusion, the alleged paradox can be reduced to the following concise formulation: the content of a statement (a) refers to another statement (b) as being true, but whose only content refers back to statement (a) as being false. This is merely a devious way of saying: the statement which I am herewith making is true but it is false, and this is my entire statement. In accordance with another sort of three-valued logic assuming truth, meaninglessness, and falsity we have here a meaningless statement.

As regards the *barber paradox* we have the *Barber of Seville* who shaves all those men of Seville and only those men of Seville who do not shave themselves. Thus, if the Barber shaves himself, then he does not shave himself; if he does not, then he does. Or: it is neither true nor false that the Barber shaves himself.

According to *Kershner and Wilcox* [1950] the flaw obtains because the Barber is defined in part, in terms of himself, and this supposed to be an inadmissible 'cyclic definition'; since the definition of the Barber involves the men of Seville of which he is one. But if the Barber is regarded not as a man of Seville, but some completely new creature introduced by this definition, the paradox disappears and the definition is admissible. In this case, he may shave himself or not, as he pleases, since the definition specifies his actions only with respect to the men of Seville, *of whom he is then not one.*

It can, however, be maintained that the paradox merely results from an inappropriate grammatical, or semantic formulation rather than from a 'cyclic definition' in terms of men of Seville, such definition being here quite permissible. The paradox therefore disappears in the following formulation: 'The Barber of Seville is one of the men of Seville, but the only man of Seville who shaves all those other men of Seville who do not shave themselves. All men of Seville including the Barber, may shave themselves or not shave themselves as they please.[133]

The Barber paradox is relevant with respect to the brain paradox if 'do not shave themselves' and 'shave themselves' are replaced by 'do not produce

---

[133] Another suitable formulation would be: The men of Seville, including the Barber, may shave themselves or not shave themselves as they please. However, only the Barber shaves those other men of Seville who do not shave themselves but wish to be shaved. The Barber is here defined in terms of the men of Seville. There is no logical error involved in the concept that men of Seville may have different attributes.

themselves' and 'produce themselves'.[134] Thus our world of consciousness is, in *Schopenhauer's* words a brain phenomenon, but the brain itself is a brain phenomenon.

The brain paradox (in the second i.e. logical sense), however, was not properly understood by *Schopenhauer*, yet it was nevertheless already clearly indicated by *Berkeley* [1713], although not explicitly designated as such, but outright dismissed by denying, in his second *Dialogue between Hylas and Philonous*, the empirically substantiated fact that mind (i.e. consciousness), as a dependent variable, is a function of the brain.

In the guise of *Philonous*, he argues as follows against *Hylas*, who had pointed out the 'origin' of 'ideas in the mind' by the brain.

Phil: The brain therefore you speak of being a sensible thing, exists only in the mind. Now, I would fain know whether you think it reasonable to suppose, that one idea or thing existing in the mind, occasions all other ideas. And if you think so, pray how do you account for the origin of that primary idea or brain itself?

Hyl: I do not explain the origin of our ideas by that brain which is perceivable to sense, this being itself only a combination of sensible ideas, but by another which I imagine.

Phil: But are not things imagined as truly in the mind as things perceived?

Hyl: I must confess they are.

Phil: It comes therefore to the same thing; and you have been all this while accounting for ideas, by certain motions or impressions in the brain, that is, by some alterations in an idea, whether sensible or imaginable, it matters not.

Hyl: I begin to suspect my hypothesis.

Phil: Beside spirits, all that we know or conceive are our own ideas. When therefore you say, all ideas are occasioned by impressions in the brain, do you conceive this brain or no? If you do, then talk of ideas imprinted in an idea, causing that idea, which is absurd. If you do not conceive it, you talk unintelligibly, instead of forming a reasonable hypothesis.

Hyl: I now clearly see it was a mere dream. There is nothing in it.

Phil: You need not be much concerned at it; for after all, this way of explaining things, as you called it, could never had satisfied any reasonable man. What connexion is there between a motion in the nerves, and the sensations of sound or colour in the mind? Or how is it possible these should be the effect of that?

In my '*Vorlesungen über das Zentralnervensystem der Wirbeltiere*' of 1927, I merely indicated my epistemologic viewpoint concerning the necessary postulate of a fictional physical brain in a few pertinent footnotes, of which the two following [*K.*, 1927, pp. 2, 315] can here be appropriately quoted:

'*Sowohl die Gedanken und Gefühle, also die innere Welt, geistige oder Geisteswelt des gewöhnlichen Sprachgebrauches wie die körperlich in Raum und Zeit ausgebreitete äußere (materielle) Welt sind Bewußtseinszustände*

---

[134] The quotation marks for 'produce' indicate the ambiguity of that term in the aspect here under consideration. *Berkeley*, as shown below in the text, uses the term 'occasions'. One could also use one of the connotations of 'manifests'. Still better, perhaps, at least in some respect, are the functional terms 'independent' and 'dependent' 'variable'.

(Vorstellung, Erscheinung). Das naturwissenschaftliche Weltbild mit seiner unabhängig von einem vorstellenden Bewußtsein vorhandenen objektiven, räumlichen, zeitlichen, kausalen Welt ist eine Fiktion. Aber nur mit Hilfe dieser Fiktion ist ein Verständnis der Erscheinungsreihen möglich.'

'Insbesondere ist es wichtig, sich zu vergegenwärtigen, daß die Wahrnehmungen oder Empfindungen (Bewußtseinsinhalte) nicht etwa in der Großhirnrinde oder überhaupt im Gehirn lokalisiert sind und zugleich wie durch einen Taschenspielertrick in die Außenwelt projiziert, d.h. exteriorialisiert werden. Umgekehrt wird erst der eigene Körper (und damit auch das Gehirn) sowie die sogenannte Außenwelt im Bewußtsein lokalisiert. Raum, Zeit und Kausalität (Kausalität-Materie-Wirken) sind Bewußtseinsattribute.'

Berkeley's argumentation, however, is of particular interest since, similarly to the formulation of the '*Barber paradox*' discussed by *Kershner and Wilcox* [1950], the brain is here conceived by *Hylas*, with respect to 'sensible things', i.e. 'matter', as not pertaining to this latter (cf. above *qua* Barber: 'of whom he is then not one').

Reverting now to *Schopenhauer*, the nearest approach to the brain paradox can be found in volume 2, pages 303–304 of his '*Welt als Wille und Vorstellung*'. This author stated that '*was erkennt*', or '*was Vorstellung hat, ist das Gehirn, welches jedoch sich selbst nicht erkennt, sondern nur als Intellekt, d.h. als Erkennendes, also nur subjektiv sich seiner bewusst wird.*'[135] '*Was von Innen gesehen das Erkenntnisvermögen ist, das ist, von aussen gesehen, das Gehirn. Dieses Gehirn ist ein Theil eben jenes Leibes, weil es selbst zur Objektivation des Willens gehört, nämlich das Erkennenwollen, seine Richtung auf die Aussenwelt in ihm objektiviert ist. Demnach ist allerdings das Gehirn, mithin der Intellekt, unmittelbar durch den Leib bedingt und dieser wiederum durch das Gehirn, – jedoch nur mittelbar, nämlich als Räumliches und Körperliches, in der Welt der Anschauung, nicht aber an sich selbst, d.h. als Wille. Das Ganze also ist zuerst der Wille, der sich selbst Vorstellung wird, und ist jene Einheit, die wir durch Ich ausdrücken. Das Gehirn selbst ist, sofern es vorgestellt wird, – also im Bewußtsein anderer Dinge – selbst nur Vorstellung.*'

---

[135] The brain, however, may quite evidently become 'conscious of itself' in Human consciousness, by a variety of percepts. First, as the head's content, by proprioception of its weight. Under unusual circumstances (cranial trauma) it could be touched by one's finger or seen in a mirror. It may also be indirectly perceived by looking at one's own EEG being recorded (etc.). The recording of the EEG, moreover, is one of the many instances belying the claim by *Bohr, Born, Frank, Heisenberg* and other physicists that it is impossible to observe under experimental conditions, arbitrarily isolated biologic systems without influencing the manipulated or non-manipulated significant variables, in the aspect under consideration to a degree which would invalidate the purpose of the investigation. Quite evidently, the recording of an EEG has an entirely negligible effect (if any) on the observed cortical events.

It cannot be said that *Schopenhauer's* argumentation, although partly valid, is entirely satisfactory, since it becomes vitiated by his main weakness, which is the reification of 'will' as '*Ding an sich*'.

E. Zeller (1814–1908), a professional philosopher of the *Hegelian* school, in his '*Geschichte der Deutschen Philosophie seit Leibniz*' (1873) criticized *Schopenhauer's* concept of the world as a brain phenomenon with the following comments: '*Der Philosoph konnte uns nicht genug einschärfen, in der ganzen objektiven Welt, und vor allem in der Materie, nichts anderes zu sehen als unsere Vorstellung. Jetzt ermahnt er uns ebenso dringend, unsere Vorstellung für nichts anderes zu halten als für ein Ereignis unseres Gehirns; und hieran wird dadurch nichts anderes geändert, dass dieses weiterhin eine bestimmte Form der Objektivation des Willens sein soll, denn wenn der Wille dieses Organ nicht hervorbrächte, könnte auch keine Vorstellung entstehen. Unser Gehirn ist aber diese bestimmte Materie, also nach Schopenhauer diese bestimmte Vorstellung. Wir befinden uns demnach in dem greifbaren Zirkel, dass die Vorstellung ein Produkt der Vorstellung sein soll.*'

A recent writer who has completely misunderstood the gist of the brain paradox as well as the 'nature' of consciousness (cf. above, section 5, p. 174), refers in a short comment on pages 184–185 of the *Schopenhauer Jahrbuch* 59 (1978) to *Zeller's* argumentation as the '*Zellersche Zirkel*'. It is evident that, as quoted by said writer, *Zeller* likewise failed to grasp the problem at issue. The alleged 'Zirkel' merely states the empirically substantiated fact that consciousness depends on the function of one of its contents, namely of the perceptual (or perceived) brain. While this may seem strange, it can hardly be contested and is, at most, like the 'clock paradox' a paradox in the first sense. In other words, although this is not explicable in terms of causality (*principium rationis sufficientis fiendi*) it remains an evident fact 'that one idea or thing existing in the mind, occasions all other ideas' (cf. above, p. 187).

As regards how to account for 'the origin of that primary idea or brain itself' we have the 'true' i.e. logical paradox in the second sense which is inherent in the fact that the brain itself is a brain phenomenon, or, in other words, that the brain 'produces' not only all phenomena of consciousness, but also itself. As a true paradox or paradox in the second sense, it becomes necessary to formulate the brain paradox in terms of the conventional 'Barber paradox' [*K.*, 1959]. This may be elaborated in the following fashion:

the *Barber of Seville* shaves all those men of Seville, and only those men of Seville who do not shave themselves. It is established that there are shaved men of Seville.

The *brain* which is functionally related to my consciousness-manifold produces, within the domain of that manifold, all those manifestations of consciousness and only those manifestations of consciousness which do not produce themselves. It is established that there are manifestations of my consciousness-manifold.

If there is a valid rule such that no man of Seville can shave himself nor be shaved unless shaved by the *Barber*, and ...

If there is an empirically established orderliness such that no manifestation of my consciousness-manifold can produce itself nor be produced unless produced by the *brain*, and ...

if the *Barber of Seville* shaves himself, which he does, whereby the validity of the rule is shown as not extending to the *Barber*, then, as the *Barber* shaving himself, he may be considered not to be one of the men of Seville. But as a person shaved by the *Barber of Seville*, he evidently may be considered a man of Seville.

if the *brain of my consciousness-manifold* produces itself as a manifestation of my consciousness, which it can do or does under certain circumstances, whereby the validity of the orderliness is shown as not extending to the brain, then the *brain* which does so produce itself as a manifestation may be considered not a manifestation of, i.e. a part of, my consciousness-manifold. But the *brain* which is so produced as a manifestation evidently is a part of my consciousness-manifold.

This particular status of the brain as being both a manifestation of consciousness *and* not a manifestation of consciousness differs from all other manifestations of consciousness which do not produce themselves. Said status was recognized by *Berkeley* in the guise of *Hylas*, but rejected by *Berkeley* in the guise of *Philonous*. Yet, although all phenomena of consciousness including the brain,[136] must be considered manifestations of the extramental orderliness x ('*Ding an sich*' *Kant*) the special status of that orderliness as manifested by the perceptual brain is evident: it manifests itself *and* all other consciousness phenomena. However, since, *qua* aspect of the orderliness x ('*Ding an sich*') the brain cannot have spatio-temporal qualities (characteristics, or structure), the 'extramental brain' remains an entirely unintelligible 'inexplicable something' in *Hume's* sense (cf. above, section 5, p. 166). This is, of course, the implicit (but not explicit) reason why *Berkeley* (*Philonous*) could not admit the non-perceived but imagined brain suggested by *Hylas*.

In contradistinction to the Barber paradox whose apparent contradiction is easily solvable, since it stays entirely in the domain of actuality, the brain paradox remains intrinsically insolvable. It postulates an imagined brain not in the domain of consciousness, but in an extramental public physical space-time system. However, since the extramental 'world' must be assumed as devoid of material or space-time characteristics, such imagined brain cannot exist. The only 'existing' brain is the actual, perceptual brain located in

---

[136] Thus *Schopenhauer*, [vol. 5, p. 319] repeats: '*An sich selbst und ausserhalb der Vorstellung ist auch das Gehirn, wie alles andere, "Wille".*' Discounting the term '*Wille*', *Schopenhauer's* remark justly states that the brain is '*Ding an sich*', i.e. an incomprehensible aspect of the 'orderliness x'.

consciousness, this brain being, in *Berkeley's* sense merely an 'idea' (i.e. a percept).

The brain paradox, by transcending from the domain of actuality (consciousness) into the extramental domain of the orderliness x therefore represents a proof demonstrating that the problem of brain-consciousness relationship is theoretically (i.e. intrinsically) insolvable. It shares this insolvability with the problem of reality (in the first sense: a thing is real if it persists or exists when it is neither perceived by senses nor by thoughts). Yet, we can find an operationally useful fictional solution of these two fundamental epistemic problems by postulating a fictional public physical space-time system (as taken for granted in natural sciences). The brain paradox can thus be 'economically' dodged, if we distinguish a given perceptual brain, which is part of the private perceptual space-time system under consideration, and a fictional physical brain, which is part of the fictional public physical space-time system. This dodge implies the fiction of postulational psychophysical parallelism which shall be taken up further below in chapter IV of volume 2.

Since the brain paradox is of particular importance for a proper understanding of the brain-consciousness problem, it seems here appropriate, at the risk of appearing repetitious, to elaborate once more upon the definition of consciousness as a private perceptual space-time system. This definition can also be re-worded as follows: consciousness is a *private transitory state* correlated with some brain activities in a Human or in this respect comparable Animal being.

By '*private*' is here meant that the occurrence of this state is exclusively experienced by the possessor of a given particular active brain, and cannot be detected either by the sense organs of another Human or Animal being, or by recording instruments. Its occurrence as a state experienced by 'other' Humans or Animals can merely be reasonably and formally inferred by 'analogy' on the basis of observed behavior, or may be 'imagined' on the basis of 'informal', ('sphairal') thought processes in everyday life. Children and Primitives may even imagine 'consciousness' (i.e. 'psyche' or 'soul') to be 'present' in plants (devoid of a nervous system) as well as 'in' non-living 'objects'.

By *transitory* is here meant that consciousness originates from 'non-consciousness' ('unconsciousness', whatever that may be) at some stage of ontogenetic brain development, becomes interrupted by periods of 'non-consciousness' and finally, ends in permanent 'non-consciousness' when the brain completely ceases to function. 'Non-consciousness' can reasonably be equated with 'nothing' or 'nothingness' (German: '*Nichts*').

By 'state' is here meant the occurrence of 'events', designated as percepts. These 'events' represent a 'manifold' or 'set' (German: '*eine Menge*'), and are characterized (1) by private space-time relationships, i.e. occurring 'here and now', and (2) by displaying orderly interrelations (i.e. interrelations characterized by 'invariants'), that can be described as different aspects of the principle of sufficient reason. Such orderly interrelations characterize the manifold of consciousness, represented by its contents, as what may be called a 'system'.

This structural definition of 'consciousness' involves a *petitio principii* insofar as it presupposes the 'consciousness' of the definer and the 'consciousness' of the hearer or reader capable and presumed to 'understand' the definition.

The abstract concepts ('ideas') 'space' and 'time', respectively 'space-time' represent 'invariants' displayed by the localization and by the succession (sequence) of actual percepts and, as *Berkeley* and *Hume* justly pointed out, do not refer to anything having independent actual 'existence'. In this respect they are indeed, in *Vaihinger's* sense, 'fictions', comparable to the abstract concepts 'triangle' or 'animal'. This, of course, also applies to the abstract concept 'consciousness'.

7. The Principle of Sufficient Reason

Despite its unavoidable deficiencies and its additional emotional distortions, Human thought has undeniably considerable operational capabilities. The most generalized of the functional rules inherent in our thinking processes seems to be manifested by the principle of sufficient reason: *Nihil est sine ratione cur potius sit quam non sit.* It must be considered a necessary axiom or postulate, incapable of being proved since it represents the basis of proof.[137] Some other generalized principles have been pointed out as (1) *homogeneity* (*entia praeter necessitatem non esse multiplicanda, Occam's* or *Ockham's Razor*, not explicitly formulated by *Occam* but implied in his teachings); (2) *specification* (*entium varietates non temere esse minuendas*);[138] (3) *continuity* (*datur continuum formarum*).[139]

In addition there are certain postulates which *Schopenhauer* has called *'metalogical truths'*. These are (1) the principle of identity, such that a concept (notion, *Begriff, Subject*) equals the sum of its predicates, i.e. a = a; (2) a

---

[137] Any attempt to prove this principle leads to the *circulus vitiosus* of requiring a proof for the requirement of a proof.

[138] This could appropriately be invoked against monistic views.

[139] *Bertrand Russell* criticized the general concept of continuity as a vague word convenient for philosophers who wish to introduce metaphysical muddles, but permissible only in precise and specific definitions as used in mathematics and physics. *Poincaré*, however, regards the philosophical concept of continuity as an expression of the principle of sufficient reason. Despite its vagueness, he states that *'la croyance de la continuité'* ... *'serait difficile de justifier par un raisonnement apodictique, mais sans laquelle toute science serait impossible'* [*Poincaré*, 1913b].

predicate cannot be both attributed and not attributed to a subject or concept, i.e. a $\sim -a$; (3) the principle of excluded middle, which states that of each two exhaustive and exclusive contradictory predicates, only one can be attributed to a subject (*tertium non datur*, excluded disjunction), i.e. a $+$ b; (4) truth is the relationship of a proposition to something distinct from it, this being its reason (*Wahrheit ist die Beziehung eines Urteils auf etwas von ihm verschiedenes, das sein Grund genannt wird*).[140] One must distinguish between logical and mathematical truth on one hand, that is conformity to formal rules accepted as certain, and empirical truth on the other hand, that is conformity with verifiable sensory experience (facts). Truth may be clearly two-valued, being either true (1) or not true (0). There are, however, in a three-valued logic, true, false and non-verifiable, i.e. problematic propositions. One may also distinguish true, false, and meaningless propositions. Again, many-valued logics involve innumerable truth values between the limiting value of complete significant conformity ('absolute truth') and that of complete error, fallacy, or falsity.

With regard to certainty, one could define certain as that what cannot be doubted, or in other words that what is such as it is. Nothing then is certain except the experienced phenomena of consciousness, namely sensory percepts, thoughts (*qua* occurring thoughts), memories (*qua* occurring memories), emotional feelings, and all these are certain while and only while being experienced. One might then say that nothing is certain except what is actual. The notions of truth, certainty, validity, correctness seem to overlap, and axioms are frequently called 'truths', although, in the strict sense by the above given definition of truth they are not. This overlap is related to the intrinsic vagueness, fuzziness and ambiguity of the meaning of words and other symbols or of language in general.

Reverting now to the principle of sufficient reason, it seems appropriate to consider its first systematic elaboration as propounded by *Aristotle*, who formulated the essential postulates for scientific procedure. He pointed out that we must begin with the given phenomena, which are to be described in

---

[140] It will be seen that according to this definition of truth, as formulated by *Schopenhauer*, axioms or postulates, even if certain, do not represent truths, since they are propositions not related to or depending on, another proposition representing their reason. Except for axioms, all other propositions *can* be true if proved by their reason. A concept or notion can be *correct* or *valid* if it subsumes qualifications under an abstraction or class according to the accepted formal rules. An object can be *real in the second sense* if it can be verified to have correlations in conformity with that which experience has led us to expect. Similarly, a given sensory percept can be correct or valid, if it corresponds to otherwise verifiable features of that what we postulate to be perceived. Obviously, these verifications will, in the end, depend on other sensory percepts or on reasoning about these percepts or both. A *relationship* can be *evident* if it clearly conforms to either propositions accepted as true, or to accepted axioms. An axiom can be a proposition regarded as directly or immediately (*unmittelbar*) certain.

suitable terms, and then go on to an elucidation of what he called the 'causes' (αἰτίαι). In doing so, he referred the phenomena to, or correlated them with, four sets of principles (αἰτίαι, ἀρχαί) which he designated as

(1) The material 'cause' or 'matter' out of which the 'thing' is made or of which the phenomena are a manifestation.

(2) The formal 'cause' or form which characterizes the phenomena.

(3) The efficient or motive 'cause' which is involved in the sequence of a material (physical) process or event.

(4) The final 'cause' which represents the 'end' or *rational* purpose of a phenomenon, process or event.

Only the third of *Aristotle's* principles corresponds to a cause in the strict sense, as further analyzed by *Hume* and subsequently by *Schopenhauer*. Until then, the relation of cause and effect had been generally confused with that of ground and consequent in logic (e.g. '*causa sive ratio*).

In his famed doctoral dissertation [1813, revised second edition 1847], *Schopenhauer* designated *Aristotle's* ἀρχαί collectively as 'the principle of sufficient reason' and distinguished four applications of that principle. Although mentioned above in section 2, page 82, they should here be repeated in view of their importance:

(1) To material (physical) changing events as *causality* (*principium rationis sufficientis fiendi*).

(2) To logical processes as ground of knowledge or *reason* (*principium rationis sufficientis cognoscendi*).

(3) To formal space-time relationships as arithmetical, geometrical, and topologic orderliness (*principium rationis sufficientis essendi*).

(4) To conscious activities as motivation (*principium rationis sufficientis agendi*).

Thus, if compared with *Aristotle's* principles, *Schopenhauer's* first application corresponds to the efficient cause, *Schopenhauer's* second and third application can be matched with the 'formal cause', and *Schopenhauer's* fourth application corresponds to the 'final cause'. *Aristotle's* 'material cause' was not accepted by *Schopenhauer*. I believe, however, that *Aristotle's* concept is valid, and I have included it in my own formulation of the principle of sufficient reason [*K*., 1961]. On the other hand, *Schopenhauer* expounds in his second and third applications two different aspects not clearly distinguished or separated in *Aristotle's* concept of formal 'causes'.

Schopenhauer justly considered the principle of sufficient reason as the principle of (a) all explanations, (b) of every and all necessity, and (c) of all relations.[141]

---

[141] *Das Prinzip aller Erklärung* [vol. 1, p. 129]; *das Prinzip aller Notwendigkeit* [vol. 2, p. 623]; *am Leitfaden des Satzes vom Grunde*, '*diesem Element der Relationen*' [vol. 5, p. 442].

My own concept of the principle of sufficient reason is based, with further elaborations, on what I consider to be the valid aspects of *Aristotle's* and *Schopenhauer's* formulations. It includes, however, the following 10 applications.

(1) In agreement with *Aristotle's* material 'causes', and in contradistinction to *Schopenhauer*, I believe that any phenomenon of consciousness must be the manifestation of some 'form', modality or 'substratum' of consciousness. This may be a sensory, an extrasensory, or a pseudosensory percept. A sensory one is manifested by diverse sorts of 'matter' (mass), or 'force', or of 'energy', e.g. a piece of solid metal, a feeling of pressure, a visual impression, a sound, etc. Extrasensory percepts are manifested by (a) thoughts, and (b) by emotions, which latter are superimposed upon either sensory percepts or thoughts, while thoughts, in turn are 'superimposed' upon other sorts of percepts. Pseudosensory percepts are hallucinations or dream percepts imitating true (or 'normal') sensory percepts, moreover eidetic imagery. These latter, pointed out by *Jaensch* [1930] are 'internal' images, usual visual, which may display the vividity and spatial configuration of actual sense impression, and occur in the waking state. Eidetic images differ from hallucinations. In contradistinction to the latter, they are clearly recognized as subjective, and may even be 'voluntarily' produced by those experiencing the images. Eidetic images occur more frequently in children and much less commonly in adults.

There are, moreover, very dim and vague images or pseudosensory percepts accompanying thoughts, which could be interpreted as blurred or abortive eidetic images, and may likewise to some extent be voluntary produced. Their obtains thus a blurred zone of transition between extrasensory thought percepts and pseudosensory percepts. It is of interest that *Hume* considered 'ideas' (i.e. here thoughts or extrasensory percepts) to be faint images or memory copies of sense impressions.

This application which refers to the occurrence of a phenomenon as such, for which a necessary 'substratum' ('physical' or 'mental' *sensu strictiori*, i.e. sensory, extrasensory or pseudosensory) must obtain, may be designated as the *principium rationis sufficientis apparendi* [*K.*, 1961, 1967a].

(2) In agreement with both *Aristotle* and *Schopenhauer*, the *principium rationis sufficientis fiendi* applies to changing material ('physical') events as causality (*Aristotle's* efficient cause). Any change is here a cause in the strict sense, involving an effect. Since, because of its importance, causality was separately considered *in extenso* (section 2 of the present chapter II), no further comments are here necessary.

(3) In agreement with *Schopenhauer*, *the principium rationis sufficientis essendi* refers to formal space-time relationship as geometrical, topological and arithmetical orderliness. It should be emphasized that these relationships represent significant parameters (*Zustandsbedingungen*) in all these causal

events pertaining to application 2. Thus, in *Schopenhauer's* discussion of a causal event in which an inflammable object is ignited by means of a concave mirror reflecting the sunlight, said causal event depends on numerous parameters such as relative position of sun, mirror, and object, moreover presence of oxygen, chemical composition of object, etc. which all pertain to application 2 and also to 3. Since chemical composition depends on molecular and atomic patterns, i.e. space-time relationships of particles respectively quanta thereby involved, there is an evident relationship to application 2.

Again, since geometrical, arithmetical (algebraic), and topologic orderliness can also be expressed in very abstract logical terms pertaining to the next application (4) we have an evident overlap with this latter, as shall again be pointed out further below.

The *p.r.s. essendi*, moreover, involves *kinetics*, in contradistinction to the *p.r.s. fiendi*, which involves *dynamics* (namely 'force' or 'energy'). It is here of interest that *Hoyle* [1975a] in his text of astronomy and cosmology elaborates on the history of the heliocentric system, but finally concludes [p. 7] that, in describing their relative motion, 'it makes no difference whether we consider the Earth to move around the Sun, or the Sun to move around the Earth'. He then adds that 'according to the physical theory developed by *Einstein* the two concepts must be regarded as entirely equivalent'. *Hoyle* fails here, however, to point out that this is only true in a very restrict kinematic sense, but absurd not only from a viewpoint of dynamics, but also with respect to *Einstein's* theories, since it would involve velocities of rotation for the universe of stars and galaxies around the earth utterly incompatible with *Einstein's* own concept of the constant c.

(4) In agreement with *Schopenhauer*, the *principium rationis sufficientis cognoscendi* refers to logical processes as ground of knowledge or *reason* (*sensu stricto*). Logic involves concepts (*Begriffe*), which represent abstractions, moreover propositions (*Urteile*) which are statements, and syllogisms (*Schlüsse*) which are conclusions based on at least two statements.

Of special importance are the logical particles or logical connectives, such as: and, or (or else; or, but not both), not, if – then, if and only if – then, except, unless, and various others, which play a substantial role in the *Boolean algebra* and the logistic systems mentioned below.[142]

---

[142] *Schopenhauer* [vol. 2, p. 123] particularly stressed the significance of the logical particles, which express the formal aspects of thought (*die das Formelle der Denkweise ausdrücken*). He mentioned, among others: '*denn, weil, warum, darum, also, da, obgleich, zwar, wenn – so, entweder – oder*'.

As regards notion (concepts, *Begriffe*), *Schopenhauer* [vol. 3, p. 20] stated that a '*Begriff enthält implicite alle seine wesentlichen Prädikate, die sich durch analytische Urteile aus ihm entwickeln lassen – die Summe dieser ist seine Definition*'.

Classical formal logic, systematized by *Aristotle* and the medieval *Scholastics*, and, as it were, culminating in Kant's critical analysis, doubtless contains many rules of permanent value. Yet, it contains a number of formal defects, which modern mathematical logicians have analyzed. Since the work of *Boole* [1854] it has been supplemented by mathematical logic or 'logistic', which also has its defects, as pointed out by *Poincaré* [1913a]. Mathematical logicians kept on 'inventing increasingly heavier and stiffer brands of logic, which others keep on tearing to pieces' [*Singh*, 1959]. Instead of two-valued logics, based on 'true' versus 'false', respectively the principle of excluded middle, several systems of three-valued and many-valued logic have been proposed.

Again, since concepts pertaining to the *p.r.s. essendi* (3) can be handled in abstract logical terms, some mathematicians have reduced mathematics to a purely logical discipline. *Poincaré* [1913a] however, rejected the identification of mathematics and logic. This latter author's view seems justified, insofar as mathematics can be said to involve an enactment of concepts pertaining to principle 3 in abstract and purely logical terms. In other words, although mathematics are more than pure logic, principles 3 and 4 overlap.

As regards the significance of reason i.e. of the *p.r.s. cognoscendi* (or 'logic'), *Hume* [1740] justly stressed that 'reason is the discovery of truth or falsehood. Truth or falsehood consist in an agreement or disagreement either to the real relations of ideas, or to real existence or matter of fact. Whatever therefore is not susceptible of this agreement or disagreement is incapable of being true or false, and can never be an object of our reason.'

With respect to the diverse aspects of reason, *Schopenhauer* pointed out that faulty reasoning results more commonly from inadequate notions (concepts, *Begriffe*) and from inadequate propositions (*Urteile*) than from the faulty application of syllogisms which he regards as being of limited value. Moreover, valid arguments need not be in the canonical forms of syllogisms. Thus, 'A is older than B, B is older than C, therefore A is older than C' is not a syllogism, since its two premises contain four terms, B being once in the place of a middle term, and once representing the minor term. It will be recalled that in a canonical syllogism there are two propositions called premisses, followed by a conclusion. The first premise, or *propositio maior* contains the major term P and the middle term M. The second premise or *propositio minor* contains the minor term S and the middle term M. In the conclusion, the subject is the minor term, and the predicate is the major term as shown in the three canonical *Aristotelian* syllogisms.

1. M – P	2. P – M	3. M – P
S – M	S – M	M – S
S – P	S – P	S – P

The validity of a syllogism depends on the nature of the propositions used as premises. These propositions are classified according to (a) quantity (universal, particular, singular, i.e. all, some, this), (b) quality (affirmative, negative, limitative), and (c) relation (categorical, hypothetical, disjunctive). Strictly speaking all syllogisms are tautologies, but may, however, by the resulting deductions and inferences, from general to particular, be helpful in formulating complex information that is not 'evident at first glance'. Induction, as e.g. stressed by *Francis Bacon* (1561–1626), on the other hand, represents inference from particular to general.

Reverting to the limitations of logic, it seems here appropriate to quote *Whitehead* [1948] who objects to 'the absurd trust in the adequacy of our knowledge' and emphasizes that there is not a sentence which adequately states its own meaning. In fact, he claims that 'there is not a sentence, or a word, with a meaning which is independent of the circumstances under which it is uttered'. He concludes that logic, 'conceived as an adequate analysis of the advance of thought, is a fake. It is a superb instrument, but it requires a background of common sense'. 'In practice exactness vanishes: the sole problem is, "does it work?" But the aim of practice can only be defined by the use of theory; so the question "Does it work?" is a reference to theory.'[143]

This limitation, of course, is related to the fact that *all* concepts (*Begriffe*), be they 'concrete' or 'abstract', by representing abstractions of invariants, do not entirely correspond to any given sensory or particular extrasensory experience. All concepts are thus, in this sense 'fictions'. This was pointed out by *Berkeley* who objected to the 'existence of abstract ideas'. *Berkeleys* view was supported by *Hume*, who considered it 'to be one of the greatest and most valuable discoveries that has been made of late years in the republic of letters'. According to *Berkeley* and *Hume*, all general ideas are nothing but particular ones annexed to a certain term, which gives them a more extensive signification. Both philosophers, however, do not seem to realize that 'particular ideas' are already abstractions respectively generalizations, from which the so-called abstract general ideas merely differ by a higher degree of abstraction (e.g. this frog – a frog – amphibian – vertebrate – animal – living being; or: this triangle – isosceles triangle – triangle – geometric figure – drawing).

---

[143] *Whitehead's* qualification of the value of logic as depending on a 'background of common sense' agrees with *Schopenhauer's* view, which I share, that epistemologic and, in general, philosophic considerations must be based on the 'concrete' data of sensory consciousness (i.e. on '*Anschauung*') and not on the empty (formal) abstractions of logic. Thus, the 'line of thoughts' provided by the systems of *Hegel, Bolzano, Frege, Russell, Wittgenstein, Reichenbach, Carnap*, leading to an empty formalism, can hardly be considered to represent a progress in philosophy since the beginning of the 19th century (i.e. in the *post-Kantian* period). In my opinion, the progress, since the 17th century is represented by the line *Locke, Berkeley, Hume, Kant, Schopenhauer, Vaihinger*.

Vaihinger likewise considers abstractions to be fictions. *Berkeley*, however, does not remain consistent, since he admits the 'idea' or, as he then preferably states, the 'notion' of 'spirit', 'soul', and 'God', all of which are highly 'abstract'. Thus, according to *Berkeley*, the existence of God is more evident than that of man.

As an aside, an amusing, although quite erroneous criticism of logical subtility expressed by *Montaigne* (1533–1592) may here be quoted. Said author [1595], in his posthumous '*Essais*' stated: '*Voire mais, que fera-t-il si on le presse de la subtilité sophistique de quelque syllogisme? "Le jambon faict boire; le boire désaltère; parquoi le jambon désaltère." Qu'il s'en mocque*' (Livre 1, chapitre XXV).

Quite evidently, *Montaigne's* argument does not represent a syllogism (cf. above, p. 197), since '*boire*' is not used as a canonical *terminus medius*. The argument, moreover, is also invalid by orthodox logical rules since the propositions are not universal but particular. The semantic formulation is, furthermore, incomplete. Properly stated: eating salted ham may motivate drinking; drinking may quench thirst; therefore the eating of ham may (i.e. *some* time) be followed by the quenching of thirst.[144]

Another quip at formal logic is contained in the well-known verses of *Goethe's Faust* (Part I) in which *Mephisto* addresses the young student seeking advice:

Mein theurer Freund, ich rat Euch drum
Zuerst Collegium Logicum.
Da wird der Geist Euch wohl dressiert,
In spanische Stiefeln eingeschnürt,
Dass er bedächtiger so fortan
Hinschleiche die Gedankenbahn
Und nicht etwa, die Kreuz und Quer,
Irrlichterliere hin und her.
. . .
. . .
Zwar ist's mit der Gedankenfabrik
Wie mit einem Weber-Meisterstück,
Wo ein Tritt tausend Fäden regt,
Die Schifflein herüber hinüberschiessen,

Die Fäden ungesehen fliessen,
Ein Schlag tausend Verbindungen schlägt.
Der Philosoph, der tritt herein
Und beweist Euch, es müsst' so sein:
Das Erst' wär' so, das Zweite so
Und drum das Dritt' und Vierte so,
Und wenn das Erst' und Zweit' nicht wär'.
Das Dritt' und Viert' wär nimmermehr.
Das preisen die Schüler allerorten,
Sind aber keine Weber geworden.
Wer will was Lebendig's erkennen und beschreiben,
Sucht erst den Geist herauszutreiben,
Dann hat er die Teile in Seiner Hand,
Fehlt leider! nur das geistige Band.

Finally it should be added that the rules of logic may become greatly modified under the influence of emotion, thereby resulting in 'dereistic' or 'hypobulic' [*Kretschmer*, 1926] thinking, as e.g. in schizophrenic logic. Hypobulic logic leads, of course, to propositions, conclusions, and inferences

---

[144] Thus, in the Munich beer halls, as I remember them from the period before and following World War I, plenty of salted pretzels were made freely available in order to motivate the drinking of plenty beer.

which are false by the standards of 'normal' logic. The significance of emotion respectively affectivity will be considered further below (p. 200) in the 6th application of the principle of sufficient reason.

(5) In addition to the logical processes pertaining to the *p.r.s. cognoscendi*, involving concepts, propositions, and syllogisms, it seems appropriate to distinguish a *principium rationis sufficientis comparationis* referring to processes of comparison between events or configurations. All phenomena are interrelated or correlated, that is to say stand in an orderly togetherness whereby continuous identity (sameness), characterized as 'itself', of a single phenomenon, identity or 'sameness' of two or more other phenomena ('itself' versus 'another'), similarity, conformity, dissimilarity, and diversity can be conceived and expressed by thought. The *p.r.s. comparationis* involves topologic mapping and the diverse sorts of transformations such as identical transformations, one-one, one-many, and many-one transformations, as well as the closed and open transformations discussed by *Ashby* [1957] and by myself [*K.*, 1961, 1967a, 1973a, 1978].

Although comparison also obtains within the *p.r.s. cognoscendi*, where e.g. syllogisms involve a *tertium comparationis*, it is perhaps appropriate to distinguish a separate *p.r.s. comparationis*, which, as it were, overlaps with other aspects (e.g. *cognoscendi* and *essendi*) of the principle of sufficient reason.

(6) *Affectivity*, a term overlapping with the term emotion, can be defined, in the aspect under consideration, as a (private) consciousness-modality (*qualité pure* in *Poincaré's* terminology) represented by axiologic valuations; e.g. pleasant, indifferent, unpleasant; good, indifferent, bad (evil). One of the best definitions is given by *Kretschmer* [1926]: '*Die Affektivität* ... '*umfasst alles, was die seelischen Vorgänge auf ihrem Wege vom einfachen Sinneseindruck und Bild über abstrakte Vorstellungen und Überlegungen bis zum Entschluss und zum motorischen Impuls an Gefühlstönen, d.h. an Wertungen für das Ich mitbekommen, und die Antriebe, die davon ausgehen.*'

Affectivity thus includes the feelings of pleasantness and unpleasantness, of pain and pleasurableness including voluptuousness, of irritation (disturbance, emotion *sensu stricto* of some psychologists) or indifference, moreover, complex feelings such as anger, fury, anxiety, fear, terror, hate, desire, will,[145]

---

[145] 'Will' is indeed a very vague term, which may subsume all manifestations of affectivity. As is well known, *Schopenhauer* considered 'Will' to be *Kant's* '*Ding an sich*'. The two main reasons for rejecting this interpretation by *Schopenhauer* are: (1) 'Will' is very definitely a manifestation of consciousness (i.e. '*Vorstellung*'). (2) Although 'will' may be a characteristic aspect of conscious intended ('voluntary') or purposeful action, it does not seem justified to equate 'will' with active phenomena of action displayed by activities which must be considered devoid of consciousness (e.g. unconscious nervous activity, activities of plants or organisms without central nervous system, and physico-chemical interactions).

love, like or dislike, and others, as well as axiologic valuation such as good, bad, or evil, morality and immorality. Feelings and affects *sensu stricto* are regarded as circumscribed processes of usually limited duration, moods as generalized conditions of usually longer duration and temperaments as the more stable overall affective pattern characteristics of an individual.

Since it is appropriate to distinguish between (a) the affective tone of the passive aspect of consciousness, that is to say of *Kretschmer's Abbildungsvorgänge* which include 'cognition', and (b) the active aspect, which is represented by motivated 'voluntary' action (*Kretschmer's Ausdrucksvorgänge*), the orderliness obtaining in the determination of the affective tone manifested in passive consciousness phenomena can be designated as *the principium rationis sufficientis affectivitatis.*

Hume [1740] justly stressed that the orderliness (or the 'rules') of affectivity are not conclusions of our reason, which merely deals with 'facts' and with the 'discovery of truth of falsehood'. It is evident that our passions or affective tones are not susceptible to such agreements or disagreements as provided by reason. 'It is impossible, therefore, they can be pronounced either true or false, and be either contrary or conformable to reason' [*Hume*, 1740].

It is of particular interest that the eminent statesman *Otto Fürst von Bismarck* (1815–1898) in volume II on page 155 of his '*Gedanken und Erinnerungen*' expresses a view in full agreement with *Hume's* analysis. *Bismarck* stated: '... *dass in der Politik und in der Religion keiner dem Andersgläubigen die Richtigkeit der eigenen Überzeugung, des eigenen Glaubens concludent nachweisen kann, und dass kein Gerichtshof vorhanden ist, der die Meinungsverschiedenheiten durch Erkenntnis zur Ruhe verweisen könnte.*'

'*In der Politik wie auf dem Gebiete des religiösen Glaubens kann der Konservative dem Liberalen, der Gläubige dem Ungläubigen niemals ein anderes Argument entgegenhalten als das in tausend Variationen breitgetretene Thema: meine politischen Überzeugungen sind richtig und die deinigen sind falsch; mein Glaube ist Gott gefällig, dein Unglaube führt zur Verdammis.*' *Bismarck's* comment, of course, applies, *mutatis mutandis*, to all axiologic evaluations.

(7) *The principium rationis sufficientis agendi* applies with respect to the active aspect of consciousness, resulting in voluntary or intended, or respectively purposeful intentional or motivated output activities (*Handlungen*, behavior, *Kretschmer's Ausdrucksvorgänge*). The relevant 'reason' is here a *motive*, involving a manifestation of affectivity. Such manifestation can be very weak, as for instance in aimless but nevertheless intentional (voluntary) body motions, or very strong, as in sustained difficult and disagreeable purposeful activities. Again, under compulsion, which then represents a very strong motive, an action may be both 'voluntary' and against one's 'will'.

It may be recalled that *Schopenhauer* included 'motives' into his *p.r.s. fiendi*, and then restricted them to a particular aspect representing the *p.r.s. agendi* (cf. above, section 2, p. 82).

Motives, moreover, may be exceedingly potent, although not accompanied by very vivid tones of like or dislike, that particular aspect of affectivity remaining 'sphairal' in *Kretschmer's* terminology. Such motives, representing, as it were, protracted strong determination are, e.g. the 'driving factors' in purposeful abstract scientific activities manifested by productive mathematicians, other scientists, etc.

It should also be kept in mind that a 'decision' corresponds to the 'emotionally' selected result in voluntary action. *Reichenbach* [1938] has pointed out that the character of being true or false belongs to statements only, not to decisions. This is, of course, in full accordance with the views of *Hume*, who stresses that actions do not derive their merit from a conformity to reason, nor their blame from a contrariety to it. Actions may be laudable or blamable, but they cannot be reasonable or unreasonable. Yet, if decisions or actions are based on faulty or hyponoic reasoning, they can also be considered inappropriate (*unangemessen*) or erratic. *Kretschmer* used the term 'hypobulic' for such actions, based on hyponoic thinking or overwhelming emotion. In everyday parlance such actions are commonly said to be 'unreasonable'.

A 'motive', moreover, may be a parameter (*Zustandsbedingung*) which can be repressed or suppressed, or, if finally selected, result in a decision initiating action.

It is of particular importance that 'purpose', 'meaning', respectively 'final causes' apply only to the applications 6 and 7 of the *principium rationis sufficientis* which are restricted to conscious beings, possessors of a brain. Thus, there is no purposeness, purposefulness, nor 'meaning' in the phenomena of unconscious anorganic or organic (living) nature, nor can purpose or meaning be attributed to the extramental orderliness x. The universe must, accordingly, be considered a purposeless and meaningless phenomenon, resulting, by 'chance', in the purposeful activities of conscious organic beings acting on motives, or, in the case of intelligent beings such as man, in purposeful abstract thinking based on motivation respectively decisions and 'programmed' by affectivity. Human emotional thought, however, tends, erroneously, to expand 'purpose' and 'meaning' into the domain of 'purposelessness' and 'meaninglessness'.

(8) *The principium rationis sufficientis cogitandi* applies to the active aspect of thought-consciousness which does not result in purposeful output, but merely in 'intentional' or purposeful thinking. *Berkeley* referred to this by stating 'whatever power I may have over my own thoughts' .

In a Human consciousness-manifold, thoughts or 'associated' series of thoughts may or may not occur. *Schiller* justly stated:'

Doch wer wird immer auch denken!
Oft schon war ich und hab' wirklich an gar nichts gedacht!

One may evidently relax with a blank 'mind' *qua* thoughts (German: *hindösen*), which is at times, quite a pleasant 'mental' state. Thus, *Schopenhauer*, who occasionally smoked cigars himself, characterized the '*Cigarro als Surrogat der Gedanken*'.

Thoughts, again, may be verbal or averbal (*nicht sprachgebundenes begriffliches Denken*, sphairal thought). They may occur quite randomly or in so-called 'free association', being determined by unconscious cerebration producing, as it were, a *Gaussian noise* of Np-events resulting in P-events of thought. On the other hand, in accordance with *Berkeley's* statement quoted above, they may become intentional, and motivated as purposeful often sustained cogitation. This active aspect of thought can be said to occur in accordance with the *p.r.s. cogitandi*, closely related to the *p.r.s. agendi*, but differing from this latter by not directly resulting in output, either by speech, writing, or other body activities. In other words, we may distinguish intentional and unintentional thought (*willkürliches und unwillkürliches Denken*) of which the former falls under the *p.r.s. cogitandi* and the latter under the *p.r.s. fiendi* as applying to random Np-events.

(9) *The principium rationis sufficientis percipiendi* represents a useful fiction adapted to the concept of a physical brain in which N-events take place. All N-events except Np-events are unconscious, only Np-events being correlated with P-events, i.e. consciousness (cf. above section 5, p. 180f.).

This fiction is based on the fact that there is, indeed an, actual and real (in the second sense) perceptual brain, of which consciousness is a dependent variable. Brain events, corresponding to the postulated N-events (electroencephalogram in Man and Animals, extra- and intracellular electrode recordings in Animals) can actually be observed, as registered by instruments. Yet, any 'observation' including that obtained by registering instruments already implies the consciousness of the Human observer.[146]

Regardless of these qualifications the *p.r.s. percipiendi* may be accepted as stating: the occurrence of Np-events is the sufficient reason for the occurrence of consciousness related to a living, functioning brain. In other words, said principle subsumes the relation of Np-events to P-events.

---

[146] It is important to realize the difference between 'observation' and 'registration'. Observation implies consciousness of the observer, registration, in the here adopted sense, is an unconscious event, presumed to take place in the fictional physical space-time system or to be performed by instruments or sense organs. A registration by an unconscious instrument becomes observed by the conscious observer. Likewise, the results of unconscious cerebration, which includes registration processes by the sense organs, can become experienced in consciousness according to the *principium rationis sufficientis percipiendi*.

(10) *The principium rationis sufficientis actualitatis* is related to the brain paradox. Since space and time represent as so-called primary qualities merely aspects of consciousness (i.e. of 'actuality'), there exists, in addition to the actual or real (in the second sense) perceptual brain, no physical brain, or, in other words, no brain except that perceived by a conscious observer as his own, or that of another organic being possessor of a central nervous system.

Yet, since continuous orderliness prevails despite disruption in, or interruption of, consciousness (mind *sensu strictiori*), an incomprehensible extramental *orderliness* x must be assumed of which consciousness, including the perceptual brain 'producing' consciousness, represents a manifestation. Thus, the *p.r.s. actualitatis* merely states: the existence of the incomprehensible because non-describable orderliness x (corresponding more or less to *Kant's* 'Ding an sich') is the sufficient reason for the occurrence of consciousness with its correlated perceptual brain.

In other words, said principle subsumes the relationship of actuality (consciousness) to an unknown and inexplicable orderliness x.[147]

Summarizing the preceding elaboration on the principle of sufficient reason with its at least 10 different applications it could also be said that this entire principle can be reduced to the fundamental formula 'if (and only if) – then'. If a conscious event occurs, it must conform to one of the 'substrata'[148] of consciousness (*p.r.s. apparendi*). If dynamic spatio-temporal condition A changes (cause), then spatio-temporal condition B (effect) results (*p.r.s. fiendi*). If formal or kinetic space-time relationships A obtain, then these relationships are correlated with a describable geometrical, arithmetical or topological orderliness subsumed under a corresponding transformation B (*p.r.s. essendi*). If A, I can deduce or infer or 'understand' B (*p.r.s. cognoscendi*). Any percept A can be compared as regards identity, similarity, dissimilarity, with itself or with any other percept B (*p.r.s. comparationis*). If sensory percepts, thought percepts or pseudosensory percepts A are experienced, they are correlated with positive, indifferent or negative affective tone B (*p.r.s. affectivitatis*). If affective consciousness events with affective tone A obtain, then the conscious being acts according to an intention (motive) B

---

[147] Transcendental neutralism, which assumes the 'existence' of the extramental orderliness x is, of course, not 'neutral monism' although, in some respect an apparent similarity obtains. Transcendental neutralism is strictly dualistic, if not pluralistic, since it assumes the existence of pluralistic disjoint consciousness-manifolds *and* the 'existence' of the extramental (neutral since neither mental nor physical and thus incomprehensible) orderliness x.

[148] 'Substratum' is here defined as that in which an attribute inheres. 'Subsumption' means that the concept, subject of a proposition, is taken under a predicate. It may be only one predicate or it may be the inclusion of a concept and that of a higher order, such as individual under species etc., this is sometimes also designated as subordination. Generally, however, subsumption and subordination are used as synonyms.

(*p.r.s. agendi*). We have thus purposive action determined by motives. If, in a given consciousness-manifold thoughts occur in accordance with affective tone C, then the intended or purposeful thoughts D occur (*p.r.s. cogitandi*). In other words, we have motivated thoughts which in turn, may or may not result into motivated actions. If, in a brain, Np-events A occur, then they are correlated with corresponding P-events (consciousness-events) B (*p.r.s. percipiendi*). If the consciousness-manifold A occurs, then it is related, as a manifestation, to an inexplicable orderliness B, which shall be disignated as the orderliness x (*p.r.s. actualitatis*).

It will be seen that, of the here enumerated 10 applications of the principle of sufficient reason, only the second, third and fourth are, to a significant degree, satisfactorily understood *qua* details. Thus, we have the causal events of classical large-scale physics and of chemistry. With respect to small-scale atomic and subatomic events, however, classical physics must be substituted by the statistical quantum theories. Again, we have the numerous operationally valid formulations of mathematics and of logic. In their practical applications, these relationships permit technological accomplishments of high order. Thus, computers may be contrived which perform mathematical and logicial operations with a speed and accuracy far surpassing, at least in a large number of (but not in all) applications, the capabilities of the Human brain.

As regards the other applications of the principle of sufficient reason, however, one is restricted to the formulation of very generalized statements, which, nevertheless, in accordance with *Hume's* concept of 'mental geography' provide a modicum of 'insight': *est quadam prodire tenus, si non datum ultra.*

Poincaré [1913b, 1963], who included the postulate of continuity into the principle of sufficient reason (cf. above fn. 139) also emphasized the significance of that principle for the calculation of probabilities. He stated that 'for that calculation to have any meaning, it is necessary to admit, as point of departure, a hypothesis or convention which has always something arbitrary about it. In the choice of that convention, we can be guided only by the principle of sufficient reason. Unfortunately this principle is very vague and very elastic, and in the cursory examination we have just made, we have seen it take many different forms. The form under which we have met it most often is the belief in continuity, a belief which it would be difficult to justify by apodeictic reasoning, but without which all science would be impossible.'

Reverting now to the significance of the principle of sufficient reason as the basis of all explanations, it appears relevant again to examine the meaning of 'explanation' which is closely related to, and may even be considered, in some aspects, to overlap with 'description'.

Craik [1952] has carefully considered 'the nature of explanation', distinguishing (1) 'a priorism', (2) descriptive procedures not including causal factors, (3) relational procedures involving probabilities, and (4) causal procedures based on the orderliness of physical interactions.

'A priorism', in that authour's interpretation, asserts certain facts and principles to be self-evident or certain. This, of course, applies to the principle of sufficient reason which is incapable of being proved and may be denied by scepticism. However, *Craik* seems to have misunderstood *Hume*, who merely pointed out the non-provability of causation, but did not deny, and even strongly supported its practical validity.

Craik stresses that 'explanation, to the man in the street, means giving the causes of things and saying why they happen'. He strongly supports this view, which he adopts, by pointing out the fact that experiment is possible at all.

To summarize my own view concerning 'explanation', this term merely signifies the 'reason *sensu latiori*' of an 'event' or 'thing' with respect to one or more of the ten aspects of the principle of sufficient reason. This, of course, implies relationships that, in the end, can be reduced to: if, and only if – then. This involves the questions what?, who?, how?, where?, when?, why?, expressed in different order by the old line: *quis, quid, ubi, quibus auxiliis, cur, quomodo, quando?* Some of these terms are slightly ambiguous: why did you do this?, why did this happen?, why does a body fall? (because it has lost its support; because it is attracted by the earth, because it is subject to gravity), why does the sum of the angles in an Euclidean triangle equal 180°?, how do you do this?, how is a Vertebrate characterized?, how did this happen, how does a body fall? etc.

It is evident that some 'explanations' or 'descriptions' are more satisfactory than others, particularly if they 'reduce' *prima facie* unknown relationships to others which appear better known or 'understood'.

With respect to the law of gravity, the first important step was taken by *Galileo*, who, before asking why bodies fall, first established, according to the *principium rationis sufficientis essendi*, that is to say, kinematically, how bodies fall. The causal, that is to say the dynamic question why bodies fall was finally 'explained', i.e. described by *Newton* (1642–1727) by means of the calculus, which was apparently independently developed by himself and by *Leibniz* (1646–1716).

Hooke (1635–1703), however, claimed that he had, before *Newton*, discovered the law of gravity. With regard to said 'law' *Kepler* had already suggested that the planets were driven by a 'force' originating in the sun. *Galileo* and *Descartes* had assumed that 'natural' motion of bodies is in a straight line. Combined with the concept of centrifugal force formulated by *Huygens* (1629–1695), this required that the planets be continually acted upon by a 'force' originating in the sun. *Huygens* and *Hooke* had both shown that for circular orbits the force must vary inversely with the square of distances in order to account for *Kepler's* third law. However, neither *Hooke* nor *Huygens* were able to derive a formula for a 'force' that would make a planet move in an elliptic orbit. This was indeed *Newton's* achievement.[149]

Concerning 'explication' and 'comprehensibility' in general which are based on the principle of sufficient reason, it is perhaps appropriate to quote the following comment by *Einstein* [1950]: 'The very fact that the totality of our sense experiences is such that by means of thinking (operations with concepts, and the creation and use of definite functional relations between them, and the coordination of sense experiences to these concepts) it can be put in order, this fact is one which leaves us in awe, but which we shall never understand. One may say the eternal mystery of the world is its comprehensibility. It is one of the great realizations of *Immanuel Kant* that the setting up of a real external world be senseless without that comprehensibility.'

'In speaking here concerning "comprehensibility", the expression is used in its most modest sense. It implies: the production of some sort of order among sense impressions, this order being produced by the creation of general concepts, and by the relation between these concepts and sense experience, these relations being determined in any possible manner. It is in this sense that the world of our sense experience is comprehensible. The fact that it is comprehensible is a miracle.'

The 'relations' to which *Einstein* refers in these 'general considerations concerning the method of science' quite evidently pertain to the principle of sufficient reason characterized by *Schopenhauer* as the principle of all relations and of all explanations. *Einstein* justly stressed here 'comprehensibility' in its most modest sense, qualified by overall incomprehensibility.[150]

Finally, with regard to the principle of sufficient reason as representing the principle of all relations, it seems appropriate to contest the following statement by *Russell* [1952]: 'A certain type of superior person is fond of asserting that "everything is relative". This is, of course, nonsense, because if *everything* were relative, there would be nothing for it to be relative to.

---

[149] History, however, seems to have failed in giving proper credit to *Hooke* and *Huygens*. *Schopenhauer* on the other hand, who acrimoniously contested *Newton's* color theory, considered *Hooke* to have discovered the law of gravitation, about which bitter controversies were carried on. *Hooke* accused *Newton* of plagiarism, while this latter, in turn, accused *Leibniz* as a plagiary of calculus. *Newton*, nevertheless, besides his mathematical formulation of gravity by means of the calculus, had postulated gravitation as a property of all bodies in the universe, thus establishing the law of universal gravitation.

[150] Cf. above: a fact, 'we shall never understand'. *Penfield* [1975], who quotes *Einstein's* remark on comprehensibility obviously not only misunderstood *Einstein* but, despite his early course in 'philosophy' at Princeton University, evidently failed to grasp the philosophical problem at issue in his elaboration on 'comprehensibility' which ends with the grandiloquent exclamation: 'I have no doubt the day will dawn when the mystery of the mind will no longer be a mystery.'

However, without falling into metaphysical absurdities it is possible to maintain that everything in the physical world is relative to an observer.'

Now, I would fain know what percept, 'thing', notion or emotion in the world of consciousness, is not 'relative', i.e. not characterized by a diversity of relationships. Actual 'existence' itself (i.e. consciousness) depends on the relationships resulting in a functioning brain.

Relationships are either variable or 'constant' (invariants). Constant relationships, as so-called 'laws of nature' provide constraints for variable relationships. Thus, the number is a constant relationship, but the actual magnitude expressed by the relationship depends upon the size of the circle, and the number depends upon the numerical system (e.g. decimal, binary or other) adopted.

Only the metaphysical and thus incomprehensible orderliness x is absolute, namely, per se, devoid of any intelligible relationship. Yet, its metaphysical 'existence' must be inferred on the basis of relationships between interrupted states of consciousness (*principium rationis sufficientis actualitatis*).

Russell's qualification about the 'physical world', as quoted above, is a rather ambiguous statement. A conscious 'observer' does not 'observe' the 'physical world' but merely concentrates his 'attention' upon certain sensory percepts which are relative to his brain. If these sensory percepts are considered to represent the 'physical world', then everything in this 'physical world' is relative to a functioning brain which, in turn, is a component of said 'physical world' (brain paradox). If *Russell*, however, assumes the 'existence' of a fictional unconscious physical world as a public physical space-time system, then everything in this physical world could become relative either to an unconscious recording instrument or, by means of the fictional *principium rationis sufficientis percipiendi*, to the brain of a conscious observer.

Again, the relationship of 'everything' to an 'observer', or respectively the relationship of events to a recording or registering instrument, are reciprocal, since the 'observer' or the recording instrument become 'related' to what is 'observed' or 'registered'.

Russell's quip about 'a certain type of superior person' is rather gratuitous in view of that author's not infrequently displayed snobbishness. It ill behooves people sitting in glass houses to throw stones at others.

III. The Idealistic Approach

1. Definition

Idealism (in its epistemologic denotation) may be defined as the tenet assuming that consciousness is the sole principle or essence of the phenomenal world. Idealism can also be defined as the tenet assuming that the material world, in the same manner as the world of thought and feeling, is exclusively a mental phenomenon. Because of the ambiguities associated with the various connotations of the term mind *sensu latiori* and *sensu strictiori* the first formulation appears preferable.

The self-evident conclusions leading to the idealistic concept, and first drawn on the basis of rigorous reasoning by *Berkeley* and by *Hume*, were dealt with in section 5 of the preceding chapter II. Despite additional elaborations by *Kant* and *Schopenhauer*, they have nevertheless remained poorly understood. Thus, Bertrand *Russell* [1948] states 'that whatever we know without inference is mental, and that the physical world is only known as regards certain abstract features of its space-time structure – features which, because of their abstractness, do not suffice to show whether the physical world is or is not different in intrinsic character from the world of mind'. *Russell* obviously failed here to realize that space-time, although represented by the so-called 'primary qualities', can no more be attributed to the extramental reality in the first sense than the so-called 'secondary qualities'. Inferences, moreover, are mental processes, namely thoughts, i.e. extrasensory percepts. Whatever we know, therefore, represents states of consciousness. The assumed physical world is only an abstraction of certain mental space-time structures, that is, only a pale state of consciousness related to other, more vivid states of consciousness. A physical event experienced by no one can be likened to a pain experienced by no one. Perceptual space and time are fundamental attributes of consciousness, in fact may be designated as the 'matrix' of consciousness, while conceptual, physical, and absolute space-time are abstractions – not forms, but states of thought-consciousness representing 'fictions'. Perceptual space-time is directly given, the others are only postulated, or, erroneously inferred. Even discounting the valid argumentations of *Berkeley*, *Hume*, *Kant*, and *Schopenhauer*, the actuality of the postulated extramental sorts of space-time may be denied by merely applying *Occam's Razor* (*entia praeter necessitatem non sunt multiplicanda*), and they can thereby be regarded as fictions. The burden of proof as regards their actuality is then left with the materialist who affirms it: *affirmanti incumbit probatio*. So far, no convincing logical argument contradicting the idealistic concept has been presented.

It should also be pointed out that *Schopenhauer*, in §1 of his '*Welt als Wille und Vorstellung*' (vol. I) also displays considerable weaknesses and ambiguities. Even the term '*Vorstellung*' (representation) is poorly chosen, and should be replaced by 'consciousness', thereby stating: '*Die Welt ist mein Bewusstsein*'. Again, the terms '*Objekt*' and '*Subjekt*' are misleading: Instead of the world being '*nur Objekt in Beziehung auf das Subjekt*', it should be stated: '*Die Erscheinungswelt ist nur Inhalt eines Bewusstseins, d.h. eines privaten Raum-Zeit-Systems.*'

Schopenhauer states, moreover, that the reasoning observer '*keine Sonne kennt, sondern immer nur ein Auge, das eine Sonne sieht, eine Hand, die eine Erde fühlt*'. He fails here to realize that the eye as well as the hand are percepts, which as such, are in no manner different from the percept 'sun'. He likewise fails to realize that eye and hand, although necessary for sensory perception, do not 'see' or 'feel', the seeing and feeling being exclusively the function of the brain. This latter, in turn, is likewise a percept.

We have here the double aspect of the brain paradox which *Schopenhauer* did not recognize. First, the empirically substantiated but 'paradoxical' (strange) *fact* that the brain, a percept, 'produces' all percepts, including itself. Secondly, the logical paradox requiring that the brain, like the Barber of Seville who is not, in the relevant aspect, a man of Seville, does not, as a mere percept, produce all percepts, but represents, in this respect no sensory percept but an extramental brain which merely can be imagined, as pointed out by *Berkeley's Hylas* (cf. chapter II, section 6, p. 187). But since an extramental reality in the first sense is devoid of space-time attributes, an extramental brain cannot exist, thereby characterizing the contradictory 'true' aspect of the brain paradox as unsolvable.

Finally, *Schopenhauer's* and *Kant's* concept of 'knowledge' or 'truth' a priori is evidently untenable. Space and time, as the 'formal' aspects of consciousness, and causality, as applying to sensory percepts, although pertaining to the orderliness of consciousness, are exclusively 'known' through actual conscious experience. Using a valid scholastic terminology used by *Albertus Magnus*, they are not '*universalia ante rem*', but '*universalia in re*', becoming 'known', however, only as '*universalia post rem*', i.e. through actual conscious experience.

2. Historical Remarks

In Western philosophy, the earliest expressions of an idealistic viewpoint are found in the available fragments of the *Eleatics* dating from about the sixth or fifth century BC especially in the work 'περί φύσεως' of *Parmenides*.[1]

In Eastern religious thinking, idealism is, intuitively and somewhat mysteriously, expressed in the Indian Upanishads which are about contemporaneous with or only slightly older than the *Eleatic* teachings.

In the Sutta Nipâta (II) of Hinayâna (Pâli) Buddhism, which presumably contains some of the original sayings of the *Buddha* (ca. 500 BC) it is stated: 'Where consciousness is, there is also mind-and-body; Mind-and-body is conditioned by consciousness.' 'Then, brethren, through rational thinking and insight arose the comprehension: "Consciousness not being, mind-and-body is not: by the cessation of consciousness comes the cessation of mind-and-body".' In many Sûtras of Mahâyana Buddhism dating from a somewhat later period, an impressive doctrine of emphatic idealism is propounded, especially in the series of the deeply symbolic and grandiose Prajñâ Pâramitâ Sûtras. The gist of *Vasubandhu's* Mahâyana treatise Vidyâ-mâtra-shâstra is expressed by the Sino-Japanese term *Yui-shiki* which signifies 'only consciousness'. The more recent Indian systems of the Vedânta, based upon the Upanishads, but reformulated by *Sankara* (*Shankara*) about the ninth century of the Christian Era, have elaborated an abstruse idealism supported by an intricate and ambiguous terminology.

Yet, as quoted by *Schopenhauer* (vol. I, p. 34) from a summary in the *Journal of Asiatic Researches* by *W. Jones*, the gist of Vedânta philosophy according to *Vyasa* seems to anticipate *Berkeley's* views: the fundamental tenet of that Vedânta school 'consisted not in denying the existence of matter, that is of solidity, impenetrability and extended figure (to deny which would be lunacy), but in correcting the popular notion of it, and in contending that it has no essence independent of mental perception; that existence and perceptibility are convertible terms'.

Present-day Western systems of idealism have been strongly influenced by *Descartes'* famed writings '*Discours de la Méthode*' and '*Meditationes de Prima Philosophia*' (1641). *Descartes* is justly designated as one of the fathers of modern philosophy since his method and the dictum '*Dubito, cogito, ergo*

---

[1] The verse: 'Τό γὰρ αὐτὸ νοεῖν τε χαι εἰναι', which is the only extant line of part 5 of *Parmenides'* poem, can be interpreted as closely akin in meaning to '*esse est percipi*' and '*cogito ergo sum*'. The *Pythagorean* physician and later author of comedies *Epicharmus (540–450 BC) is likewise quoted as having said:* Νοῦς ὁρῆ καὶ νοῦς ἀκουει τἀλλα κψφὰ καὶ τυ φλα.

St. Augustine, whose elaborations on time and its beginning in the *Confessions* (XI, chapt. 13 et passim) as well as in the *City of God* (XII, chapt. 16 et passim) are mere paraphrases from *Plato's Timaeus*, also brings, in the, *City of God* (XI, chapt. 21) the following remark, presumably adapted from the then available philosophical literature: '*Quia ergo sum si fallor, quo modo esse me fallor, quandum certum me esse si fallor?*' – '*Sicut enim novi esse me, ita novi etiam hoc ipsum posse me.*'

sum' based on his treatises have opened, as it were, a new approach. *Descartes* himself must be considered a matter and mind dualist and the weaknesses of his system have provoked many criticisms. One of his later compatriots, I believe *Voltaire*, is said to have stated: '*il commence par tout douter et finit par tout croire*'. As regards the 'thinking', *Schiller* voiced his objection in the distich:

> *Denk' ich, so bin ich. Wohl! Doch wer wird immer auch denken!*
> *Oft schon war ich und hab' wirklich an gar nichts gedacht!*

Finally, concerning the 'I think, therefore I am' as proof of the self, ego or I, *Descartes*' assertion represents merely a *petitio principii*. The general principle of the *Cartesian* approach, however, is fundamental for any system of idealism, although the original formulation must be considered unsatisfactory.

3. The Modified Cartesian Approach

Avoiding both the reference to the self and the emphasis on the thinking, *Descartes*' sentence *cogito ergo sum* must be replaced by the initial statement: there is consciousness (*percipitur atque nonnunquam cogitatur*).[2]

It can next be stated that this consciousness is differentiated and yet represents, while in being, a unified, individual manifold. Components of this complex are optic and tactile sensations organized as percepts, furthermore acoustic, olfactory, and gustatory percepts. In addition, there are vague feelings, emotions, 'internal images', abstractions ('universals') and thoughts. One of the most fundamental properties of thought, as emphasized by various authors, is its power of predicting events. This abbreviated enumeration, omitting the details given in the more elaborate description of consciousness outlined in section 5 of chapter II (p. 168f.), and discounting the sophistication of specialized psychological terminology, appears sufficient for the present intent.

The consciousness-manifold is integrated into a unit by its space-time structure. It could also be said to represent a unified perceptual space-time matrix with many compresent modalities which run the entire gamut from vivid and well-localized sensations to pale, poorly localized abstractions and ideas.[3]

---

[2] Although the form of the passive verbal voice is here used, the meaning should be that of a deponent verb, and, moreover, that of a *verbum impersonale*: there are percepts and sometimes thoughts (German: *es wird empfunden und es wird zuweilen gedacht*).

[3] Consciousness has thus been occasionally designated as 'experienced integration' or EI [*Fessard*, 1954]. Since this definition refers only to one aspect of consciousness, I do not believe that it is particularly helpful. Moreover, the degree of integration may vary considerably, as e.g. under the influence of hyponoic and hypobulic factors, in dreams, and under pathologic conditions.

Optic, tactile and related modalities of human consciousness are as a rule vivid, well localized, and characterized by spatial configuration. Acoustic and olfactory modalities may be vivid, but are less accurately localized and lack spatial configuration. Internal mental images, thoughts and emotions are poorly localized and likewise lack spatial configuration. With some exceptions, e.g. as regards strong emotions, most of these latter modalities display a low degree of vividity. Nevertheless, even thoughts have a certain localization, being referred to a region of space corresponding to the interior of the body (outside or dorsally to the visual space); they are very vaguely localized in the head, so vaguely in fact, that the impression of a localization in the heart or the diaphragm, as assumed by some of the popular views of antiquity, did not seem unreasonable. A similar vagueness of localization occurs with regard to some types of referred or visceral pain – even dental pain appears occasionally to be localized in the wrong tooth or even in the wrong jaw.

R. Semon (1859–1918), one time Professor of Anatomy at the University of Jena, who introduced and elaborated the concept of mneme, and coined the term engram, emphasized in his posthumous treatise 'Bewußtseinsvorgang und Gehirnprozeß' [1920] certain quantitative connotations of consciousness, such as intensity and vividity, concerning both the particular modalities and the integrated consciousness manifold as a whole. Awareness may be clear and distinct, or dim, faint, and hazy.

As intensity and vividity approach zero, consciousness vanishes unnoticeably. Kretschmer [1926] has stressed this twilight zone which will again be considered below in discussing the 'unconscious' of psychoanalysts. Slater [1950] states in this respect: 'Many people think of consciousness as something that is either there or not there. But it is not like that at all.' In agreement with Kretschmer's view I would rather emphasize that although an event can be more or less conscious, we must still consider consciousness as a phenomenon alternating between manifestation and complete interruption and extinction: awareness, despite considerable differences in degree, allowing for an indistinct vanish, is either there or not there.

In psychological terminology, consciousness modalities have been referred to as qualities, and vividity has been designated as 'attention'. Spatial relationships have been classified as 'extensity', and temporal relationships as 'protensity'. Thus the following so-called dimensions of consciousness are enumerated: quality, attensity, intensity, extensity, and protensity. Although this formulation can be considered a good pun, I do not believe that it is particularly helpful to expand or adulterate the meaning of the term 'dimension' which should rather be restricted to characterize space-time and mathematically related concepts.

The temporal structure of consciousness seems to have a certain primacy over the spatial structure; all modalities are integrated into a common flow of events. This temporal flow expresses itself in the sequence of sensory events as well as in the association of abstract ideas and in the sequence of complex motor patterns involving a configuration of many different consciousness modalities.

Empty perceptual space-time does not exist except as an abstract notion; awareness of such space-time depends always on a consciousness-modality whose attribute is, of necessity, a space-time relationship. Consciousness could, in fact, even be defined as an occupied or filled space-time continuum.

Conversely, it should be clear that the term consciousness by itself is a rather vague generalization. Empty consciousness per se has no existence except as an abstract notion, as a generalized term for the phenomenal world. Consciousness merely signifies: something (thought, sensation, image, 'object') within a given particular perceptual space-time framework. In this respect, the dictum *'esse est percipi'*, based on *Berkeley's* Treatise [1710], can be fully upheld. Consciousness can thus be defined as any pattern of events in a perceptual space-time system, and this definition is essentially identical with the shorter formulation: *esse est percipi*. The most concise and simplified definition of consciousness would probably be this: consciousness is the stuff of our world.[4]

If it is recognized that perceptual space-time is the fundamental attribute of consciousness, the controversy concerning *Kant's* concept of 'a priorism' loses its significance: perceptual space-time is present whenever consciousness occurs. Its distinctiveness, i.e. sharpness of definition, shows considerable variations and such variations may even be conceived in terms of both phylogenetic and ontogenetic evolution.

A similar deproblematization obtains with regard to the mathematical concepts: *Euclidean* and *non-Euclidean* spaces as well as relativistic space-time are useful and significant abstractions referring to certain orderly relationships derived from perceptual space-time which, in turn, might be best designated as an *'Euclidoid* mollusk-like (or ameboid) field'; the vague center of localization for its frame of reference is located within the body. This 'mollusk' represents an integration, within its three spatial dimensions, of the different spatial modalities such as visual, tactile, acoustic, and thought space, as well as similar others.

The definition or description of perceptual time is exceedingly difficult, and attempts at a rational formulation have not been very successful. Time represents a vectorial property of consciousness phenomena, comparable to an apparently irreversible flow. The present has no duration, the past has vanished, and the future has not appeared. How is it then possible to ap-

---

[4] Thus my father, *L. Kuhlenbeck* [1903, p. 19] stressed that *'Dasein ist Bewusstsein'*.

prehend duration? It should, however, be realized that, since empty perceptual space-time has no existence, duration represents an attribute of experienced events, constituting the conscious present of psychologic terminology. Duration would thus be linked to the gestalt qualities of percepts. It is possible that *Mach* [1922] had this aspect of time in view when he considered 'times' as sensations or elements, but time and space, in my opinion, should not be equated with other aspects of sensation and represent, hierarchically, a category of higher order. Many authors have also justly stressed that a mnestic component is involved in our perceptions of duration and succession, such that earlier events are fused with later events, and organized into a composite perception.

Time is measured by rhythmical or cyclic processes (events) representing public data, such as the rotation and revolution of the earth. We obtain thus, as sidereal time units, seconds, hours, days, and years. Absolute time, as postulated by *Newton*, was supposed to flow at a uniform rate: '*Tempus absolutum, quod aequabiliter fluit.*'

In perceptual time, our appreciation of duration is by no means uniform, depending on the total situation. 1 minute may seem to be a very long time, and under different circumstances, hours or days may seem to pass very rapidly.

In addition, *Schopenhauer* [1850] pointed out that appreciation of time changes with aging. Time, on the whole, seems to flow more slowly during infancy and youth, gradually accelerating its course: '*Man kann demzufolge annehmen, daß, in der unmittelbaren Schätzung unseres Gemüthes, die Länge eines Jahres im umgekehrten Verhältnisse des Quotienten desselben in unser Alter steht: wann z.B. das Jahr 1/5 unseres Alters beträgt, erscheint es uns 10 Mal so lang, als wann es nur 1/50 desselben ausmacht.*'

In his treatise *Biological Time* [1937] *Lecomte du Noüy* has elaborated these views, without, however, referring to *Schopenhauer's* contributions to the subject. *Lecomte du Noüy* states [p. 164/165]: 'A year seems longer to a child of five than to a man of fifty because it represents only the fiftieth part of the life of the older man. This would imply a notion of time based on memory, and a permanent subconscious confrontation of the time which flows with the time elapsed since birth.'

Lecomte du Noüy assumes chemical modifications of the organism with age. In this regard, he demonstrated, as *Korschelt* [1924] had done before, a progressive loss of proliferative and regenerative power with age, and formulated a concept of 'biologic time'. At different ages, repair of wounds, or cicatrization, proceeds at a different rate: it takes different lengths of time to accomplish the same amount of work as e.g. expressed by one square centimeter of a wound. In this respect, everything occurs as if sidereal time flowed four times faster for a man of fifty than for a child of ten.

Lecomte du Noüy plotted the curve representing the perceptual value for one year of each age according to the principle formulated by *Schopenhauer* (whom he does not mention) and superimposed it on the curve computed from the relative rate of cicatrization. The abscissae have the same value (age), the ordinates are adjusted, so that the different figures remain proportionate. Although there is no complete coincidence, the similarity of the two hyperbolic curves is striking. It is possible that, in terms of the materialistic view, biochemical processes play a role. *Lecomte du Noüy* cites experiments by *Piéron* showing that increase in body temperature modifies perceptual time appreciation. An acceleration in the temporal standard, corresponding to a shortening in appreciation of time, is said to occur with increase of temperature.[5]

Another aspect of biologic time is related to the specific average life duration of organisms. In the rat, for instance, metabolic rate was found to be thirty times as rapid as in Man, and the span of life one thirtieth. Three years of rat life thus correspond to ninety years of Human life. When, in accordance with this representative fraction, rat and Man of equivalent age were compared, they were found to be in like phases of life span. As regards the neurologic aspect, such correspondences were found in the phases of the growth of the brain in weight, in the cessation of cell division in the cerebellum, in the time of attainment of the full thickness of the cerebral cortex, and in the appearance of the cell bodies of full size in various localities. On the basis of my own observations I reported on various histologic age changes in the rat's brain and their relationship to comparable changes in the Human brain [*K.*, 1954b].[6]

Awareness of temporal relationships may concern duration of an event, or timing (phase situation) within a cycle, or awareness of the cyclic process of a total pattern. The designations '*Zeitgedächtnis*' for awareness of duration, and '*Zeitsinn*' for awareness of relationship to such cycles have been suggested [*Stein*, 1951]. Expressed in materialistic terminology, physical time and its relationships can be recorded by neural mechanisms. This formulation does not presuppose consciousness.

---

[5] *Hoagland* [1951] discusses similar observations in a report on *Consciousness and the Chemistry of Time*. Various other authors (e.g. *Haldane*) have likewise commented upon chemical events as a time standard and it is well known that the rate of a chemical reaction is increased by a rise in temperature. According to *van't Hoff's* rule, the velocity of chemical reactions is usually twofold or more for each rise of 10 °C in temperature. Physical time standards, of course, are now provided by the registration of the frequencies displayed by atomic events.

[6] Further comments on aging of the nervous system as well as on aging in general can be found in section 9 (p. 714f.), volume 3/I of the author's *Central Nervous System of Vertebrates* [*K.*, 1970]. Said section also includes remarks on the concept of biological time which *Comfort* [1956, 1964] attempted to disregard on the basis of erroneous arguments.

In addition to its space-time structure, the consciousness complex displays furthermore a certain structure of its contents, insofar as many modalities are grouped around, or are closely related to, an indistinct center, the self or the ego group. This center cannot be clearly delimited but emerges, with fluctuations through broad boundary zones, into the peripheral group of sensations or percepts known as the external world.

The well-localized, spatially configurated and vivid, relatively permanent and stable percepts representing the body[7] may be considered as the peripheral portion of the ego complex, i.e. 'my' body. The poorly localized, spatially not configurated consciousness modalities such as thoughts, memories, emotions, which thus appear as predominantly temporal modalities, constitute 'my' mind *sensu strictiori* and are also frequently termed psychic processes in contradistinction to the spatially configurated percepts designated as objects or as material.

The brain with its peripheral input and output, that is to say the nervous system included in the body, insofar as this brain 'produces' or 'mediates' the phenomenon of a consciousness manifold, represents, figuratively speaking, said manifold's 'center of gravity' or, more correctly that manifold's 'central locus' respectively 'neighborhood' experienced as the transitory 'self'. Said brain, which is experienced by proprioception (through its weight) as content of the 'self''s head, and, under various unusual circumstances, by other senses or by instruments (EEG etc.) differs thus, in a most relevant manner, from all extraneous brains which may be perceived outside the 'self''s' body, and pertain to other organisms. It is evident that consciousness phenomena presumed to be correlated with such 'extraneous' brains occur in private space-time systems entirely 'outside' or 'disjoint' from the perceiving 'self' [cf. also K., 1978, p. 348].

The unique status of the brain 'producing' or 'mediating' a given 'self' with respect to this latter is also evidenced by the problems of organ transplantation which have resulted from recent advances in transplantation surgery.

In contradiction to all organ transplants, including that of the heart, the concepts of donor and recipient would become reversed, if brain or head transplants were feasible. Thus, a person may be the recipient of another

---

[7] *Schopenhauer* [vol. 1, pp. 52–53] considers the body to be the '*unmittelbares Objekt*' (direct or immediate object) representing the '*Ausgangspunkt der Erkenntnis*' (point of origin of knowledge). Avoiding the term 'object', and modifying *Schopenhauer's* terminology, the body may be conceived as the complex of percepts here indicated in the text, and including the perceptual brain. This complex 'mediates' all sensory and extrasensory percepts. The body with its brain thus indeed represents the locus of origin of all experiences whatsoever occurring in the consciousness manifold related to said brain.

heart, kidney, etc., or even of an artificial organ. *Per contra*, assuming that the at present hardly possible transplantation of a Human brain (or head) could be accomplished, such brain or head with its 'self', i.e. such 'person would become the recipient of a donor body [cf. *K*, 1970, pp. 702–704]. As an aside, it may be said that the title of a pretentious publication by *Popper and Eccles* [1977], namely *The Self and its Brain* obviously reverses the actual relationships or, in the vernacular, 'puts the cart before the horse'. If the useful fictional concept of a 'self' is adopted, one may then speak of 'the brain and its transient self'.

Further analysis reveals the intrinsic vagueness of the ego – or self – complex. Any part of the body can be lost or removed so long as the remainder stays alive as an integrated whole. Any particular thought, sensation, emotion or memory can be considered unessential with respect to the I. The limits of the ego or self complex may thus be more and more narrowed, until at last nothing remains but an imaginary point representing the 'center of gravity' (better 'center of emphasis') or zero point (comparable to an intersection of perceptual space-time coordinates) of the entire consciousness complex: '*ein imaginärer Punkt hinter allem Erlebtem*' [*Kretschmer*, 1926]. As already mentioned above (p. 171), *Schopenhauer* and some other philosophers distinguish in consciousness a perceiving subject and a perceived object, but this distinction cannot be upheld on convincing grounds. Any consciousness modality is a given fundamental phenomenon which unifies in itself both the attributes of objectivity and subjectivity. The tree as I see it in space at a certain distance from my body is, while I am aware of it, as much 'I' as my body or my thoughts. *Lord Byron* expressed this insight in the poetical form:

> Are not the mountains, waves and skies a part
> Of me and of my soul as I of them?

The self thus 'fluctuates' (*Kretschmer*) between 0 and ∞; it can be considered a mere fiction or at best an abstraction symbolizing the centralized structure of an individual consciousness manifold.

In Western philosophy, the non-existence of a substantial self was stressed by *Hume* [1739] who conceived the ego as a mere aggregate of mental states and formulated the bundle theory of the self as a sheaf or 'collection of different perceptions which succeed each other with an inconceivable rapidity, and are in a perpetual flux and movement'.

Hume, of course, did not deny the significance of that aggregate of mental states representing the fictional 'self' and correctly derives it from memory, that is to say in present terminology from engram complexes, whereupon so-called 'identity' depends. Memory contributes to the 'self's' production, 'by producing the relation of resemblance among the perceptions. The case is the same, whether we consider ourselves or others.'

In this respect, *Hume* (*Of the Passions*, part I, section XI) states that the idea or rather impression of ourselves is always intimately present with us, and that our consciousness gives us so lively a conception of our own person, that it is not possible to imagine that any thing can in this particular go beyond it. It is evident that not only memory but also especially affectivity plays a significant role in generating the 'impression of ourselves', that is to say the operationally valid fiction of a 'self', and *Hume* justly reverts here to a discussion of the 'self' in his Book II *Of the Passions*.

Popper [*Popper and Eccles*, 1977], who completely failed to understand *Hume's* argumentation, quotes out of context, statements from *Hume's* Book II in order to show contradictions in that author's concept of the 'self' which is said to be denied in Book I and asserted in Book II.

However, in the former, *Hume* justly states that we have no idea of the self *after the manner it is here explained by some philosophers*, namely as its existence and continuance in existence both *qua* perfect identity and simplicity. This does not conflict with diverse statements in Book II that 'ourself is always intimately present to us'. This positive assertion *Hume's* is by no means the same position which is attributed in Book I to 'some philosophers', and which he there justly declares to be manifestly contradictory and absurd. Again, in the 'Appendix' to his *Treatise of Human Nature*, *Hume* [1740] states: 'When I turn my reflection on *myself*, I never can perceive this *self* without some one or more perception. It is the composition of these, therefore, which forms the self.'

While *Popper's* attempt seems, *prima facie*, based on complete misunderstanding of *Hume's* view, one might perhaps also wonder whether it does not represent an intentional misrepresentation in order to save the hopeless concept of an essential self.

In this connection, it seems appropriate to quote an important passage from the Samyutta Nikâya of Hînayâna Buddhism:

> The wandering ascetic *Vacchagotta* came to the *Buddha* and enquired from him:
> – 'Master *Gotama*, what have you to say about the existence of the Self?'
> At these words the Exalted One was silent.
> – 'How then, Master *Gotama*? Is there no such thing as the Self?'
> At these words the Exalted One still remained silent.
> Then *Vacchagotta* the Wanderer rose up and went away.
> Soon after he was gone *Ânanda* asked the Exalted One why he did not reply to the questions asked by *Vacchagotta*.
>   Then the Exalted One said:
> – 'If, when asked "does the Self exist?" I had replied "the Self exists" I would have sided with the

recluses and brâhmins who
proclaim immortality.'
    'But if, when asked the question "does
the Self not exist?" I had replied
"No! the Self does not exist", I would
have sided with those recluses and brâhmins who are complete nihilists.'
    'Again, *Ânanda*, if asked "does the Self exist?"
would that reply be consistent
with my knowledge that all things
are impermanent?'
– 'No, Lord, it would not'.
– 'Again, *Ânanda*, when asked
"then does not the Self exist?", I would
have added to the bewilderment of *Vacchagotta*,
already bewildered. For he would have
said, "formerly I had a self, but now
I have one no more".'

Mr. *Popper* should have done his homework by pondering upon the here quoted saying of the *Buddha*.

The 'self', however, which in *Hume's* words, 'is always intimately present to us', may become manifested at the level of very dim, sphairal consciousness, that is to say remain 'subconscious', and at times even fades into 'unconscious cerebration' (cf. vol. 2, chapter IV, section 10). On the other hand, the 'self' may become vividly manifested as a component of consciousness in so-called 'self-awareness', strongly influencing behavior.

Again, what is called 'personality' or 'character' with reference to the overall behavioral pattern, is a feature of Human nature evidently closely related to 'self-awareness'.

Schopenhauer, following *Kant*, distinguished an innate and unchangeable 'intelligible character' from an 'empiric' one, which latter again, is said to evolve as so-called 'acquired character'. Discounting *Schopenhauer's* metaphysical interpretation, which I do not share, of the 'intelligible character', one may evidently distinguish, as regards the so-called character, nature and nurture, namely a genetically determined component, which, although not immutable, displays considerable permanence, and a component determined by environment and teaching or conditioning. 'Nature' represents here the genetically determined brain mechanisms which may become modified by pathologic changes (e.g. dementia paralytica) or crude interference (e.g. lobotomy) and 'nurture' represents the programming, effected by engram complexes, determining the relevant behavioral activities of the given mechanisms.

Although much of what *Schopenhauer* elaborates on character and personality remains valid despite the weaknesses of his metaphysical 'will' concept, his assertion that the 'character' is always inherited from the father, and the 'intelligence' from the mother is contradicted by the obtaining rules of genetics and represents an evident error.

With regard to the problem of the 'self', *Mach* [1922], in his provocative '*Analyse der Empfindungen*' (9th ed.), has again elaborated on this theme and forcefully supported the concept of nonreality of the self: '*Das Ich ist unrettbar.*' He designates the ego simply as a 'practical unit'. The first edition of *Mach's* treatise appeared *in 1886. Forel* [1922; 1st ed., 1894] expresses on this subject a view agreeing with that of *Mach*. Other authors, e.g. *James* [1890], likewise subsequently pointed out that there is no direct knowledge of an experiencing self.

In Eastern religious thinking, the doctrine of non-self (termed *Anâtman* in Sanskrit) is one of the three fundamental tenets (*Trividyâ*) of Buddhism, and characterizes this religious philosophy as an essentially protestant reaction against Brahmanism which exalts the concept of a substantial self or Âtman. The tenets of Trividyâ, presumably dating back to the sixth century BC, are: *Anâtman, Anitya* (non-permanence: all phenomena are transitory), and *Duhkha* (immanent suffering).

4. Methodologic Solipsism

Consciousness phenomena occur as an individual manifold which, with the necessary qualifications and restrictions, we may designate as the (ephemeral) self. In this respect, since all experiences are exclusively restricted to the self, it represents a completely isolated 'island universe'. Paraphrasing a statement by *Eddington* it can also be said that any knowledge of things where we are not, and of things when we are not, is our inference, consisting of consciousness-modalities, including memories, here and now. In shorter formulation this may be expressed as follows: our knowledge of things that we are not is solely an inference, couched in the symbolism of our consciousness, from things that we are.

The idealistic approach, as exemplified by the *Cartesian* method, is therefore of necessity solipsistic, but only as far as its starting point is concerned. The intrinsic orderliness of events expressing itself in experience, analogies and deductions leads us to the conviction that phenomena of consciousness, similar to those representing our self, pertain to other human beings as well as to animals endowed with a nervous system akin to ours. Concerning lower vertebrates, such as fishes, or in the case of invertebrates, this assumption becomes more and more uncertain as we descend the morphologic or phylogenetic scale. It is hardly possibly to assert with any degree of justification whether rudimentary consciousness phenomena should or should not be attributed to an ameba, to plants or even to individual cells.

Although methodological solipsism[8] can be considered the only rational starting point for epistemological argumentation, there is no need for extensive constructions overemphasizing this solipsistic aspect, such as *Driesch* [1912, 1924] has elaborated in his '*Ordnungslehre*' und '*Metaphysik*'. Dogmatic solipsism, on the other hand, represents the extreme opposite to dogmatic behaviorism; both need not to be taken seriously.

According to *Sherrington* [1950] 'mind is always an inference from behavior'. This statement does not appear acceptable as a general proposition. Consciousness or mind *sensu latiori*, and mind *sensu strictiori* (thoughts etc.) are definitely not an inference but, on the contrary, the most certain, in fact the only direct experience; however, direct experience is exclusively restricted to the individual 'self'. Nonetheless, consciousness (or mind), attributed to other living organisms on the basis of convincing evidence, is indeed always an inference from behavior. *Sherrington's* statement is thus a valid particular proposition. Behaviorism, ignoring consciousness and exclusively substituting behavioral responses, assumes that since mind is an inference from behavior, and psychology is a study of mind, psychology can be reduced to a study of behavior. This argumentation must be regarded, in terms of classical logic as a *fallacia de dicto secundum quid ad dictum simpliciter*. It is true, of course, that as regards mental processes of animals, which lack comprehensive speech or language, we are essentially restricted to the behavioristic approach. The physician, however, is primarily interested in human psychology.

Again, according to *Sherrington* [1950] 'it would seem that though there is matter which exists apart from mind, we know of no instance where mind exists apart from matter; that is, if we define "mind" as we agreed to do'.

If we define mind as consciousness it might be said, on the contrary, that 'matter' (spatially configurated sensory consciousness modalities) never exists apart from consciousness. It must obviously be granted that such 'matter' may not be related to other living organisms to which mind should be

---

[8] In a chapter on solipsism, *Russell* [1948] states that said concept is impossible to believe, 'and is rejected in fact even by those who mean to accept it'. He then adds: 'I once received a letter from an eminent logician, Mrs. *Christine Ladd Franklin*, saying that she was a solipsist and was surprised that there were no others. Coming from a logician, this surprise surprised me. The fact that I cannot believe something does not prove that it is false, but it proves that I am insincere and frivolous if I pretend not to believe it.' Mrs. *Ladd Franklin* evidently meant methodological solipsism, and it is hard to believe that *Russell* did not understand this. His comment can thus be considered insincere and frivolous. Despite his considerable merits and his eminence as a logician, *Bertrand Russell* unfortunately displays lack of candor and insincerity in a number of other instances [cf. e.g. the comments in *K.*, 1961, p. 174, fn. 9; p. 470, fn. 144]. The quip aimed at *Russell*, and coined by an irate Britisher, seems therefore not inappropriate: 'There is much less to that fellow than meets the eye.'

attributed by inference from behavior. Moreover, many reflex activities of living organisms presumably take place without consciousness and it is most likely that even complex and seemingly very 'purposive' actions may be completely unconscious in some instances. It should be stressed that inferences from behavior cannot be considered as always valid, or in other words: *a posse ad esse non valet consequentia*.

Yet, in agreement with *Sherrington's* dictum, 'it can reasonably be assumed that 'mind' (i.e. consciousness) exclusively occurs as a special type of function (transformation), performed by a brain which consists of perceptual 'matter'. All other sorts of perceptual matter, anorganic or organic, are devoid of concomitant consciousness (i.e. mind) of their own. In this respect, *Sherrington's* dictum, as just quoted above, can be fully upheld. This, again, is in agreement with the well-founded view that 'mind' (i.e. consciousness) cannot be attributed to reality in the first sense, i.e. to the extramental orderliness x.

5. Introspection

The idealistic approach is both solipsistic and introspective. Considerable haziness prevails with regard to the term introspection which has been defined as observation directed upon the mental states and operations of the self. *Sensu latiori* all percepts, including those leading to the concept of matter, are mental, that is consciousness modalities. Thus the whole of physics is based on inference derived from introspection. The naive materialist describes an introspective process while disclaiming or forgetting that it is introspective.

In a narrower sense the term introspection may be restricted to the observation of poorly localized and spatially not configurated consciousness modalities such as thoughts, emotions, and sensations, that is of extrasensory percepts or mental states *sensu strictiori*, although it is difficult to draw an accurate boundary line. It is true, nevertheless, that certain consciousness modalities are absolutely private and cannot be verified by another observer, while other consciousness modalities are, to a certain extent and indirectly, simultaneously or successively shared by a number of persons. This particular aspect of the orderliness of events is expressed in the concept of *public data* which will be discussed below. Objective validity *sensu stricto* is non-existent, but *sensu latiori* objective validity can be said to represent a subjective validity extended to public data, that is a validity which can be simultaneously or successively corroborated by several observers. This validity concerns especially but not exclusively the consciousness modalities displaying distinct spatial and temporal configuration as well as a certain stability, thus permitting comparisons expressed as measurements, and recording. It concerns, however, *all* sensory percepts. These are either directly experienced phenomena or non-perceived so-called interphenomena[9] registered or recorded by instruments whose reading provides the required sensory percepts.

6. Public Data

All actual, direct experiences are restricted to the 'self', that is to any one individual consciousness manifold. Thus, consciousness in one individual is never directly, but only indirectly related to the consciousness in another individual namely through a set of relationships or 'norms' which have been designated as public data [*Russell*, 1948; and other authors].

According to *Russell's* definition a public datum 'is one which generates similar sensations in all percipients throughout a certain space-time region, which must be considerably larger than the region occupied by one human body, say, half a second – or rather it is one which would generate such sensations if suitable placed percipients were present'.

Since this definition, which correctly stresses 'sensations', i.e. sensory percepts, is couched in the language of materialism and implies a reification of public data in terms of physicalisms, it requires, for the present discussion, a modification based on premises which differ from *Russell's* formulation.

As defined from the idealistic viewpoint, a public datum is a sensory consciousness modality (sensory percept), which, on the basis of convincing grounds, I can assume to occur, in a transposed but essentially similar form, in a number of other consciousness manifolds pertaining to that same number of other sentient beings, related to me through my private perceptual space-time coordinates. It should be emphasized that these space-time coordinates refer to the other sentient beings solely insofar as these form an 'external' or 'material' part of my own consciousness manifold. There is no direct space-time relation between my consciousness field, which is a private space-time manifold (or system) and such fields pertaining to other sentient beings, whose consciousness manifolds represent entirely separate (disjoint), likewise private space-time systems. I could not draw a spatial vector to connect well-localized

---

[9] The term 'interphenomena', apparently introduced by *Reichenbach*, and also used by *Whittaker* and others, evidently subsumes two denotations. Interphenomena in the first sense are not directly perceived by the Human senses but indirectly perceived through their registration by instruments. Interphenomena in the second sense are neither directly observed through the senses nor registered by instruments but merely inferred on the basis of logical or mathematical reasoning, i.e. by extrasensory percepts (e.g. various atomic or subatomic events, or events in a hypothetical 'black hole').

and configurated percepts, i.e. 'matter', in my consciousness, with similar percepts in another field of consciousness. In other words, a set of public data, e.g. a tree, lies in altogether different spaces in my field of consciousness and in that of my neighbor, although I can trace or imagine a line from that tree to his eyes and his brain. But all this refers solely to my own field of consciousness. If I conceive the tree as related to other fields of consciousness, it loses, as far as I am concerned, its perceptual spatial character and becomes an abstract relationship, namely a set of public data. In a slightly different formulation, public data may thus also be defined as a set of orderly relationships between certain events, namely sensory percepts, in my consciousness field and inferred similar events in the consciousness fields of presumed other sentient beings.

The perceptual space-time field which we experience (our 'self') and those perceptual space-time fields of which we have knowledge through inference (our fellow sentient beings) are each four-dimensional. But these dimensions are not the same in any two different individual fields, that is, each individual represents a perceptual space-time universe of its own. There are thus, comparable to the abstract dimensions of mathematics, innumerable different (perceptual) spatial and temporal dimensions. With regards to public data, a certain 'parallelism' ['psychopsychical parallelism', cf. *K.*, 1961, p. 31, §7] may obtain between these different dimensions, so that numerous events 'appear' to be simultaneous and of similar spatial relationships in a number of different individual consciousness fields. In a way, using a somewhat bold simile, I may compare the field of consciousness of my neighbor, that is his world, to *Alice's* world behind the looking-glass.

The purely mental construction of an imaginary, but for all practical purposes indispensable physical world is thus mainly based on the abstraction, symbolization and analysis of public data. In other words, the postulate of a physical world in a public physical space-time, 'reduced', as it were, to the so-called primary qualities, is an operationally valid fiction in *Vaihinger's* sense, indispensable for an intelligible description and formulation of the experienced phenomena (cf. the comments in *K.* [1927] p. 2, fn. 2 quoted above in chapter II, section 6, p. 187).

Many public data are not only well localized but also spatially configurated (visual, tactile and proprioceptive body-sense percepts), but some others, such as sounds, odors and tastes are not spatially configurated and are only vaguely localized. All events experienced in consciousness as public data can also be registered and recorded by instruments which, in turn, represent public data and thereby, directly or indirectly, permit measurement.

Qua percepts, all public data are experienced as sensory phenomena, including the interphenomena (cf. above, section 5, fn. 9, p. 224) in the first sense displayed by the reading or output of instruments.

Münsterberg [1900] claimed that a given 'psychic' datum (i.e. a percept) could be experienced by only one person, while a given 'material' datum could be experienced by many – in other words, that 'psychic' data are private, and 'material' (physical) data public. *Münsterberg* failed here to realize that material data *qua* sensory percepts are likewise entirely private.[10]

Ziehen [1924], on the other hand, claimed that *Münsterberg's* criterion for 'psychic' and 'material' data cannot be considered entirely valid. *Ziehen* pointed out that sensations, such as fear, concepts, such as duty, and abstractions, such as π, which must all be considered psychic processes *sensu strictiori*, can, in a given situation be simultaneously or successively experienced in essentially similar form by a number of persons. *Ziehen*, however, failed to realize that the conscious events which he mentioned as occurring in persons other than the observer can only be inferred on the basis of such persons' observable behavior, manifested as material (physical) events, i.e. as sensory percepts of the observer. Thus, both *Münsterberg* and *Ziehen* missed the essential point at issue.

Since the brain, of which consciousness is a function, consists of perceptual matter, the paramount significance of public data is self-evident. Perceptual matter corresponds, of course, to *Berkeley's* 'ideas perceived by the senses' (cf. further below, p. 256). Such 'ideas' can be registered by instruments which, in turn, represent 'ideas perceived by the senses'. In other words, 'material events' act upon each other in accordance with the principle of causality. 'Extrasensory percepts', such as concepts, thoughts, and emotions, are both (or 'simultaneously') public and private data. Public insofar as they can actually or potentially be registered by instruments *qua* 'material' brain events (Np-events, e.g. EEG tracings), and private insofar as they are experienced in, or 'contents' of, a consciousness-manifold.

It seems evident that the difficult concept of public data has four different aspects, namely (1) as experienced sensory percepts, i.e. as perceptual matter or sensory P-events, which include the primary as well as the secondary qualities of *Locke*; (2) as highly abstract, nondescribable relationships between sensory percepts in different, disjoint consciousness manifolds; (3) as the fictional physicalisms (mass, energy and their interactions) in public physical space-time; (4) as the fictional R-events *sensu latiori* (including the N-events and Np-events superimposed upon a particular sort of biologic R-events), or as the 'primary qualities' in *Locke's* sense.[11] Quite evidently, (3)

---

[10] *Poincaré's* [1909] *qualités pures: 'Les sensations d'autrui seront pour nous un monde éternellement fermé.'*

[11] These 'primary qualities' were justly recognized by *Berkeley* and *Hume* as being likewise 'secondary', i.e. 'mental', but are here, in *Vaihinger's* sense, taken to represent the fiction of public physicalisms, indispensable for an intelligible description and 'understanding' of the given phenomena.

and (4) are merely different semantic formulations for 'physical events', including cosmology and cosmogony.[12]

From the viewpoint of fictional psychophysical parallelism, and reduced to the simplest terms, public data represent here all R- and N-events (including Np-events), while private data are all P-events.

7. Symbolization; Positivism

While the well-localized, spatially configured modalities of consciousness, including many of their reciprocal relationships, are rather easily symbolized, and identified by the concepts of matter and physical events, most other modalities as well as the overall classification of consciousness processes present considerable difficulties in this respect. The confusion resulting from this situation manifests itself in the ambiguous, indiscriminate or enigmatic terminologies referring to these consciousness phenomena. This aspect of fuzziness prevails along the whole line of psychological cogitation, from the abstruse nomenclature of the Vedânta through the often very questionable concepts underlying certain modern psychological theories and tests to the obscure speculations of various mutually dissenting schools of psychoanalysis.

Kant recognized the subdivision of conscious activities into '*Erkennen, Fühlen und Wollen*' (cognition, affection and conation), established by other authors of that period; this useful classification was long upheld in standard treatises of psychology but has become superseded by the subsequent trends.

From an analysis of conscious experience psychology has shifted to the study of many other problems, such as behavior, the effect of physiological processes upon conscious phenomena, and the so-called unconscious of the psychoanalysts.

In his *Medical Psychology, Kretschmer* [1926] has presented an excellent practical subdivision of the consciousness-manifold. Like all systematizations of this type, it is of necessity, in some respects arbitrary, and subject to the intrinsic haziness of generalized thinking, but can be considered to be the most reasonable at the present time. It may be summarized as follows:

(1) Soul (psyche) is the name given to consciousness.

(2) Consciousness has a tendency to resolve itself by a grouping around two poles, namely the 'I' (ego, self), and the 'external world'. The zones of consciousness corresponding to the ego and to the external world complexes have ill-defined boundaries and overlap with wide, fluctuating border zones.

---

[12] The proper interpretation of cosmologic and cosmogonic events from the idealistic viewpoint was given above in chapter II, section 5, page 178.

(3) Consciousness phenomena display an interaction of ego and external world; the ego is influenced by the external world: limning processes (*'Abbildungsvorgänge'*, also translated as portrayal processes or reproductive processes), or can act upon the external world: expression processes (*'Ausdrucksvorgänge'*).

(4) To these limning processes and expression processes affectivity must be added as a third category of consciousness phenomena. Affectivity comprises all modalities which occur in the ego as an emotional component, superimposed on or blended with simple sensory impressions and perceptions, abstract concepts, reflections, decisions and resulting motor impulses. In other words, affectivity comprises all valuations and motives arising therefrom. Affectivity thus includes simple feelings such as pleasure and pain, like and dislike, enthusiasm and indifference, and complex emotional states such as love, anger, fear, hatred, desire, and others. The emotional modality may be positive, negative, nearly indifferent, or mixed (ambivalent).

Kretschmer's subdivision into limning processes, expression processes, and affectivity may be considered, but only to a certain degree, as analogous to the old psychologic classification distinguishing cognition, conation and affection. To *Kretschmer's* subdivisions must be added the concepts of intensity and vividity [*Semon*, 1920]. All complex consciousness phenomena, such as e.g. artistic or scientific activities, represent patterns of consciousness modalities involving attributes pertaining to all these subdivisions. Excessive influence of affectivity modifies limning as well as expression processes, and results in the 'hyponoic' and 'hypobulic' mechanisms of *Kretschmer's* terminology.[13] It appears, however, illegitimate to separate thought completely from feeling. This point was set forth by *Craik*.

Bertrand Russell emphasizes that mathematics has the advantage of teaching the habit of thinking without passion. It is true that affectivity plays a less apparent role in this scientific activity and is altogether eliminated from the relationships between the abstract mathematical concepts. Yet, the creative mathematician will be driven into his activity by his inner urge (affectivity) and will be impressed, as *Russell* affirms, by the beauty and exactitude of his science, while an uninterested student compelled to take up this subject will experience a negative emotional modality. Conversely, *Russell* [1927] states that the mathematician or physicist 'is liable to feel a kind of intellectual nausea when he finds himself among the uncertain and vague speculations of the less scientific sciences' such as physiology and psychology.

Through certain limning processes events may be reproduced in an attenuated, less vivid transposition by means of memories and abstractions,

---

[13] Hyponoic mechanisms correspond to *Bleuler's* autistic or dereistic thinking.

especially by those of verbal symbolism. These processes display a compelling tendency toward symbolic representation or duplication of significant patterns of consciousness modalities and their relationships. A most remarkable development of such limning processes manifests itself in scientific thought. Science or philosophy in general consists of a totality of knowledge, organized or classified essentially following the three principles emphasized by *Kant* and *Schopenhauer*: homogeneity (*entia praeter necessitatem non esse multiplicanda, Occam's Razor*), specification (*entium varietates non temere esse minuendas*), and continuity (*datur continuum formarum*). This results, as it were, in a reflection, image (*Abspiegelung*), or model of the entire phenomenal world in the symbolism of abstract concepts (ideas, '*Begriffe*'). In this respect, the remark by *Francis Bacon* in his treatise '*De dignitate et augmentis scientiarum*' (1623) may be quoted: '*Ea demum vera est philosophia, quae mundi ipsius voces fidelissime reddit et veluti dictante mundi conscripta est, et nihil alius est quam ejusdem simulacrum et reflectio, neque addit quidquam de proprio, sed tantum iterat et resonat.*'

With regard to the terms 'ideas' or 'concepts' in their denotation as 'abstractions' ('*Begriffe*'), *Schopenhauer* (vol. 1, p. 78) justly characterizes the latter as '*Vorstellungen von Vorstellungen*'.

Occam's principle and the principle of specification are of particular importance because both represent the application of the principle of sufficient reason to the assumption of entities. Both are, in fact, merely additional formulations of the *principium rationis sufficientis*.

As regards the various systems of knowledge providing abstract models of the phenomenal world, the views stressed by *Auguste Comte*, and resulting in the doctrine of positivism, might be briefly mentioned in this connection. *Comte* assumed three stages of philosophical cogitation: The theological, in which anthropomorphic will and purposes were assumed in order to explain natural events; the metaphysical, in which the theological explanations were replaced by depersonalized concepts, and finally the positive, in which simple description represents the highest form of knowledge. In other words, if an event is exhaustively described with all its implications, it is presumed to be fully understood.

The term 'description', however, is highly ambiguous. It may refer to definition, to an enumeration of spatial configurational features, moreover to an 'explanation' of either 'meaning'[14] or 'mode of action'. Explanation involves several sorts of procedures, such e.g. as (a) suitable symbolization of data by abstraction and generalization (these two overlap); (b) reduction of

---

[14] Again, the term 'meaning' is vague and ambiguous. *Ogden and Richards* [1946], in their treatise *The Meaning of Meaning*, give no less than 16 representative definitions. Cf. also the discussion in *K.* [1961, §59, pp. 260–277].

one group of concepts to another group of concepts, and (c) subsumption of the data under the principle of sufficient reason in one of its diverse aspects. This last procedure (c) is perhaps the most significant one and leads to that peculiar kind of mental (*sensu stricto*) experience characterized by the '*qualité pure*' of 'insight'. Procedure b on the other hand, may lead to the common type of 'explanation' by which 'unfamiliar' things, events, or relationships are stated in terms of familiar ones. This again may overlap with 'definition', concerning the 'what' which represents the 'referent', indicated by the definition. Explanation then concerns the 'how' and 'why'. Yet, in describing a mechanism, the 'how' also may include not only its structure but also the 'why' of its action. Again there is a difference in the questions: how do you do this?, and why do you do this?

It will thus be evident that 'positivism' referring to 'description' becomes a rather ambiguous term with different connotations and denotations.

Rigorous positivists substitute 'description' for 'explanation' and maintain that scientific procedure can never explain, but only describe, by an appropriate conceptual shorthand, our perceptual experiences. It is said that only the description 'how' but not the determinative 'why' can be understood.

Haeckel [1906], in his '*Lebenswunder*', objects to the term '*Beschreibende Naturwissenschaft*' (e.g. morphology) as contrasted with '*erklärende Naturwissenschaft*' (e.g. physics). He also disputes the claim of noted scientists such as *R. Virchow* (1821–1902) and *G. R. Kirchhoff* (1824–1887) that complete 'description' is the ultimate aim of natural sciences. It is evident that *Virchow* and *Kirchhoff* interpreted 'description' as including dynamic formulations in accordance with the *principium rationis sufficientis fiendi* (causality), while *Haeckel* distinguished mere description of facts ('*Beschreibung der einzelnen Tatsachen*') from explanation, which, in his opinion, must refer to 'causes' ('*Erklärung durch die bewirkenden Ursachen*'). The difference in opinion concerns here merely arbitrary questions of semantics.

Pure morphology refers essentially to the *principium rationis sufficientis essendi*. Systematics, respectively taxonomy, refer to both *principium rationis sufficientis cognoscendi et essendi*, to which, likewise, mathematics refer. Logic refers exclusively to *principium rationis sufficientis cognoscendi*. The *principium rationis sufficientis fiendi* (causality) plays no role at all, or at least only a very marginal one, in these sciences. One can hardly talk of 'causal mathematics' or 'causal logic' although dynamic (causal) factors can be formulated in mathematical or logical terms,[15] and can be introduced into 'explanations' of morphologic and taxonomic relationships.

---

[15] For instance the application of logic in the form of *Boolean algebra* to electrical circuit processes by *Shannon* [1938].

In an extreme formulation, positivism contends (1) that scientific assertions are meaningless if they cannot be directly verified by experiments, and
(2) that questions inherently unanswerable through our senses are meaningless questions.

This type of positivism has been adopted by a number of contemporary
physicists, mathematicians and logicians, especially by those quantum theo-
rists denying causality. In support of this denial, it has been pointed out, inter
alia, that no experiment can prove causality. To this, it can be replied that
experiments are not undertaken in order to prove causality, but on the
contrary because our thought mechanisms presuppose causality, which, as
elaborated above in section 2 of chapter II, cannot be proved. The ex-
perimenter, explicitly or implicitly (subconsciously, intuitively), investigates
the relationships between phenomena on the basis of the dynamic principle of
causality, even if he denies this latter.

I disagree thus with said extreme brand of positivism, since I believe that
descriptions must be correlated with the principles of orderliness emphasized
by *Kant, Schopenhauer*, and others; in this respect, *Planck* [1931] emphasized
the significance of causal thinking and the irrelevance of positivism in the
analysis of physical events. Some further remarks about positivism will be
included below in the discussion of the views of *Mach*, who may be considered
a strict positivist.

As regards allegedly the inherently meaningless questions unanswerable
through our senses, it will be recalled (cf. chapter II, section 1, p. 4) that
Planck, in a manner still more explicit than in a similar statement by *Einstein*,
formulated the following two canons of natural philosophy:

(1) There is a real outer world which exists independently of our act of
knowing.

(2) The real outer world is not directly knowable.

My own formulation is only slightly different and can be condensed in the
following two sentences:

(1) There is a real orderliness x independent of (my, our, or any)
consciousness.

(2) This independent reality is both transcendental and transcendent. It
remains therefore unknowable.

This formulation differs from that of *Planck* by omitting the term 'outer'
which I consider meaningless, and by omitting the term 'world' which I
consider somewhat inappropriate because of too many possibly misleading
denotations and connotations. Said two propositions contain the gist of
transcendental neutralism which shall be discussed with further details in the
final section 10 of the present chapter. It can here, however, already be stated
that, although in some respects comparable to so-called 'neutral monism',
transcendental neutralism is definitely dualistic, since it assumes two funda-

mentally different realities, namely the actuality (reality in the second sense) of pluralistic consciousness (innumerable disjoint consciousness manifolds), and the unknowable but necessarily obtaining reality in the first sense, 'existing' independently of consciousness (i.e. when there is no consciousness). Said reality, devoid of the space-time attributes of consciousness, and therefore neither 'mental *sensu strictiori*', nor 'material' ('mental *sensu latiori*'), i.e. 'neutral', can only be conceived as 'orderliness x'.

Although I consider myself a positivist since I believe that epistemologic argumentation must begin with an analysis of the given (conscious) perception, with particular emphasis on sensory percepts or on the basis of what *Schopenhauer* called '*Anschauung*',[16] or '*anschauliche Vorstellungen*', it is evident that, in the view of extreme positivists, transcendental neutralism represents the answer to a meaningless question, respectively a meaningless answer to a question unanswerable through our senses. In contradiction to such positivists, I maintain that said answer provides the best attainable 'insight' (of which extreme positivists are lacking) into the unsolvable problem of 'existence'.

Depending on initial viewpoint and emphasis, numerous positivistic systems can be constructed. Such positivistic systems in the wider sense include the doctrines of *Avenarius*, of *Husserl*, and of existentialist authors who, which a certain justification, stress the contents rather than the formal aspects of thought experience. All these systems are, in *Kretschmer's* terminology, limning processes; all the cited systems may thus, to a certain extent, reproduce some aspects of the phenomenal world, although I have failed to be impressed by their results. Positivism in some of its more sophisticated presentations might be termed an incomplete or inconsistent idealism and figuratively speaking, leads, I believe, into a blind alley. Moreover, the argumentations of extreme positivists do not seem to be particularly well adapted to an analysis of the relationships between brain and consciousness, which is the theme of my inquiry.

In this respect I believe that the concepts of fictional physical matter[17] and of consciousness (mind) are[18] highly useful, practical, and logically unobjectionable. I have therefore chosen both the materialistic and the idealistic

---

[16] The following comments by *Schopenhauer* are here of interest: '*dass der Kern aller Erkenntnis die anschauliche Vorstellung ist*' [vol. 2, p. 93]. '*Der gegebene Stoff jeder Philosophie ist demnach kein anderer als das empirische Bewusstseyn*' [vol. 2, p. 96]. '*Nur soviel lässt sich behaupten, dass jedes ächte Philosophem zu ihrem Kern, oder ihrer Wurzel, irgend eine anschauliche Auffassung haben muss*' [vol. 3, p. 121].

[17] Cf. the definition of 'matter' as fictional R-events in section 5, page 180 of chapter II.

[18] Cf. the definition of mind *sensu latiori* as consciousness in chapter I, page 2, chapter II, section 5, page 172, and as P-events in chapter II, section 5, page 180.

approach, purposely ignoring an extreme positivistic approach, although I am not unfamiliar with such positivism and its claims.

All abstract systems are subject to the inherent haziness of generalization and symbolization, even if they significantly reproduce certain aspects of relationships. Symbols may be regarded as mnestic shades of more vivid and substantial consciousness modalities. If we attempt to penetrate beyond the realm of relatedness linked to direct experience, we find ourselves in a predicament somewhat similar to that of the inhabitants of *E. A. Abbott's* 'Flatland' with regard to the properties of three-dimensional space.

Nevertheless, despite the shadowy aspect of abstract symbols, their instrumental value yields powerful effects. This is well expressed in a mathematical poem by *Clarence R. Wylie, Jr.*, entitled 'Paradox', which appeared in the July 1948 issue of the *Scientific Monthly*; it was used as motto by *R. B. Kershner* and *L. R. Wilcox* for their interesting text *The Anatomy of Mathematics* [1950]:

> Not truth, nor certainty. These I forswore
> I my novitiate, as young men called
> To holy orders must abjure the world.
> "If ..., then ...", this only I assert;
> And my successes are but pretty chains
> Linking twin doubts, for it is vain to ask
> If what I postulate be justified,
> Or what I prove possess the stamp of fact.
>
> Yet bridges stand, and men no longer crawl
> In two dimensions. And such triumphs stem
> In no small measure from the power this game,
> Played with the thrice-attenuated shades
> Of things, has over their originals.
> How frail the wand, but how profound the spell!

In this connection it is also important to keep in mind the relevant comments by *Einstein* [1954, 1959] in his lecture 'Geometry and Experience' [19]; 'How can it be that mathematics, being after all a product of human thought which is independent of experience, is so admirable appropriate to the objects of reality? Is human reason then, without experience, merely by taking thought, able to fathom the properties of real things?'

To these questions it can be answered that mathematics [cf. §64, 'significance of Mathematics' in *K.*, 1961, pp. 288–302] doubtless originated from experience, namely from observation which became translated into logical propositions by the orderliness óf Human thought. Again, the orderliness of actuality (objects of reality in the second sense) as well as the orderliness of the

---

[19] Lecture given under the title *'Geometrie und Erfahrung'* before the Prussian Academy of Sciences, January 27, 1921.

brain mechanisms (pertaining to actuality) can be conceived as a manifestation of the orderliness x. In this respect, the old saying, attributed to *Plato*, and often quoted to me by my father, has indeed a profound meaning representing a metaphorical 'truth':

"Ἀεὶ Θεὸς γεωμετρεῖ'.

On the other hand, as regards fathoming the properties of real things, it is necessary to distinguish (a) real things in the second sense, that is to say actual experienced material events, (b) thought models of such events, and (c) real things in the first sense. It is evident that these latter, representing the orderliness x, remain intrinsically unknowable and unintelligible. With respect to the events (a) and their thought models (b), the large number of both known and unknown 'causes' respectively parameters ('*Zustandsbedingungen*') must be kept in mind, whereby constraints, such as boundary conditions or boundary values are imposed upon the abstract mathematical formulations. While these latter are absolutely certain and indisputable, their application to reality (in the second sense), although indispensable and, in general, astonishingly valid, is not. This was clearly recognized by *Einstein*, who, with remarkable insight, stated: 'As far as the propositions of mathematics refer to reality, they are not certain; and as far as they are certain, they do not refer to reality.'

8. Imperfect Idealists: Th. Ziehen, E. Mach, Bertrand Russell

The treatment of the space-time problem is, in my opinion, the main criterion of any genuine idealistic viewpoint. Idealism does not recognize the existence of any space-time outside of consciousness and maintains that material objects only exist through being perceived. Time may thus be defined as that aspect of consciousness wherein consciousness phenomena appear as a succession of events. Space is accordingly that aspect of consciousness in which phenomena display simultaneous (compresent) reciprocal relations, characterized as location and, in many instances, as spatial configuration. Matter can then be defined as the causal (dynamic) aspect of spatially configurated events in this perceptual space-time.

The fiction of a physical space-time is postulated by materialistic theories of epistemology so that orderly relationships independent of consciousness may be expressed in the language of consciousness. But, as far as epistemologic analysis is concerned, physical space-time can be considered an unnecessary auxiliary construction which may be well dispensed with if the abstract principle of orderliness is substituted. The elimination of physical space-time in idealistic epistemology could be compared to the elimination of ether in relativistic physics.

Among the many authors dealing with epistemological subjects, *Th. Ziehen*, *E. Mach*, and *Bertrand Russell* have expounded, in a particularly penetrating way, several important aspects of the idealistic approach without however, reaching conclusions fully consistent with a genuinely idealistic interpretation. These writers are of special interest by reason of their scientific background: medicine, physics, and mathematics.

Theodor Ziehen (1862–1950), a successful psychiatrist at the University of Jena, and a very competent brain anatomist, author of the encyclopedic, but unfortunately not completed *Anatomie des Zentralnervensystems* (1899–1934) in *Bardeleben's* Handbook, changed his career to philosophy and became Professor of Philosophy at the University of Halle. In his numerous epistemological publications, whose gist is well summarized in '*Grundlagen der Naturphilosophie*' [1922], the phenomenal world, termed the '*Gignomene*', is conceived as a mental experience. We do not experience the sun in the concept of the physicist, but merely as a complex of sensations from which we infer that there exists a celestial body in the interpretation of the astronomer. This well-known and obvious argumentation, coinciding with the formulation of *Bertrand Russell* quoted above in the definition of the idealistic approach, is emphasized as the fundamental idealistic principle ('*idealistisches Grundprinzip*').

Ziehen then distinguishes one particular class of 'gignomena' which he calls '*Empfindungsgignomene*' representing that which I prefer to call sensory percepts, from '*Erinnerung oder Vorstellung*', namely from that which I prefer to call extrasensory percepts.[20]

Ziehen then postulates an objective and a subjective component of sensations, that is to say of his '*Empfindungsgignomene*' The subjective or N-component is related to the function of sense organs and nervous system, the objective or R-component (reduced component) is independent of the activity of a nervous system. The orderliness of N-components is that of consciousness and is designated as the orderliness of 'parallel laws' (*Parallelgesetze*). The orderliness of R-components is that of causal laws.

---

[20] It will be seen that '*Vorstellung*' in *Schopenhauer's* terminology corresponds to *Ziehen's* entire '*Gignomene*', while *Ziehen's* '*Vorstellung*' essentially corresponds to *Schopenhauer's* '*Begriffe*', i.e. '*Vorstellungen von Vorstellungen*'.

It is of interest that *Hume* distinguished the following sorts of Human perceptions: (a) impressions, and (b) ideas. Impressions are characterized by greater vividity, and include both what I designate as sensory percepts and as the affectivity or the emotions of extrasensory percepts. *Hume's* 'ideas' are the thought concepts as well as the memories pertaining to extrasensory percepts, i.e. essentially *Ziehen's* '*Vorstellungen*'. It will also be recalled that *Berkeley* distinguished 'ideas imprinted on the senses' (sensory percepts) as the 'real things', and those excited in the imagination as 'images of things' (extrasensory percepts). Both sorts, however, exist in the mind 'and in this sense are ideas' [*Berkeley*, 1710].

The task of 'natural philosophy', according to *Ziehen*, is the reduction of the *'Gignomene'*, namely the elimination of the N-components, whereby the general attributes of the R-components in the given *'Gignomene'* are ascertained. *Ziehen's* R-components essentially correspond to what could be called physicalisms, namely to the concepts of mass (inertia), energy, and electric charge in an 'objective', i.e. public space-time system, as conceived by the contemporary physicists. He is, however, compelled to admit that both the 'static' and the 'dynamic' model of R-components remain insufficiently clarified.[21] However, he very definitely attributes space-time properties to his R-components,[22] and claims that the *'Lokalität'* and the *'Temporalität'* of the *'Gignomene'* (i.e. of consciousness) is based (*'beruht'*) on the space-time attributes of the R-components. He claims, moreover, that *'Lokalität'* essentially (*'im wesentlichen'*) pertains to the *'Empfindungsgignomene'* (i.e. the sensory percepts) while *'Temporalität'* pertains to all gignomena. He evidently fails here to distinguish between spatial localization and spatial configuration; while all percepts, sensory and extrasensory are spatially localized, however vaguely or, *per contra*, distinctly, not even all Human sensory percepts are spatially configurated.

Turning now to *Ziehen's* N-components, it is evident that he failed to take into account several relevant points: (1) the nervous system, including the brain, would also, according to his concepts, consist of R-components; (2) the relevant function of the components of the nervous system is the transmission of signals, transduced by the sensory (afferent) nerve endings and processed by the brain; although, as activities of the nervous system, we would here have N-components according to *Ziehen*, most of these activities remain unconscious and do not display the orderliness of *Ziehen's* 'parallel laws'; (3) only some but by no means all activities of N-components are concomitant with consciousness, thereby resulting in the *'Gignomene'*.

It can thus be said that *Ziehen's* theory, for which he coins the term binomism (*Binomismus*), represents a modified version of psychophysical parallelism. Since *Ziehen* assumes causal processes in a physical space-time

---

[21] '*So muss unbedingt zugestanden werden, dass sehr viele wesentliche Fragen noch nicht endgültig beantwortet worden sind; nur einige grobe Umrisse des allgemeinen Weltbildes zeichnen sich etwas deutlicher ab.*'

[22] *Ziehen*, who apparently failed to understand *Berkeley's* and *Hume's* convincing arguments with regard to the so-called 'primary qualities', but merely criticizes the much less conclusive arguments elaborated by *Kant*, states '*dass auch den R-Bestandteilen Lokalität zukommt, und wenn diese Lokalität auch in einzelnen Punkten von derjenigen der Empfindungs-gignomene abweicht, so besteht doch andererseits eine sehr weitgehende Analogie*'. He then adds: '*Um aber jede Verwechselung zu vermeiden, habe ich vorgeschlagen, die lokalen Eigenschaften der R-Bestandteile als "lokativische" zu bezeichnen. Auch für die Temporalität kommen wir zu dem Schluss, dass sie den R-Bestandteilen selbst zukommt.*'

independent of consciousness, his R-components correspond to the concept of matter, despite his objections to the term matter and regardless of his assertions that the term matter does not convey any definite meaning.

From the idealistic standpoint, *Ziehen's* views represent materialism and can thus be rejected as an inadmissible extrapolation from consciousness into the independent orderliness of which consciousness is an expression. Yet, *Ziehen's* approach includes many valuable arguments. In accordance with modified criteria, the distinction of R- and N-components can be upheld (1) by substituting the term 'events' for 'components' and (2) by distinguishing two sorts of N-events, namely N-events not correlated with consciousness, and Np-events correlated with consciousness. Conscious events, in turn, that is to say *Ziehen's* '*Gignomene*', then represent a third sort of events, namely P-events (parallel events). Instead of *Ziehen's* '*Binomismus*', we have thus a '*Trinomismus*', or a 'trialistic' model of R-events, N-events, and P-events as elaborated on page 180, section 5 of chapter II. It is evident that the weakness of *Ziehen's* concept results from an insufficient analysis of what he called N-components.

One could, in fact, even speak of a quadrinomismus, if, since not all N-events but only Np-events are correlated with P-events (consciousness), the distinction between N-events and Np-events is emphasized. On the other hand, it should be recalled that not only R-events, but all N-events (including Np-events) are physicalisms, which might be called R-events *sensu latiori*. R-events *sensu strictiori* are, of course, only those physicalisms which, acting upon sensory endings, become by these latter transduced into N-events (i.e. 'signals'). The relevant cut, of course, is that between P-events, which are actually experienced, and Np-events representing physicalisms, i.e. R-events *sensu latiori*, which, on the basis of P-events are merely imagined and must be considered fictions.

One may, of course, also observe N-events in one's own brain or in other brains by means of the EEG. But, if so observed, then these N-events represent P-events of the observer, who merely interprets said P-events as representing the fictional N-events.

Again, from still another viewpoint, all physicalisms or R-events *sensu latiori* represent public data as discussed in section 6 of chapter III.

Nevertheless, in its modified formulation, *Ziehen's* distinction of N- and R-components does provide, within the postulated fictional materialistic concept, a useful model of the anorganic and the organic world, including physiological psychology. This model is well suitable for an analysis of the manner in which temporal and spatial relationships, that is events in the postulated fictional physical world, are coded in terms of mental processes.

Ziehen's analysis of the organic world, in his 1922 treatise as well as in his later epistemologic writings, is obsolescent insofar as he dealt with the problems of evolution and heredity before the significance of the nucleic acids was generally understood, and before the subsequent progress in macromolecular chemistry and communication respectively information theory opened the way for a better understanding of biological problems. His overall conclusions, however, were, already in 1922, entirely valid, and summarized as follows: '*Der Weltbegriff, den wir auf die Untersuchung der anorganischen Natur gegründet hatten, ist durch die Untersuchung der organischen nicht umgestossen, ja nicht einmal wesentlich modifiziert worden. Die Komplikationen und damit die Erklärungsschwierigkeiten haben ausserordentlich zugenommen, aber die letzten Elemente und daher die letzten Erklärungsprinzipien sind dieselben geblieben*'.

Ernst Mach (1838–1916), an Austrian physicist of considerable merit, became in the last phase of his academic career, Professor of the Philosophy of Science in Vienna. His name as a physicist is at present widely known through the *Mach number* (ratio of air speed to speed of sound), significant in problems of suprasonic flight.

In his fundamental epistemologic treatise '*Die Analyse der Empfindungen und das Verhältnis des Physischen zum Psychischen*' [posthumous 9th ed., 1922], *Mach* elaborates the thesis that our world is built up of sensations or perceptions[23] (*Empfindungen*) which he interprets as elements. Matter is not conceived as anything given, but merely as a 'thought symbol' for a relative stable complex of sensory elements. He suggests that the laws of physics may be formulated as functional relations between perceptions such as warm, hard, color sensations, and others; he includes among these elements space and time in terms of space perceptions and time perceptions: '*Farben, Töne, Wärmen, Drücke, Räume, Zeiten usw. sind in mannigfaltiger Weise miteinander verknüpft und an dieselben sind Stimmungen, Gefühle und Willen gebunden.*' He emphasizes, however, that, since the world must be interpreted in terms of functional relations between these elements, it cannot be regarded as a mere sum of these sensations.

Mach intended to use a terminology suitable for a unified language of science and characterized by the most economical formulae ('*Ökonomie des Denkens*'). All metaphysical propositions were to be eliminated and he regarded both materialism and idealism as metaphysical propositions which cannot be stated in terms of a genuine scientific problem. These tendencies and opinions of *Mach* have been further developed in the voluminous writings of authors belonging to the so-called *Vienna Circle* and associated groups.

---

[23] This, of course, is merely a paraphrase of *Hume's* statement [1739, vol. 1, part IV, section II]: 'We may observe that all what we call a *mind*, is nothing but a heap or collection of different perceptions, united together by certain relations, and supposed, though falsely, to be endowed with a perfect simplicity and identity.'

Concerning the Unity of Science Movement which is closely related to logical positivism, *Craik* [1943] has advanced the following criticism: 'There is a good deal of evidence that the precise definitions of the symbolic logicians and the logical positivists do not, in fact, cover very much of the range even of sensory experience.[24] As *Haldane* [1938] remarks, logistic 'will only work for material that has certain highly abstract properties, which are rather less frequently and much less completely exemplified in the real world than logicians would like us to believe'.

This remark is very appropriate and characterizes the intrinsic weakness of all philosophical systems based on empty abstractions or on mere syntax language (e.g. those of *Hegel, Carnap, Bertrand Russell, Wittgenstein, etc.*).

---

[24] That simplified purely logical concepts are often inadequate as models for real events (real in the second sense) is clearly evidenced by the well-known chicken paradox: what came first, the chicken for the egg?

From the viewpoint of evolution, we might assume in physical space-time an uninterrupted causal line from inanimate matter to the present-day chick. This line might lead through prebiotic and prokaryote organic structures, eukaryote protozoan-like structures, various metazoan forms, and amphibian-like forms, to sauropsidan and finally chick characteristics. Whether by micro- or macromutations, we might assume a large number of either disjoint, e.g. 'sudden' or of practical infinitesimal steps. It would furthermore presumably be arbitrary to designate, toward the end of this process, any single cyclic step, such as fertilized egg or hatched individual, as the first hen egg or the first chick.

Or again: *Achilles* cannot overtake the tortoise. This venerable paradox, proposed about 470 BC by *Zeno of Elea*, actually resolves itself into a modification of the expression: $(1 + 1/2 + 1/4 + 1/8 + 1/16 \ldots) < 2$. The imaginary *Achilles* obviously cannot catch up the imaginary tortoise if the required time, by an imaginary process of gradual fractionalization, amounting to a progressive slowdown, is brought to a virtual stop. More accurately, such a series would have 2 (for any other value applying to the particular case) as its limit. Mathematicians have given a number of different explanations and solutions. Thus, although *Achilles* and the tortoise allegedly occupy, in the same number of distinct successive moments, the same number of distinct points (whatever this may mean), *Achilles* could yet travel further than the tortoise because, in accordance with *Cantor's* concept of an infinite class, a whole does not have more terms than one of its parts.

Again, the gist of *Gödel's* much discussed paper '*Über formal unentscheidbare Sätze der Principia Mathematica und verwandter Systeme*' [M. H. Math. Phys. *38:* 173–198, 1931] may be interpreted as a demonstration that (1) if a logistic system is consistent, then it is incomplete, and (2) that the consistency of a logical system cannot be established by any reasoning in conformity with the rules of that particular system.

It is now well recognized by many mathematicians that theorems of logic and pure mathematics represent tautological systems. Although the notion of tautology does not entirely coincide with *Kant's* concept of *a priori* synthetic judgements, it is very closely and significantly related to *Kant's* concept. From the neurological viewpoint, theorems of logic and pure mathematics are both synthetic and *a priori* insofar as they merely represent functional expressions of a given neural structure. In addition, it may be pertinent to quote here *Bertrand Russels's* dictum that pure mathematics is the subject in which we do not know what we are talking about, nor whether what we are saying is true.

Craik [1943] also justly comments that 'admittedly the phenomenologists give a somewhat more sophisticated statement of their position, and evade all questions as to where sense data exist, what status they have, or how they are related to each other or to us'.

This very interesting remark points out the fallacy that sensations respectively percepts could independently exist as combining and recombining 'elements', without spatio-temporal relationships to a given consciousness-manifold pertaining to a perceptual ('real' in the second sense) brain, said manifold being a 'gestalt property' of the manifested correlated percepts. The fallacy of 'floating' and 'status-less' percepts is the opposite to that which postulates a perceiving 'soul', 'mind', 'spirit', 'self' or 'subject' as the perceiver.[25]

Notwithstanding *Mach's* endeavor to minimize or even to deny the conformity of certain aspects of his views with the idealistic concept as outlined above, several significant agreements obtain. This conformity concerns the world as a combination of percepts (sensations), the essential identity of psychic and physical phenomena, the concept of matter as a mere abstraction, the principle of orderliness (functional relationships in *Mach's* terminology), and the non-existence of a substantial self.

Considered from the idealistic approach, *Mach's* thesis displays several weaknesses. In his attempt at epistemological analysis, *Mach* rejects the methodological solipsistic approach and does not recognize the import of individual consciousness manifolds, although he emphasizes the fundamental significance of sensations. Yet, as just stated above, the term sensation conveys a meaning only if conceived as a modality within a given consciousness field. Such modalities are inconstant, variable and transient, appearing, disappearing and reappearing. Furthermore, sensations or percepts not sensed by any one are no sensations and cannot either be hypostatized as elements constituting a world independent of consciousness nor can they be reified as integrals simultaneously or successively entering into or withdrawing from functional relationships pertaining to a number of different consciousness fields.

A non-sensed sensation is a *contradictio in adjecto*; a vanished sensation has lost identity as well as entity, and may be conceived as disintegrated into a complex of orderly relationships.

Mach conceives space and time ('*Räume und Zeiten*') as a plurality of percepts or elements ('*Raumempfindungen*' etc.) comparable to other elements

---

[25] The statements 'no percept without a perceiver' or 'no object without a subject' are merely valid if referring to percepts as components of a consciousness manifold respectively private perceptual space-time system. This latter, as such, has no existence or actuality, except for its correlated and organized percepts.

of his terminology. Contrarily, according to the idealistic interpretation, perceptual space-time is not a sensation, but the fundamental attribute of all conscious phenomena. It may also be expressed as the 'background' of all sensations.

Eliminating consciousness, only non-qualifiable orderly relationships remain; insofar as these may concern similar events in different consciousness manifolds, such relationships can be designated as public data which, however, have little resemblance with the reified perceptions ('*Empfindungen*') or elements of *Mach*.

It is feasible, in conformity with the principles included in *Kretschmer's* concept of limning processes, to devise a model of the phenomenal world in *Mach's* terminology. However, the resulting system, despite many constructive, valid and intellectually stimulating features appears as a rather chaotic fabric of elements; but in any case, it represents an interesting thesis:

> 'For let Philosopher and Doctor preach
> Of what they will, and what they will not – each
>   Is but one Link in an eternal Chain
> That none can slip, nor break, nor over-reach.'
> (*FitzGerald's Omar*, 1868, LXXVII)

It is perhaps possible to accept *Mach's* contention that his doctrine is neither idealism nor materialism, although this must remain a matter of opinion; emphasizing the concept of (hypostatized) elements, *Mach's* views may be described as an expression of neutralism. However, *Mach's* system is encumbered with many ambiguities; the very different and even contradictory opinions about his doctrine, expressed by different authors, are thus easily understandable. Despite *Mach's* repeated protests, diverse features of his system might be interpreted as identical with certain aspects of *Berkeley's* and *Hume's* views. On the other hand *Mach* acknowledges, as regards his concept of the ego, its close agreement with the *anâtman* (*anattâ*, Pâli) doctrine of Buddhism [1922, p.291]. There is, moreover, a further evident, although distant kinship between *Mach's* elements and the attributes designated as *khandhas* (Pâli) or *skandhas* (sanskrit) in Buddhism, especially as interpreted in the positivistic teachings of Southern or Pâli-Buddhism (Hinayâna).

Bertrand Russell, despite various considerable weaknesses, is justly regarded as an eminently lucid writer, both in his style and in his thoughts. His approach to the problems of epistemology follows, on the whole, the argumentation designated by *Ziehen* as the fundamental idealistic principle. Nevertheless, his views seem to imply the assumption of a physical space-time independent of consciousness. While his concepts cannot be considered idealism they certainly do not represent naive materialism. *Russell* tends towards a construction of neutral monism or neutralism: 'Mental events and their qualities can be known without inference, but physical events are known only as regards their space-time structure. The qualities that compose such events are unknown – so completely unknown that we cannot say either that they are or that they are not different from the qualities that we know as belonging to mental events.' The traditional separation of mind and matter is considered untenable; the two may be brought together, not by subordinating either to the other, but by displaying each as a logical structure composed of what may be called 'neutral stuff'.

From the idealistic viewpoint one might reply that mind *sensu latiori* (i.e. consciousness) is experienced; its structure is thus not composed of 'neutral stuff' but of sensations, percepts, feelings, thoughts etc., while the logical structure of matter is an abstract construction, referring to the orderly relationship of certain events experienced in consciousness. Therefore matter, which actually consists of sensory percepts or of thoughts about matter, should be subordinated to mind *sensu latiori*, i.e. consciousness.

With regard to *Russell's* 'neutralism', which, except for the space-time problem is closely similar to my own concept of transcendental neutralism, it should again be emphasized that the term 'neutral monism' is erroneous, because said 'monism' in no way eliminates the evident dualism of (1) consciousness, and (2) unconscious 'existence', or in other words, the dualism of (1) a mental (conscious) world, and (2) an extramental world. The fundamental difference between these two 'worlds' is obvious.

I shall briefly refer to a few additional pertinent statements by *Bertrand Russell*, and endeavor to show that in a somewhat modified formulation, these statements may be perfectly consistent with the idealistic concept.

We can, according to *Russell*, adopt the view that all our perceptions are causally related to antecedents which may not be perceptions. Since in our premises causal relations were strictly defined as the *principium rationis sufficientis fiendi*, I would rather express *Russell's* statement as follows: we can adopt the view that all our perceptions are related to an unknown which is not perception. This relationship cannot be regarded as causal nor as functional in a mathematically expressible sense, but merely logically as an undefined 'relation' according to the *principium rationis sufficientis actualitatis*.

Again, according to *Russell*, 'the spatial relations of physics hold between electrons, protons, neutrons, etc., which we do not perceive; the spatial relations of visual percepts hold between things that we do perceive, and in the last analysis between colored patches'.

While the second half of this statement is incontestable, the first half may be reformulated in the following fashion: our observation of certain phenomena reveals an orderliness which, on the basis of inferences and when expressed in the symbolism of our consciousness, can be conceived in fictional terms of spatial relations between electrons, protons, neutrons, etc.

It should here be added that we may indeed 'perceive' electrons and protons with respect to their 'tracks', and even neutrons with respect to their collision effects, as discussed and illustrated in section 1 of chapter II.

In summing up a discussion of 'space in psychology', *Russell* states: 'When I have the experience called "seeing a table", the visual table has, primarily, a position in the space of my momentary visual field. Then, by means of experienced correlations, it has a position in a space which embraces all my perceptual experiences. Next, by means of physical laws it is correlated with a place in physical space-time, namely the place occupied by the physical table. Finally, by means of psychophysical laws it is related to another place in physical space-time, namely the place occupied by my brain as a physical object.'

The first two sentences of this statement, again, are incontestable. From the strictly idealistic viewpoint, the remainder of the statement might have the following formulation: Next, by means of abstract reasoning I am able to construct the fictional concepts of physical laws and of a physical space-time in which I assume a physical table, correlated with my visual table, to be located. Finally, I may introduce the supposition of a psychophysical law, relating the postulated physical table to another place in physical space-time, namely the place occupied by my brain as an assumed physical object.[26]

9. Summary and Critique of Idealism

In the preceding sections I have presented my own interpretation of the idealistic approach, stressing some of the points which, in my opinion, appear particularly relevant. I do not, however, contend that any of these views are either original or new; all the arguments or ideas reviewed were either explicitly or implicitly expressed, although perhaps in more or less different context, in different formulations and sometimes with different conclusions, in the writings of *Descartes, Spinoza, Locke, Hume, Berkeley, Kant, Schopenhauer* and *Vaihinger*. As regards the numerous more recent authors, I have particularly referred to *Ziehen, Mach*, and *Bertrand Russell*. There is furthermore a certain resemblance between the concept of an individual consciousness manifold which I am emphasizing, and *Leibniz'* highly ambiguous notion of a monad, presumably borrowed from *Giordano Bruno*.

The resulting formulation of transcendental neutralism, which recognizes the dualism of a mental (conscious) and extramental (non-conscious) 'world', is, nevertheless, as I believe, a new and independent synthesis of the valid epistemologic viewpoints contained in the writings of *Locke* (1632–1704),

---

[26] This 'psychophysical law', involving psychophysical parallelism, is evidently the fictional *principium rationis sufficientis percipiendi*.

George Berkeley (1684–1750), *Hume* (1711–1776), *Kant* (1724–1804), *Schopenhauer* (1788–1860), and *Vaihinger* (1851–1933). Reduced to the simplest terms, it could be said that *Locke* firmly established empiricism (or positivism *sensu strictiori*), *Berkeley* showed that there is no physical 'matter', *Hume* showed that there is no 'mind' as a substantial 'self' or 'spirit', thus independently rediscovering the *anâtman principle* of Buddhism, and *Kant* emphasized the distinction between phenomena (consciousness, perception, '*Erscheinung*', '*Vorstellung*') and independent reality in the first sense.[27] *Schopenhauer* recognized that our world of consciousness is a brain phenomenon, and *Vaihinger* elaborated a notable concept of *fictionalism*, suitable for coping with the intrinsically unsolvable brain paradox.

Summarizing the conclusions resulting from the idealistic approach, we may now formulate the following propositions:

(1) The given, experienced, or phenomenal world consists exclusively of more or less definitely localized consciousness modalities constituting a temporal flow; certain classes of these modalities display, in addition, a definite spatial (geometric or topologic) configuration. Time and space can be assumed to be exclusive attributes of consciousness; perceptual space-time, accordingly, might be the only actually existing space-time. All consciousness modalities are interrelated in an orderly manner and manifest an enduring orderliness throughout a continual succession of consciousness events, whereby nothing remains permanent (πάντα ῥεῖ, *Heraclitus*).

(2) Consciousness modalities occur within a solipsistic individual consciousness manifold, which is not directly related to merely inferred other similar consciousness manifolds. Indirectly, however, different consciousness manifolds are interrelated through orderly relationships or 'norms' which may be designated as public data. The orderliness manifesting itself as public data must be conceived as not pertaining to the domain of space-time but can, by introducing a fiction in *Vaihinger's* sense, be imagined as representing 'physicalisms' in a postulated public physical space-time system. Each individual consciousness manifold is characterized by its own set of private perceptual space-time dimensions.

(3) Within an individual consciousness manifold, no definite limit between self and not-self or between ego and external world can be maintained.

---

[27] *Kant*, particularly in the first edition of his '*Kritik der reinen Vernunft*' stressed the significance of space and time as the given 'forms' or 'attributes' of consciousness. This, however, although less clearly formulated, is very definitely and implicitly indicated in the treatises of *Berkeley* and *Hume*. *Kant's* 'proofs' concerning that topic, moreover, are weaker than the argumentations of his cited predecessors and suffer from an untenable concept of 'knowledge *a priori*'.

Ego and non-ego are fluctuating concepts which may be arbitrarily assigned to certain groups of consciousness modalities.

(4) There is furthermore no essential difference between mind (*sensu strictiori*) and matter. The term mind in this denotation comprises poorly localized and spatially not configurated extrasensory consciousness modalities such as feelings, memories, and thoughts; the term matter covers well-localized and mostly spatially configurated sensory consciousness modalities representing the body and the external world.

Although the boundary between the mental and the physical may thus be regarded as artificial, it is possible, by postulating a fictional physical space-time, to express the orderliness of relationships between modalities of the latter class in terms of physical laws determining the character and duration of so-called objects of perception without any reference to the fact that they are perceived: 'In the establishment of such laws the propositions of physics do not presuppose any propositions of psychology or even the existence of mind' (*Bertrand Russell*).

(5) Modalities classifiable as material, seem, however, to play a special role in consciousness insofar as verifiable experience shows that the occurrence of consciousness depends upon the function of the brain which is, in the above sense, a 'material' complex. We may nevertheless state that consciousness is not localized in the brain, but that the body, including the brain, and the external world become localized in consciousness. We face in this respect the repeatedly mentioned brain paradox apparently involving a vicious circle[28] which can be expressed as follows: consciousness is a brain phenomenon, but the brain itself, as we know it, is a phenomenon of consciousness; or more pointedly: consciousness is a brain phenomenon, but the brain itself is a brain phenomenon.

---

[28] This vicious circle represents a *circulus in definiendo*, the material brain, a notion or potential percept, that is a brain phenomenon, being defined in terms of itself. Cyclic definitions are exemplified by the well-known barber paradox, in which the *Barber of Seville* is defined as follows: he shaves all those men of Seville and only those men of Seville who do not shave themselves. It is then asked 'who shaves the *Barber of Seville*?'; if the *Barber* shaves himself, then he does not shave himself, and if he does not, then he does. It has been said that whatever involves all of a collection must not be one of the collection. We have furthermore classes which are members of themselves and others which are not members of themselves. But is the class composed of those classes which are not members of themselves a member of itself or not? Thus, we again obtain the logical paradox. *Whitehead* and *Russell* attempt to solve such difficulties by their axiom of reducibility, which, however, has not been generally accepted. Definitions by recursion, as developed by *Peano* and *Frege*, or by the set theory of Zermelo, have been substituted.

As regards the well-known barber paradox (cf. section 6 of chapter II), the apparently precise logical definition does not sufficiently account for the functional configuration of the

Continued on p. 246

(6) In the terminology of the idealistic approach, the problem of brain-consciousness contingency may finally be formulated as follows: within a consciousness manifold, modalities are related to one another and simultaneously depend upon, or represent a function of, a certain grouping of some of these modalities (brain); this latter grouping, in turn, is the essential condition for the manifestation of consciousness which thus has gestalt character and emerges as an integrated unit. If the spatial, compresent structure of the consciousness manifold is considered, the static ('structuralistic') aspect is emphasized; if the temporal structure is primarily considered the active ('functionalistic') aspect is stressed. It will be noted that in this formulation, since its abstract wording does not define the brain as a material object, the circulus vitiosus exhibited under 5 is avoided.

The idealistic viewpoint as expressed in present-day Western thinking has been put on a firm foundation in the important treatises of *Berkeley* [1710, 1713]. His argumentation that material objects only exist through being perceived, can, in my opinion, be fully upheld. In this respect, *Berkeley's* writings assume a significance which may be likened to that of *Euclid's* elements. It must nevertheless be admitted that a compelling logical proof cannot be given as regards either non-existence or existence of an independent physical world. Even *Berkeley* concedes this: 'If therefore it were possible for bodies to exist without the mind, yet to hold they do so must needs be a very precarious opinion' (Principles, 1710; XIX); 'That a substratum not perceived, may exist, unimportant' (Principles, LXXVII); '*Hyl*: . . . But thus much seems pretty plain, that it is at least possible such things may really exist; and as long as there is no absurdity in supposing them, I am resolved to believe as I did, till you bring good reasons to the contrary.

Phil: What! is it come to this, that you only believe the existence of material objects and that your belief is founded barely on the possibility of its being true? Then you will have me bring reasons against it: though another would think it reasonable, the proof should lie on him who holds the affirmative' (First Dialogue of *Hylas* and *Philonous*, 1713).

Under these circumstances it remains thus a matter of personal opinion or judgement to decide which view appears more reasonable. Since a decision or

---

situation which involves a principle of hierarchy. Thus, within the domain of the gestalt-like aspect, the *Barber of Seville*, in his function as the *Barber*, assumes a position which is apart from that of the other men of Seville such that all the implications of the definition do not apply to this position.

In the formulation under 6, the brain paradox is, I believe, avoided by the definition of the relation as a function, that is in this case as a gestalt-like dependence between elements of a set. It should again be emphasized that this formulation does not imply or postulate the existence of physical matter.

choice giving assent to one of the alternatives involves by definition an act of will, we have here an illustration of the dictum '*voluntas est superior intellectu*' set forth by the British Franciscan and Scholastic *John Duns Scotus* (1266[?]–1308), famed as *Doctor subtilis* and teacher of *William of Occam*, who in turn was renowned as *Doctor Invincibilis*.

Yet, as emphasized by *Hume* [1750] in his '*Enquiry*', two objections, based on strict reasoning, seem conclusively to demolish the concept of 'matter' in the physical sense. The first objection consists in this, that said concept, 'if rested on natural instinct, is contrary to reason, and if referred to reason, is contrary to natural instinct, and at the same time carries no rational evidence with it, to convince an impartial enquirer'. The second objection goes farther, and represents said concept as contrary to reason: 'At least if it be a principle of reason, that all sensible qualities are in the mind, not in the object. Bereave matter of all its intelligible qualities, both primary and secondary, you in a manner annihilate it, and leave only a certain unknown, inexplicable something as the cause of our perceptions; a notion so imperfect, that no sceptic will think it worth while to contend against it.' Instead of 'cause' I would, of course, say: 'as the *principium rationis sufficientis actualitatis* of our perceptions'. *Hume*, moreover, failed clearly to indicate that the 'primary qualities' involve space and time, although this is implicitly contained in his and in *Berkeley's* views. It was *Kant's* merit to have recognized that space and time are the 'formal aspects' of consciousness, although his elaborations on that topic include various weaknesses.

The objections directed against *Berkeleian* idealism seem to me rather weak and often irrelevant. *Jeans* [1943] for instance asserts: '*Berkeley* maintained that as the effects A on the mind side of the mind-body bridge are purely mental, their causes B on the body side must also be purely mental. In brief, as A is an idea, 'and an idea can be like nothing but an idea', therefore B also must be an idea, or of course a set of ideas.'

'The argument is obviously double-edged, and just as effective when reversed. For if B must be of the same nature as A, it is equally valid to argue that A must be of the same nature as B. Since A ('*sic*') is purely material, the argument would now prove that our mental processes must be material in their nature, as the materialists claim.'

Jeans presents here an inaccurate version of *Berkeley's* statement. According to this latter author: 'Ideas imprinted on the senses are real things, or do really exist; this we do not deny but we deny (1) they can subsist without the minds which perceive them, or (2) that they are resemblances of any archetypes existing without the mind: (1) since the very being of sensation or idea consists in being perceived and (2) an idea can be like nothing but an idea' (Principles, XC). In other words, *Berkeley* merely states that a percept is a modality of consciousness which obviously cannot exist as such apart from consciousness, and therefore cannot be likened to anything lacking the attributes of consciousness.[29] As regards causes, *Berkeley* states that 'the causes of our sensations are not things immediately perceived and therefore not sensible' (First Dialogue).

The allegedly 'double-edged argument' construed by *Jeans* appears to me irrelevant and artificial; it might be answered as follows: Consciousness (A) is directly experienced, and is, by definition, mental (*sensu latiori*); the nature of matter existing apart of consciousness, an inference, is queried; matter is therefore x. The argument, if valid, would thus prove that x, the unknown, equals A, the known. This, however, contradicts the assumption of matter apart of consciousness. Conversely, we may, for the sake of argument, concede the existence of matter (B) as postulated by the materialists. Even under such premises, a consciousness modality could not, in the definition of causality, be the causal effect of a material process. If, again, we grant this miracle or if we substitute instead a quasi-mathematical functional relationship of matter and mind, it is still not possible to claim that our mental processes are or 'must be material in their nature', since 'material' is postulated to mean 'apart of consciousness', and the argument proves to be invalid.

Another argument of *Jeans* reads: 'Whatever capacity a red flower may have for producing a sensation of redness in a man's mind, it has also a capacity for reflecting red light whether there is anyone to see it or not, as may be very simple proved by photography. This capacity is obviously a primary quality, being "utterly inseparable from the body in what state soever it be", and *Berkeley's* argument cannot touch it.' One is here reminded of *Boswell's* anecdote recounting *Dr. Johnson's* rebuttal of *Berkeley's* views: 'I never shall forget the alacrity with which *Johnson* answered, striking his foot with mighty force against a large stone, till he rebounded from it, "I refute it thus!".'

Quite evidently in the dualistic materialistic view, the sensation 'red' is a P-event, related to R-events transduced into N- respectively Np-events. The frequencies, wavelengths or photon energies postulated by physics and the

---

[29] It is thus by no means an argument of refuting idealism to stress that 'what we perceive exists and has the qualities that it is perceived to have '[*Moore*, 1922], since this is exactly what *Berkeley* states. Again, to cite another commonly proffered objection: 'the worst that can be said of it, is that it is not also real, i.e. that it does not exist when it is not object of someone's perception, not that it does not exist at all. This comment is interpreted to be another argument against idealism, but actually expresses a fundamental statement of idealism, although with the somewhat awkward terms 'object of someone's perception'. It would be better to say: 'that it does not exist in space-time when it is not a consciousness modality in a consciousness manifold'.

Additional arguments supporting *Berkeley's* fundamental thesis against objections by various writers, including *Bertrand Russell*, are given in *K.* [1961, §31, pp. 122–129].

postulated physiologic N- or Np-events in the nervous system can hardly be assumed to be red. What color would then have the (invisible) electromagnetic radiations not recorded by N- and Np-events? Would they have the 'color' black?[30] But black and white are conscious experiences. Although loss of consciousness is occasionally called a 'blackout', no 'color' black is perceived by the unconscious Human being nor in dreamless (unconscious) sleep.

However, from the idealistic viewpoint, *Jeans'* argument might be answered by stating that there is indeed an orderly relationship between our percept of a red flower and our percepts of its photograph which could even be a kodachrome. This relationship can be expressed in terms of reflection of red light; but the concepts 'red' and 'light' refer to sensations which together with their pertinent temporal and spatial relationships, have actuality only in consciousness. What this relatedness represents outside of consciousness, we cannot know: 'objective scientific redness' postulated by *Jeans* must be considered a self-contradictory hypostatization. In his First Dialogue between *Hylas* and *Philonous*, *Berkeley* has, in my opinion, successfully coped with an extensive series of similar arguments.

Another frequently encountered objection concerns the 'jerky life' of what we assume to be material objects, 'suddenly leaping into being when we look at them'. It is taken for incongruous that things are every moment annihilated and created again. *Berkeley* writes in effect: 'The objects of sense exist only when perceived: the trees therefore are in the garden, or the chairs in the parlour, no longer than while there is somebody to perceive them. Upon shutting my eyes, all the furniture in the room is reduced to nothing, and barely upon opening them it is again created' (Principles, XLV). This statement seems absurd only because the notions of an independent physical space-time and of so-called primary qualities, that is, of matter, are firmly ingrained in our reasoning processes. A materialistic physiologist distinguishing primary and secondary qualities might find nothing incongruous in the assertion that each time we open our eyes and see, we 'paint the world in colors', provided there is light and we are not color-blind, or, in other words, that material objects suddenly leap into color when we look at them. If we assume that there is no other space-time than perceptual space-time, it will no longer appear absurd that material objects come into being only when perceived. Moreover, thoughts, memories as well as feelings arise into being and vanish; their 'jerky life' is commonly taken for granted. Although the furniture in the room – except for the chair I sit on or the table I touch – is reduced to nothing *qua* material objects when I shut my eyes, orderly relationships involving these

---

[30] Invisible ultraviolet (and infrared) radiation is indeed popularly sometimes designated as 'black light'.

vanished percepts persist with respect to my consciousness-manifold, but, in the idealistic view, these relationships are outside the domain of space-time, cannot be qualified, and therefore remain unknown. Conversely, in the peculiar but fundamental phenomenon of awareness designated as consciousness, orderly relationships of an unknown or rather unknowable nature become 'physical', that is compresent, successive, localized and, in part, spatially configured, just as they become colored, hard or soft, warm or cold, and in some instances, sonorous and odorous.

Berkeley also emphasizes that we perceive distant objects not only when we are awake but also in dreams, and they may then have the same appearance of distance. Regarding this statement, *Craik* [1943] raises the objection that *Berkeley* chooses his situation so as to avoid the issue of the truth or falsity of a perception and its relation to consistency. According to *Craik*, *Berkely* 'ignores the fact that a person's dreams are not, in fact, internally consistent for long, and even when this occurs, they are not consistent with any other person's except on the rarest occasions'.

Despite my genuine esteem for *Craik's* brilliant treatise, I believe that, in this connection, his argument is not relevant to the problem. It is, nevertheless, of significant interest to compare the consciousness phenomena in a vivid dream with those of the waking state.

First, it should be emphasized that from the idealistic viewpoint, the 'external world' in such dreams, with all its objects, consists exactly of the same 'stuff' which represents, in the waking condition, the 'physical world', namely of localized and, in part, spatially configured consciousness modalities. Conversely, the 'stuff of the world' (*Bertrand Russell*) is mental *sensu latiori*, and remains identical[31] whether I dream or whether I am awake. In both instances I am conscious in accordance with the definition of consciousness adopted as the base of this thesis, that is I experience awareness.

However, there are indubitably substantial differences between the dream-world and the world of the waking state. The most important difference, which was well stressed by *Bertrand Russell*, involves the circumstance that 'material objects' in a dream are private data while those in the waking state represent public data.

Next, there is, as pointed out by *Craik* and others, a lack of consistency and continuity in the relationship of dream events to events of the waking periods. 'Physical events' in a dream may furthermore display correlations unconformable to those in waking experience. Thus, for instance in bodily flight-dreams, the law of gravity appears modified or abolished. Nevertheless,

---

[31] Identical, since consciousness events in both the waking and the dreaming state represent, in the fictional physical model, cerebral P-events correlated with Np-events.

events in dreams are presumably related in an orderly manner to other events in waking consciousness. It may be said that memories are activated into percepts and combined into new as well as old patterns. Affectivity most likely plays an important although perhaps not exclusive role in these processes and may be mainly responsible for the 'hyponoic mechanisms' of *Kretschmer's* terminology, which are very manifest in dream events, and comprise such processes as imaginal agglutination, asyntactical sequence, condensation, substitution, and symbolization. Thought processes in dreams are likewise modified and assume a pronounced catathymic aspect.[32]

Despite gross exaggerations and not infrequent absurdities,[33] the interpretation given by the psychoanalysts can be accepted as valid in principle, at least for certain categories of dreams. Manifestations of affectivity which are prevented from adequate expression may vanish from consciousness, but the orderly relationships involving the emotional processes persist and can again become manifest in dreams as well as in the overall behavioral pattern.

Such 'relationships' constitute the 'unconscious mental activities' of psychoanalytic terminology. Despite its semantically inappropriate designation, this concept appears well supported by observation, and of significant practical value. It must be reiterated, however, as *Kretschmer* pointed out, that an unconscious psychic or mental activity is a *contradictio in adjecto* (unconscious consciousness). What fails to be conscious, that is what is in no way directly experienced, cannot be termed psychic or mental. It may be defined, in materialistic terminology, as a physical brain process or, in idealistic terminology, as a set of unknown relationships, incomprehensible, because devoid of space-time characteristics.

Consciousness assumes different degrees of distinctness or vividity. *Kretschmer* resorts here to an adaptation of visual terms. He refers to a focal point of consciousness with ill-defined surrounding concentric zones in which consciousness is progressively less distinct and fades imperceptibly into nothingness, unconsciousness or extra-consciousness. For the periphery of consciousness he suggests, modifying a concept of *Schilder*, the term sphere, also translated as 'sphaira'. Sphairal psychic processes thus occupy the border-zone of consciousness and are exceedingly vague and obscure. Many of the factors significant in the realm of psychoanalysis, however, remain beyond the sphaira in the domain of the unconscious.

---

[32] Further elaborations on nature and significance of dreams are given in the present author's contribution to the *Festschrift Hübscher* [*K.*, 1972].

[33] The interpretations of psychoanalysts are presented, with considerable details, in a publication by *Hadfield* [1969] to which the interested reader may be referred. It is entitled *Dreams and Nightmares*. Another such publication is that by *Thomas* [1979]: '*Träume – selbst verstehen.*'

Depending on the viewpoint, the dream world and the everyday world are similar and dissimilar. As regards the similarities, both are consciousness phenomena in which a mental (*sensu strictiori*) and a physical world are displayed in perceptual space-time, that is, dream world and everyday waking world both consist of the same 'stuff'. Both evidence an inherent orderliness based on 'relationships' or – in the materialistic view on physical (physiological) processes. The entire phenomenal world which we experience, waking or dreaming, represents thus a strictly determined, orderly phantasmagory. In this respect, and despite *Bertrand Russell's* disapproval, the view of *Heracleitus*, of *Leibniz* and of *Schopenhauer* may be considered plausible, although with some modifications: it could be said that in everyday waking life we are all dreaming, but that the dreams we all have are based on identical orderliness, have essentially similar structure, and are to a large extent 'public':

> 'We are such stuff
> As dreams are made of, and our little life
> Is rounded with a sleep.'
> (*Shakespeare*, Tempest IV, I)

These lines are possibly a paraphrase from *Pindar's Phythian Ode* (VIII, 95):

> 'ἐπάμεροι· τί δέ τις; τί δ'οὔ τις; σκιᾶς ὄναρ ἄνθρωπος.'

Sophocles' Ajax likewise contains a comparable passage where, in one of the opening dialogues with *Athena, Ulysses* avows:

> 'ὁρῶ γὰρ ἡμᾶς οὐδὲν ὄντας ἄλλο πλὴν
> εἴδωλ' ὅσοιπερ ζῶμεν ἢ κούφην σκιάν.'

In *FitzGeralds* version of *Omar the Tentmaker*, this feeling is expressed in the quatrain:

> 'For in and out, above, about, below;
> 'Tis nothing but a Magic Shadow-show;
> Play'd in a Box whose candle is the Sun,
> Round which we Phantom Figures come and go.'
> (XLVI, 1859)

In the Diamond Sûtra (Sino-Japanese: Kongô-kyô, Chinese: Ching-kang-ching or Kin-kong-king) of Mahâyâna Buddhism, very similar statements are found. This scripture is one of the key treatises of the Prajñâ Pâramita series.[34] The extant Sanskrit text of the Diamond Sûtra, Vajracchedika (The Diamond-Cutter), appears to be less complete than the classic Chinese translation by *Kumârajîva* about 400 AD. The following three passages may be quoted:-

---

[34] *Prajñâ Pâramitâ* signifies the cardinal virtues (*pâramitâ*) of deep insight (*prajñâ*, *pradschna*; German: '*Erkenntnis*', '*Einsicht*').

'Every form or quality of phenomena is transient and illusive. When the mind realizes that the phenomena of life are not real, the Tathâgata[35] may then be clearly perceived.'

'Thus, you shall be delivered from an immeasurable, innumerable and illimitable world of sentient life; but, in reality, there is no world of sentient life from which to seek deliverance. And why? Because in the minds of enlightened disciples there have ceased to exist such arbirary concepts of phenomena as an entity, a being, a living being, or a self.'

'In what attitude of mind should it be diligently explained to others? Not assuming the permanency or reality of phenomena. And why? Because the phenomena of life may be likened unto a dream, a phantasm, a bubble of foam, a shadow, the glistening dew, a flash of lightning, and a cloud. Thus should we contemplate the world.'

The various quotations represent, of course, essentially an emotional attidude towards events, and may furthermore be considered mere assertions. However, I believe that these assertions agree with an analysis of the facts. Moreover, as regards many relevant statements of Buddhist philosophy, it can be said that these views are based on a logical analysis in full accordance with more recent views of *Hume* or contemporary ideas of *Mach*.

Idealism can be considered a logical interpretation of the phenomenal world as it actually exists for a sentient being such as Man. Unlike materialism which is based on the concept of a substratum assumed only by inference, it is based on the most certain, in fact on the only direct knowledge, that is on conscious experience: all phenomena represent modalities of consciousness.

Various attitudes and methods are required in order to construct, in the symbolism of thought, a model of the phenomenal world upon this foundation: *a priorism*, which, as I believe, appears less significant than often assumed, scepticism remaining within reasonable limits, descriptive, relational, and causal theories. The pattern into which these different attitudes will be blended must of necessity remain a question of individual judgement.

A discussion concerning the significance of idealism (again in its epistemologic denotation) for an approach to the problems of (axiologic) values,

---

[35] The honorific *Thathâgata*, one of the diverse appelations of preeminence referring to the *Buddha*, has been interpreted in several ways by the Buddhist commentators, since an ambiguity of the Sanskrit language is involved. If derived from *tathâ-gata*, the meaning is: 'he who has gone', *scilicet* the way of all *Buddhas*. If derived from *tathâ-âgata*, the meaning is 'he who has so come' ('he who has come thus'), *scilicet* in accordance with the sequence of *Buddhas* as manifestation of the cosmic law. The Chinese and Sino-Japanese translations *Ju-lai* and *Nyo-rai* conform to *tathâ-âgata*. Another honorific is *Bhagavat* (the Exalted One, 'der *Erhabene*'). *Buddha* is the participium perfectum passivum of *budh*, to awake, to know, and has the active meaning: 'the awakened one' or 'the wise one'. The *Buddha* himself, in his sermons (*sûtras*), used the term *Tathâgata* frequently as a substitute for the first personal pronoun.

especially to ethics and aesthetics, obviously remains outside the scope of the present discussion which concerns idealism only insofar as this view is related to the problem of epistemology with regard to brain and consciousness.[36]

In this respect idealism has both an advantage and a disadvantage. The advantage, in my opinion, is the insight into the problem of consciousness provided by this approach and the realization that consciousness cannot be conceived as a causal effect of material processes.

Nevertheless, in dealing with the phenomenal world, we are faced with orderly events which we designate as material and which include the nervous system and its functions. There can be little doubt that the (transitory) existence of a state of consciousness depends upon the activities of the brain. In studying the structure and the functions of this organ, the terminology of idealism is poorly suited and the symbolism of physics appears appropriate. For an understanding of morphology, anatomy, physiology and pathology of the nervous system the fiction, or if we prefer, the working concept of a physical world with a public space-time structure conceived in terms of mathematics, and in which physical events take place, become a necessary practical postulate.

An attempt may be made, by means of a postulational (i.e. fictional) psychophysical parallelism, to combine the idealistic and the materialistic approach. This will be discussed in the next volume and chapter of my disquisition. There still remains, however, one pertinent question related to the scope of this presentation. Granted that configured events in a space-time structure, that is matter, do not exist independently of consciousness, what persists when there is no consciousness? In other words, what is the nature of reality? It cannot be 'mental' since consciousness represents an ephemeral and transitory phenomenon. Neither can it be 'physical' since 'matter' merely represents a particular aspect (public data) of consciousness.

Reverting to the previously discussed meaning of the concept 'reality' (chapter II, section 5, p. 161), it should here be repeated, that, as defined by *Russell* [1952], said term has evidently at least two denotations: 'A thing is real if it persists at times when it is not perceived; or again, a thing is real when it is correlated with other things in a way which experience has led us to expect.' The above question, of course, concerns the first of these two definitions of reality, which, as might well be mentioned, were already given by *Schopenhauer* in his '*Skitze (sic!) einer Geschichte vom Idealen und Realen*' [1851]. I prefer to use the designations reality in the first sense and reality in the second sense with respect to *Russell's* two definitions.

---

[36] The conclusions resulting from transcendental neutralism with regard to axiology (ethics, aesthetics) shall be discussed in chapter VII, vol. 3, of this treatise.

10. Transcendental Neutralism

Since consciousness arises, fades and arises again in orderly continuity, an independent x outside of consciousness must be granted as representing reality in the first sense according to the definition adopted in the preceding paragraph. Thought operates with abstractions embodied in words, subject to the orderliness of grammar and logic. *George Boole* showed in his treatises on the mathematical analysis of logic [1847], and on the laws of thought [1854], that mathematics is, at least in some respects, reducible to logic. *Bertrand Russell* and *Whitehead, Couturat, Jevons, Hilbert, Peano, Frege, Zermelo* and others have successfully elaborated on this reduction of mathematics. Words are consciousness modalities of mnemic nature, symbolizing other consciousness-modalities: sensations, patterns, feelings, and awareness of relationships. In order to have meaning, that is symbolic equivalence, words must, in the last end, have a reference to direct experience, that is to consciousness. Words, despite their many shortcomings, are thus more meaningful and carry further than the highly abstract notations of symbolic logic, although the great value of this later procedure, especially in analyzing the formal aspect of thought processes, can hardly be denied. Whatever persists beyond consciousness must thus be regarded as inexpressible, indefinable, and unknowable. Even the word 'persists' becomes meaningless, since reality, beyond the domain of space-time relationships, cannot be conceived in any temporal term such as duration. Many philosophers have nevertheless considered this 'reality' as intelligible, that is as apprehensible by the intellect only, or as purely conceptual. What remains, in this sense, intelligible if we exclude consciousness, is at most only a vague abstraction of relationships which may be expressed as 'orderliness', 'laws' or 'norms' (*Dharma* in Sanskrit terminology). From one of the Prajñā Pâramitâ Sûtras of Mahâyâna Buddhism, the following passages may be quoted: 'The *Lord Buddha* addresses *Subhûti*, saying: "What think you, *Subhûti*, can the *Tathâgata* be perceived by means of any physical phenomena?" *Subhûti* replied: "Not indeed, *O Bhagavat*! the *Tathâgata* cannot be perceived by means of any physical phenomena. And why? because what the *Tathâgata* referred to as physical phenomena are not in reality physical phenomena. Physical phenomena are merely a figure of speech."'

The *Lord Buddha* addressed *Subhûti*, saying: 'Do not affirm that the *Tathâgata* thinks thus within himself: I ought to promulgate a system of law or doctrine. Have no such erroneous thought! and why? Because if a disciple would think so, he would be manifestly unable to understand the purport of my instruction. *Subhûti*, regarding the promulgation of a system of Law or doctrine, there is in reality no system of Law or doctrine to promulgate, a system of Law or doctrine is indeed merely a figure of speech.'

For the materialist, the problem is simple: in the old-fashioned view, reality consists of atoms, conceived as small inertial entities, acting in absolute space and time according to physical and chemical laws. Present-day materialists will instead assume much more complex 'events', either statistically 'determined' or causal, within a structure of physical space-time which may be *non-Euclidean*.

For the idealist, the problem, as stated above, is most difficult and practically insolvable. *Berkeley* formulates it as follows: 'We perceive a continual succession of ideas, some are anew excited, others are changed or totally disappear. There is therefore some cause of these ideas whereon they depend, and which produces and changes them. That this cause cannot be any quality of idea or combination of ideas, is clear from the preceding section. It must therefore be a substance; but it has been shown that there is no corporeal or material substance (it remains therefore that the cause of ideas is an incorporeal active substance or spirit)' (Principles, XXVI).

'(But whatever power I may have over my own thoughts, I find the ideas actually perceived by sense have not a like dependence on my will.) When in broad daylight I open my eyes, it is not in my power to choose whether I shall see or no, or to determine what particular objects shall present themselves to my view; and so likewise as to the hearing and other senses, the ideas imprinted on them are not creatures of my will. (There is therefore some other will or spirit that produces them.)' (Principles, XXIX).

While the gist of these statements can be accepted, several objections might be raised concerning the terminology.

Since, for the purpose of this presentation, and following *Schopenhauer*, a narrower definition of causality was adopted, it cannot be said that as such, ideas that is consciousness modalities or percepts, are 'causally' related to an inferred reality existing outside of consciousness. Moreover, the terms 'substance', 'spirit', and to a certain extent also 'will', may be challenged because of their various denotations and connotations conducive to excessive vagueness or ambiguity. *Berkeley* moreover, failed to distinguish between (a) the relationship of actual consciousness, i.e. of a private perceptual space-time system characterized by the 'succession of ideas' (percepts) to some other will or spirit that produces them, and (b) the relationships of 'ideas' to one another. In other words, he failed to distinguish (a) the relationship of actuality to reality in the first sense, from (b) the orderliness obtaining within the domain of actuality (consciousness). The relationship (a) involves the *principium rationis sufficientis actualitatis*, and the relationship (b) involves all other empirically ascertained aspects of the principle of sufficient reason. As regards the relationship between the succession of sensory percepts (public data), the *principium rationis sufficientis fiendi* (causality) is of particular importance, supplemented by the fictional *principium rationis sufficientis per-*

cipiendi (relationship of Np-events to P-events, i.e. fictional psychophysical parallelism).

The well-known theological interpretation set forth by Bishop *Berkeley* is in part based upon the ill-defined significance of his concepts of incorporeal spirit, substance, etc., leading to a μετάβασις εἰς ἄλλο γένος, and, in addition, represents a non-valid extrapolation, namely: since sensible things really exist, they are necessarily perceived by an infinite mind (*sic secus*, Second Dialogue between *Hylas* and *Philonous*). It will be noted that 'reality', in this instance, corresponds to the second definition of the term 'real' as given above. The argument lacks cogency inasmuch as the concept of an infinite mind appears self-contradictory. We can only conceive mind *sensu latiori* as identical with consciousness, and mind sensu strictiori as a subset (thoughts etc.) of consciousness modalities. On the basis of what we can know or infer, mind is thus strictly a very limited *functio animalis* characterized by a perceptual space-time structure, and depending on certain transitory relationships which obtain in that space-time, manifesting themselves as an organic body with a nervous system. This limited *functio animalis* can hardly be assumed to be the predicate of a postulated infinite substance. *Berkeley's* conclusions should thus preferably be reformulated to state that ideas (consciousness modalities) arise and succeed each other in a constant and orderly manner, and that, in toto, their manifestation appears to be related to an unknown orderliness.

Kant analyzed the functions of reason which, according to his view, consist in relating or synthesizing the data of sense. He endeavored to define by what right and within which limit reason may interpret such data. Space and time are shown to be forms of sensibility. Our thought processes follow certain principles which he designated as categories, classified as pertaining to quantity, quality, relation and modality. The formal principles are considered transcendental, that is pertaining to the necessary condition of human experience, as determined by the constitution of the mind itself, and transcending what is determined by the contingent particularity of experience, but not transcending all human knowledge. Within the realm of theoretical knowledge, we cannot know things-in-themselves, but only phenomena.

Kant's analysis is of great and lasting fundamental value; nevertheless, it suffers from excessive rigidity and reconditeness, often leading to ambiguity. The separation of the formal aspect of experience from actual experience remains, to a certain extent, artificial and is subject to the inherent fallibilities of abstractions. *A priorism* of the transcendental formal elements is, I believe, overstressed by *Kant* and some of his followers; this undue emphasis leads to spurious problems (*Scheinprobleme*) and illusory controversies. In addition, the rigid concept of time as the sole form of the 'inner sense' has led to the widespread dogmatic assertion that mind *sensu strictiori* has no place in space. One can maintain, however, that even mind *sensu strictiori* is localized in perceptual space-time; I grant that it is poorly or indistinctly localized and that it has no spatial configuration. There are, of course, additional definitions of mind, not considered in my discussion because I regard these concepts as devoid of significance, e.g. mind as an essential self, or as the subject which perceives,[37] in contradistinction to the object; furthermore mind as a metaphysical substance which pervades all individual minds (consciousness manifolds), and is contrasted with matter or material substance. There is finally still another exceedingly vague definition of mind referring to cerebral activities preparing, initiating and controlling the complicated forms of behavior which 'we cannot explain in terms of reflexes or automatisms' [Fessard, 1954]. This double-bottomed definition blurs the clear distinction between material processes in fictional physical space-time and conscious processes in actual perceptual space-time. The implication of this definition will be considered in vol. 2 in the discussion of conscious and unconscious cerebration.

Perceptual space-time is the given form of experience and has no empty existence outside of an actual particular experience, which occurs 'here and now'.

It is thus neither a priori nor a posteriori with reference to experience. The abstract concept of empty space-time is merely a mnemic consciousness modality referring to experienced space-time relationships and is thus truly a posteriori.

Our thought processes take place in accordane with a certain orderliness which includes the principle of sufficient reason, and, moreover, all consciousness modalities can be conceived as occurring in a constant and orderly manner. However, an infant will hardly be able to formulate geometrical or

---

[37] It has been claimed that 'when one perceives something, one perceives something, and that what one does perceive cannot be the same as the perception of it'. This argumentation leads to the concepts of subject and object, as postulated by Schopenhauer and others. It might be asked, however, who is the 'one', or, as it could also be worded, what is the subject, I or self? In a perceptual space-time system, there is a given percept, and that percept is, of course, identical with itself, that is, the percept is the percept. In other words, I am (or 'one is') a perceptual space-time system, and part of this system is the given percept. Still in other words, if I see a tree, that visual tree is part of me, or I am that tree, as long as the tree is my percept, or is part of my perceptual space-time system, just (as transitorily) as an emotion or a thought is part of me, that is 'my' thought or 'my emotion'. Instead of saying esse est percipi, the formulation can be reversed to 'percipi est esse'. Percipi should be emphasized as 'being a percept' rather than 'being perceived'. This, I believe, is the most appropriate formulation of the equivalent dicta: 'existence and observability are coextensive', and 'the meaning of a proposition is the means of its verification'. When we come to the ultimate given phenomenon, to the 'Urphänomen' of consciousness, then, and only then, observer and observed are one, namely the individual consciousness manifold or perceptual space-time system. There is, of course, no observation without an observer, no inference without an inferrer, and no percept without a perceiver. But observation, inference, and percept are merely modalities of a consciousness manifold.

logical propositions, although it will potentially do this after aquiring experience and the necessary degree of maturity in due course of time. On the other hand, a *Wistar* rat will presumably never be able to perform such mental operations, although it could be taught to run a maze or recognize a triangle, and a plant presumably does not experience consciousness at all. In this respect, the following statement of *Sherrington* [1950] seems rather appropriate: 'Most life is, I imagine, mindless'.

It appears justified to assume certain intrinsic prerequisites upon which the possibility of specific actual conscious experiences is contingent and which, in *Kant's* attempt of interpretation, represent the gist of his *a priori* concept. In materialistic terminology, such prerequisites could be conceived in terms of neural structures and functions; some aspects of these structures and functions might even be interpreted in terms of circuit algebra just as this algebra is applied to electronic computers.

In summary, comparing *Kant's* presentation with that of *Berkeley*, I believe that *Berkeley's* analysis of matter is superior to that by *Kant*, and I concur in this opinion with *Mach* [1922, p. 299]. However, *Kant's* doctrine is far more versatile, universal and comprehensive than *Berkeley's* philosophic system. While this latter author's interpretation of reality, strongly influenced by obvious hyponoic factors, is unsatisfactory, *Kant's* interpretation may be considered sound, provided that the designation 'thing in itself' is not construed as referring to anything having attributes of consciousness (mind), matter, or particularity. Still, in view of some of the denotations and connotations of the term 'thing', *Kant's* expression for what remains as independent reality apart from consciousness does not appear particularly well chosen.

Schopenhauer (vol. 1, p. 53) stated that '*Kant's grösstes Verdienst ist die Unterscheidung der Erscheinung vom Dinge an sich*'. This, however, was already anticipated by *Hume* (cf. above, section 9, p. 247). *Kant*, nevertheless, clearly pointed out that the relevant characteristics of consciousness (actuality, phenomena, '*Erscheinung*') are space and time, not pertaining to reality in the first sense ('*Ding an sich*'). Discounting *Kant's* poorly chosen inappropriate term '*Ding*', i.e. 'thing' with regard to reality in the first sense, *Kant's* derivation of said 'reality' is, moreover, based on faulty logic, as *Kant's* critics (e.g. *Schulze, Schopenhauer*, and others) clearly pointed out. *Kant* postulated his '*Ding an sich*' as the 'cause' of our perceptions by a conclusion referring to the 'law of causality'. Yet, he had rightly shown that 'causality' is a relationship exclusively pertaining to the interconnection of perceptions ('*Erscheinungen*'), or, in other words, to the world of consciousness. Thus, the principle of 'causality' cannot be invoked to derive consciousness from 'something' which is not consciousness. *Kant* seems, nevertheless, to have felt his inconsistency, to which he referred in his *Prolegomena* at the end of §53: '*Denn wenn die Ursache in der Erscheinung nur von der Ursache der Erscheinungen, sofern sie als Ding an sich selbst gedacht werden kann, unterschieden wird, so können beide Sätze wohl nebeneinander bestehen, nämlich, dass von der Sinnenwelt überall keine Ursache (nach ähnlichen Gesetzen der Kausalität) stattfinde, deren Existenz schlechthin notwendig sei, ingleichen andererseits, dass diese Welt dennoch mit einem notwendigen Wesen als ihrer Ursache (aber von anderer Art und nach andern Gesetzen) verbunden sei; welcher zweier Sätze Unverträglichkeit lediglich auf dem Missverstande beruht, das, was bloss von Erscheinungen gilt, über Dinge an sich selbst auszudehnen und überhaupt beide in einem Begriffe zu vermengen.'*

It is evident that *Kant's Ursache von anderer Art* represents the principle which I have pointed out as the *Principium rationis sufficientis actualitatis*. The formulation of this principle eliminates the mistake of confusing causality '*in der Erscheinung*' with the relationship of '*Erscheinung*' to orderliness x.

In his comments on *Schelling, Schopenhauer* [*Nachlass*, ed. *Grisebach*, vol. 3, p. 133] adds the highly pertinent remark: '*Der Erscheinung des Menschen in der Zeit liegt etwas zum Grunde was ausser aller Zeit, wie ausser allen Bedingungen der Erscheinung liegt: will man dem sonst richtigen Begriff von jenem Etwas diese Bedingungen anpassen, so erhält man monstra.*' *Schopenhauer*, of course, should have said: '*was ausser aller Zeit und aller Räumlichkeit liegt*' (i.e. 'something' beyond or without any space-time relationships).

Schopenhauer has propounded a noteworthy fictional solution of the problem of reality by postulating that *Kant's* 'thing in itself' is will. In *Schopenhauer's* concept of an individual mind or self, the body represents the direct object for the percipient subject. The perceiving self, on the other hand, is regarded as directly related to reality. In the voluntary motions of the body, we have thus a direct awareness of or insight into the nature of action: activity of the body is an objectivated act of will. Thus, *Kant's* 'thing in itself' is interpreted as will, which is conceived by *Schopenhauer* as 'blind', that is as unconscious. The will attains consciousness only by means of a brain phenomenon.

It is interesting to note that *Sperry* [1952], a neurobiologist, has recently reemphasized the significance of motor patterns for an insight into mental processes. This author states that 'an analysis of our current thinking will show that it tends to suffer generally from a failure to view mental activities in their proper relation, or even in any relation, to motor behavior. The remedy lies in further insight into the relationship between the sensori-associative functions of the brain on the one hand, and motor activity on the other.' The approach suggested by *Sperry*, although differently formulated, based on different premises, and leading to a different argumentation, is nevertheless essentially *Schopenhauer's* approach.

Following *Schopenhauer's* reasoning, we might go farther and state that, in looking for universal principles which do not supposedly postulate consciousness, we find as the two ultimate abstractions orderliness and action.

In the hypothetic physical world, action can be conceived as magnitudes of movement, related to the dimension of energy $(g \cdot cm^2 \cdot sec^{-2})$ which again equates with 'matter' or mass $(E = Mc^2)$.[38]

In the phenomenal world of consciousness, everything represents conscious activity. This, as action, and stripped of all other qualities and relationships, can perhaps figuratively be conceived as will in the sense of *Schopenhauer's* attempt at interpretation. If this is assumed, then will or action may be equated with energy which, in turn can be equated with matter. *Einstein's* equation $E = Mc^2$ would thus represent a vindication of *Schopenhauer's* thesis.

However, several objections to *Schopenhauer's* solution could be maintained. The subdivision, as it were, of the consciousness manifold into unperceived although percipient subject, and perceived object, is of dubious validity, and, I believe, untenable; but, in reference to the problem at issue, this question is perhaps irrelevant.

Moreover, the concept of will can be challenged. Will may be considered to represent the dynamic aspect of consciousness activities, but is also defined as desire, purpose, intention, and choice or decision. Will, referring to a factor or component of more or less complex consciousness activities, cannot be experienced as a separate, individual phenomenon. *Russell* [1952] stresses this point and reaches the conclusion that, as a separate occurrence or as a faculty, the concept of will is a delusion which this author spurns as 'a metaphysical superstition'. I am disinclined to follow *Russell* that far, and believe that will may be considered a significant abstraction denoting a definite aspect of consciousness phenomena, regardless whether *Schopenhauer's* interpretation is deemed acceptable or not.

My own misgivings about this interpretation concern the following two points: (1) will is an exceedingly vague term denoting emotional tones or aspects of both expression and limning processes: it subsumes intentional body motions as well as mere desires, moreover planning as well as negation, pleasure as well as suffering, (2) in all these denotations and connotations will is very definitely and exclusively a conscious percept ('*Vorstellung*') and cannot be postulated to have any 'existence' apart from consciousness; thus, it

---

[38] This equation can, of course, also be expressed as $E = M$, if c is taken as the unit value. Moreover, this latter formulation involves interesting consequences, such as exceedingly small natural units of lengths and time, of an order of magnitude related to small-scale phenomena in the atomic domain [cf. *Bachem, A.*, Brain astigmatism. Am. Scient. *40:* 497, 1952].

cannot possibly represent the 'thing in itself' of *Kant*, nor the orderliness of extramental (non-conscious) existence. Thus, even if it is granted that will (action) is experienced in its most elemental or relatively purest form in voluntary motor activity – and this is open to doubt –, it still remains a consciousness phenomenon with perceptual space-time properties. If will is taken as an abstraction, it still retains a very definite temporal implication. Finally, if will is fictionally posited as an abstraction for reality, this concept does not take into consideration the ultimate principle of orderliness. *Schopenhauer's* interpretation, I believe, refers thus rather to the temporal aspect of an overall principle of orderly action in the phenomenal world, corresponding perhaps to the energy concept of physics. However, to quote *Bertrand Russell* again: 'None of our beliefs is quite true; all have at least a penumbra of vagueness and error.'

Assuming that reality is transcendental but intelligible – which is by no means certain –, I shall now summarize my own viewpoint.

Reality may be conceived as neither mental (*sensu latiori*), i.e. conscious, nor material in terms of physics and is devoid of, or beyond, space-time relationships. Transcendental neutralism could then be formulated as follows:

There is an orderliness x such that consciousness modalities, characterized by private perceptual space-time relationships, become manifested, in an orderly[39] manner, within a large number of discrete (disjoint) intermittent (interrupted) and transitory consciousness manifolds displaying gestalt properties in reference to their constituent modalities. In other words, events become localized, compresent, and successive by means of the phenomenon known as consciousness. Each consciousness manifold is characterized as an individual space-time system by its own set of private space-time dimensions.

This orderliness x involves a norm x' such that in a consciousness manifold M certain patterns of modalities a, b, c, etc. have configurated perceptual space-time relationships that can be defined in terms of physics; these relationships can be inferred to be valid for corresponding modalities a', b', c', etc. and a'', b'', c'', etc', in a series of other but similar consciousness manifolds M', M'', ... etc., related to M and to each other within the domain of the postulated norm.

It can also be said in this respect that there is a norm x', such that a transposable pattern a, b, c, ... is manifested as public datum within a set of different private perceptual space-time systems pertaining to the domain of that norm.

---

[39] 'Orderly' means here: interrelated in accordance with the various aspects of the principle of sufficient reason applicable to the manifestations of consciousness phenomena.

We may conversely state that public data, comprising the set a, b, c, ... and many other sets, interrelate the private perceptual space-time systems (or consciousness manifolds) M, M', M", ... etc.

The term 'public datum' has several connotations as defined in the preceding section 6 on public data (p. 224). These connotations may be subsumed under two main categories: First, as indirectly shared consciousness phenomena represented by events either perceived through the sense organs or recorded by instruments accessible to sensory 'reading' (German: 'ablesbar'). Secondly, in a more abstract sense, namely as norm x', public data denote the unknowable relationship between said category of shared consciousness modalities.

Moreover, it should be emphasized that public data do not exclusively comprise the spatially configurated sensory consciousness modalities definable in terms of physics but include all sensory percepts which, in turn, are likewise definable in terms of physics and chemistry.

Finally, all consciousness modalities within a given private perceptual space-time system display orderly relations with regard to spatially configurated public data manifested as a correlated nervous system. Insofar as these spatially configurated consciousness modalities representing the nervous system are definable in terms of physics, all consciousness modalities whatsoever can, with respect to their relations to the nervous system, be defined in terms of physics (physics in the wider sense, that is, as physiological or physicochemical neural events, or in corresponding terms of circuit algebra).[40]

In this respect, it is also of particular importance that, while all conscious events are correlates (open transforms) of some brain events, not all brain events (which remain public data recordable by instruments perceivable by an observer) are correlated with conscious events.

Again, the identity of an intermittent consciousness manifold, despite complete interruption of its manifestations, is based (1) on its correlation with a particular given perceptual brain, and (2) on mnestic processes (engraphy) of said brain's potentially observable neural mechanisms. These processes result in the experience of the 'self's' 'identity'.

Since the brain, as directly (e.g. proprioception, touch in an open cranial wound,[41] etc.) or indirectly (e.g. through EEG) perceived by the senses, is a material ('physical') object, of whose function consciousness represents a

---

[40] Cf. the hypothetical case described by *Bertrand Russell* and discussed further below in volume 2 section *1* of chapter IV.

[41] Cf. e.g. the case *Angelmeier* mentioned in the important paper by *Fritsch and Hitzig* [1870] and briefly discussed in volume 5/I, pages 753–754 of the present author's series *The Central Nervous System of Vertebrates* [*K.*, 1977].

dependent variable,[42] it becomes evident that public data, of which the perceptual brain is one, are of particular and fundamental importance.[43]

To summarize the difficult and highly relevant topic here under consideration, it could also be said, in other words, that actual (concrete) public data are experienced sensory percepts, including the reading of instruments which register interphenomena. Abstract public data, as conceived by thought (namely by extrasensory percepts) are physicalisms (fictional matter *sensu latiori*, including R-events, N-events and Np-events). All public data, except certain sorts of merely inferred interphenomena, can be detected by instruments which, in turn, provide sensory percepts.

---

[42] Since the perceptual (actual) brain thus 'produces itself' we have here the brain paradox (cf. chapter II, section 6) which, although anticipated by *George Berkeley*, *Schopenhauer*, and *Zeller*, was neither properly understood nor adequately formulated by these authors. *Berkeley*, however, had almost recognized the relevant point at issue which he merely disregarded because of his theological interpretation necessitated by his ecclesiastic status.

[43] *Sherrington's* [1951] comment that by means of the brain 'the finite mind obtains indirect liaison with finite minds around it' can be interpreted as an intuitive recognition of the brain's status *qua* public datum. Public data, moreover, could be conceived as representing the *harmonia praestabilita* postulated by *Leibniz*, whereby the disjoint consciousness manifolds, roughly comparable, at least in some respects, to the 'monads', borrowed by *Leibniz* from *Giordano Bruno*, become interrelated. Again, the *harmonia praestabilita* assumed by *Leibniz*, corresponds to that what can be designated as the 'psycho-psychical parallelism' elaborated in §8, pages 31–32 of the present author's monograph *Mind and Matter* [*K.*, 1961].

References

Abbot, E. A.: Flatland. A romance of many dimensions (Dover, New York 1952).

Abelson, J.: Recombinant DNA: examples of present-day research. Science *196:* 159–160 (1977).

Abelson, P. H.: Recombinant DNA legislation. Science *199:* 13 (1978).

Abramson, H. A.: Problems of consciousness. Transactions (Five conferences sponsored by Josiah Macy Jr. Foundation) (New York, 1951, 1952, 1953, 1954, 1955).

Alexander, S.: Space, time, and deity. 2 vols. (Macmillan, London 1920; Dover, New York 1966).

Alfvén, H,: Plasma physics, space research, and the origin of the solar system. Science *172:* 991–994 (1971).

Alfvén, H.; Elvius, A.: Antimatter, quasi-stellar objects, and the evolution of galaxies. Science *164:* 911–917 (1969).

Alvarez, L. W.: Recent developments in particle physics. Science *165:* 1071–1091 (1969).

Aristotle: Movement of animals. Original text and translation; et al. opera. Loeb Classical Library (Heinemann, London 1945).

Ashby, W. R.: Design for a brain (Wiley, New York 1952); 2nd ed. (1960).

Ashby, W. R.: An introduction to cybernetics (Wiley, New York 1956); 2nd ed (1957); 3rd ed. (1958).

Avenarius, R.: Kritik der reinen Erfahrung (Fues, Leipzig 1888).

Avery, O. T.; Macleod, G. M.; McCarty, M.: Induction of transformation by a desoxyribonucleic fraction isolated from pneumococcus type III. J. exp. Med. *79:* 137–158 (1944).

Baker, R.: Simon Newcomb's astronomy for everybody (Blakiston, Philadelphia 1932).

Berkeley, E. C.: Giant brains or machines that think (Wiley, New York 1949).

Berkeley, E. C.: Symbolic logic and intelligent machines (Reinhold, New York 1959).

Berkeley, E. C.: The computer revolution (Doubleday, New York 1962).

Berkeley, G.: A treatise concerning the principle of human knowledge (1710; Dent, London 1946).

Berkeley, G.: Three dialogues between Hylas and Philonous, in opposition to sceptics and atheists (1713, 1725; Everyman's Library, Dent, London 1946).

Bismark, O., Fürst von: Gedanken und Erinnerungen. 3 vols. (Cotta, Stuttgart 1898, 1922).

Bochner, S.: Eclosion and synthesis. Perspectives on the history of knowledge (Benjamin, New York 1969).

Bohr, N.: Das Quantum Postulat und die neuere Entwicklung der Atomistik. Naturwissenschaften *16:* 245–257 (1928a).

Bohr, N.: The quantum postulate and the present development of atomic theory. Nature, Lond. *121:* 580–590 (1928b).

Bohr, N.: Kausalität und Komplementarität. Erkenntnis *14:* 293 (1937).

Bondi, H.: Cosmology (Cambridge Monographs in Physics, Cambridge 1952).

Bonin, G. von: Types and similitudes. Philosophy Sci. *13:* 196–202 (1946).

Boole, G.: The mathematical analysis of logic (Macmillan, Cambridge 1847, Blackwell, Oxford 1948).

Boole, G.: An investigation of the laws of thought, on which are founded the mathematical theories of logic and probabilities (1854; Dover, New York, n.d.).

Boring, E. G.: The physical dimensions of consciousness; 1st and 2nd ed. London (Constable, Dover, New York 1933, 1963).

Born, M.: The restless universe (Dover, New York 1951).

Born, M.: Natural philosophy of cause and chance. (Waynflete lectures delivered in the College of St. Mary Magdalen, Oxford in Hilary Term 1948, together with an essay 'Symbol and Reality'.) (Dover, New York 1964).

Boughn, S.: Detecting gravitational waves. Am. Scient. 68: 174–183 (1980).

Brain, W. R.: Speech and thought; in Laslett, The physical basis of mind (Blackwell, Oxford 1950).

Brain, W. R.: Mind, perception and science (Blackwell, Oxford 1951).

Brain, W. R.: The physiological basis of consciousness. A critical review. Brain 81: 426–455 (1958).

Brain, W. R.: The nature of experience (Oxford University Press, Oxford 1959).

Brain, W. R.: Some reflections on brain and mind. Brain 86: 381–402 (1963).

Brain, W. R.: Perception. A trialogue. Brain 88: 697–710 (1965).

Brancazio, P. J.: The nature of physics (Macmillan, New York 1975).

Brandt, J. C.; Maran, S. P.: The new astronomy and space science reader (Freeman, San Francisco 1977).

Bullock, T. H.; Bern, H. A.; Hagadorn, I. R.; Smith, I. E.: Structure and function in the nervous system of invertebrates. 2 vols. (Freeman, San Francisco 1965).

Burns, B. D.: The uncertain nervous system (Arnold, London 1968).

Buscaino, V. M.: Basi neurologiche dei fenomeni di coscienza. Acta neurol. 6: 1–4 (1951).

Cajal, S. R. y: Histologie du système nerveux de l'homme et des vertébrés. 2 vols. (Maloine, Paris 1909, 1911).

Cajal, S. R. y: Charlas de Café. Pensamientos, anécdotas y confidentias; 3rd ed. (Espasa-Calpe, Buenos Aires 1944).

Chandrasekhar, S.: An introduction to the study of stellar structure (Chicago University Press, Chicago 1939).

Chandrasekhar, S.: The 'black hole' in astrophysics; in Brandt, Maran; The new astronomy and space reader, pp. 208–209 (Freeman, San Francisco 1977).

Cherry, E. C.: The communication of information. Am. Scient. 40: 540–664 (1952).

Cherry, E. C.: On human communication. A review, a survey, and a criticism (Science Editions, New York 1961, 1968).

Child, C.: Patterns and problems of development (Chicago University Press, Chicago 1941).

Ciba Foundation Study Group 20: Functions of the corpus callosum (Little, Brown, Boston 1965).

Clara, M.: Das Nervensystem des Menschen; 3. Aufl. (Barth, Leipzig 1959).

Comfort, A.: Ageing. The biology of senescence; 1st and 2nd ed. (Holt & Rinehart, New York 1956, 1964).

Craik, K. J. W.: The nature of explanation (Cambridge University Press, Cambridge 1943, 1952).

Crick, F. H. C.: The structure of the hereditary material, part 3, chapter II: The physics and chemistry of life. Scient. Am. ed., pp. 118–133 (Simon & Schuster, New York 1955).

Dantzig, T.: Number. The language of science; 4th ed. (Macmillan, New York 1954).

Darnell, J. E. Jr.: Implications of RNA·RNA splicing in evolution of eukaryote cells. Science 202: 1257–1260 (1978).

Davies, P. C. W.: Space and time in the modern universe (Cambridge University Press, Cambridge 1977).

Davies, P. C. W.: The tailor-made universe. Science 18/5: 6–10 (1978).

De Broglie, L.: Matière et lumière (Albin Michel, Paris 1937).

De Broglie, L.: Matter and light. The new physics (Norton, New York 1939).

De Broglie, L.: Physics and microphysics (Pantheon, New York 1955).

Delafresnaye, J. F.: Brain mechanisms and consciousness. Symp. Council for International Organizations of Medical Sciences (Blackwell, Oxford 1954).

Delgado, J. M. R.: Aggression and defense under cerebral radio control; in Clemente, Lindsley, Aggression and defense, pp. 171–193 (University of California Press, Berkeley 1967).

De Morgan, A.: A budget of paradoxes (Dover, New York 1954).

Descartes, R.: Discours de la méthode (1637; Cousin, Paris 1824).

Descartes, R.: Meditationes de prima philosophia (1641; Cousin Paris 1826).

Dirac, P. A. M.: A new basis for cosmology. Proc. R. Soc. A *165:* 199–208 (1938, 1939).

Dirac, P. A. M.: Principles of quantum mechanics (Clarendon Press, Oxford 1947).

Dirac, P. A. M.: The evolution of the physical picture of nature. Scient. Am. *208/5:* 45–53 (1963).

Dreyer, L. E.: A history of astronomy from Thales to Kepler (Dover, New York 1953).

Driesch, H.: Ordnungslehre (Diederichs, Jena 1912).

Driesch, H.: Philosophie des Organischen (Engelmann, Leipzig 1921).

Driesch, H.: Metaphysik (Hirt, Breslau 1924).

Dühring, E.: Robert Mayer, der Galilei des 19. Jahrhunderts (1880; Repr. Wiss. Buchges. Darmstadt 1972).

Dunning, J.; Paxton, H. C.: Matter, energy and radiation (McGraw-Hill, New York 1941).

Ebbecke, M.: Physiologie des Bewusstseins in entwicklungsgeschichtlicher Betrachtung (Thieme, Stuttgart 1959).

Ebbinghaus, H.: Abriss der Psychologie (Veit, Leipzig 1919).

Eccles, J. C.: The neurophysiological basis of mind (Clarendon Press, Oxford 1953).

Eccles, J. C.: Facing reality. Philosophical adventures by a brain scientist (Springer, New York 1970).

Eccles, J. C.: The understanding of the brain; 2nd ed. (McGraw-Hill, New York 1977).

Eddington, A. S.: The nature of the physical world (Cambridge University Press, Cambridge 1928).

Eddington, A. S.: Space, time and gravitation (Cambridge University Press, Cambridge 1929).

Eddington, A. S.: The philosophy of physical science (Cambridge University Press, Cambridge 1939).

Eigen, M.: Der Zeitmassstab der Natur. Jb. Max-Planck-Ges., 1966, pp. 4–67.

Einstein, A. (1905): see Lorentz et al. (n.d.)

Einstein, A.: Geometrie und Erfahrung (Springer, Berlin 1921).

Einstein, A.: The world as I see it (Covici, Friede, New York 1934).

Einstein, A.: The meaning of relativity (Princeton University Press, Princeton 1945).

Einstein, A.: Out of my later years (Philosophical Library, New York 1950).

Einstein, A.: Ideas and opinions (Crown Publishers, New York 1954); 2nd ed. (1959).

Einstein, A. and Infeld, L.: The evolution of physics (Simon & Schuster, New York 1938).

Elliot, H. C.: The shape of intelligence. The evolution of the human brain (Scribner's, New York 1969).

Ey, H.: La conscience (Presse universitaire de France, Paris 1963, 1968).

Eysenck, H.: Sense and nonsense in psychology (Penguin Books, Baltimore 1962).

Fessard, A. E.: Mechanisms of nervous integration and conscious experience; in Delafresnaye, Brain mechanism and consciousness, pp. 200–248 (Blackwell, Oxford 1954).

Feynman, R. P.: The development of the space-time view of quantum dynamics. Science *153:* 699–708 (1966).

Feynman, R. P.: Structure of the proton. Science *183:* 601–610 (1974).

Flechsig, P.: Gehirn und Seele (Veit, Leipzig 1896).

Flechsig, P.: Anatomie des menschlichen Gehirns und Rückenmarks auf myelogenetischer Grundlage. I (Thieme, Leipzig 1920).

Flechsig, P.: Meine myelogenetische Hirnlehre (Springer, Berlin 1927).

Fooden, J.: Breakup of Pangaea and isolation of relict mammals of Australia, South America, and Madagascar. Science *175:* 894–898 (1972).

Forel, A.: Einige hirnanatomische Betrachtungen und Ergebnisse. Arch Psychiat. *18:* 162–198 (1887).

Forel, A.: Das Sinnesleben der Insekten (Reinhardt, München 1910).

Forel, A.: Gehirn und Seele (Kröner, Leipzig 1922).

Forel, A. Le monde social des fourmis du globe, comparé à celui de l'homme (Kundig, Genève 1921–1923).

Frank, P.: Between physics and philosophy (Harvard University Press, Cambridge 1941).

Freedman, D. Z.; Nieuwenhuizen, P. van: Supergravity and the unification of the laws of physics. An approach to relating the basic forces. Scient. Am. *238/2:* 126–143 (1978).

Frege, G.: Die Grundlagen der Arithmetik (Marcus, Breslau 1884, 1934).

Frese, W.: Bauplan der 'nackten Viren' erstmals entziffert. Max-Planck-Ges. Spiegel Nr. 4; pp. 3–6 (1978).

Frisch, K. von:: Bees, their vision, chemical senses and language (Cornell University Press, Ithaca 1950).

Frisch, K. von: The dancing bees (Harcourt Brace, New York 1953).

Fritsch, G.; Hitzig, E.: Über die elektrische Erregbarkeit des Großhirns. Arch. Anat. Physiol. wiss. Med. *37:* 300–332 (1870).

Gabor, D.: Theory of communication. J. Inst. Electr. Eng. *93:* 429 (1946); *94:* 369 (1947); quoted from Cherry (1952).

Gabor, D.: Holography 1948–1971. Science *177:* 299–313 (1972).

Gamow, G.: One two three ... infinity. Facts and speculations on science (Viking, New York 1947).

Gamow, G.: The creation of the universe (Viking, New York 1952).

Gamow, G.: The evolutionary universe; in Gingerich, Cosmology, pp. 12–19 (Freeman, San Francisco 1977).

Gegenbaur, C.: Vergleichende Anatomie der Wirbeltiere. 2 vols. (Engelmann, Leipzig 1898).

Gell-Mann, M.; Rosenbaum, E. P.: Elementary particles. Scient. Am. *237/4:* 56–70 (1977).

George, F. H.: The brain as a computer (Pergamon Press, Oxford 1962).

Gingerich, O.: Cosmology (Freeman, San Francisco 1977).

Goldschmidt, R.: Die Lehre von der Vererbung (Springer, Berlin 1927).

Goldschmidt, R.: Portraits from memory. Recollections of a zoologist (University of Washington Press, Seattle 1956).

Goodfield, J.: Playing god. Genetic engineering and the manipulation of life (Random House, New York 1977).

Gott, J. R., III, Jr.; Gunn, J. E.; Schramm, D. N.; Tinsley, B. M.: Will the universe expand for ever?; in Gingerich, Cosmology, pp. 82–93 (Freeman, San Francisco 1977).

Greiner, W.; Hamilton, J.: Is the vacuum really empty? Am. Scient. *68:* 154–190 (1980).

Gurwitsch, A.: Die mitogenetische Strahlung (Springer, Berlin 1923).

Gurwitsch, A.: Die histologischen Grundlagen der Biologie (Fischer, Jena 1930).

Hadfield, J. A.: Dreams and nightmares (Penguin Books, Harmondsworth, Middlesex 1969).

Haeckel, E.: Generelle Morphologie der Organismen. 2 vols. (Reimer, Berlin 1866).

Haeckel, E.: Natürliche Schöpfungsgeschichte (Reimer, Berlin 1898).

Haeckel, E.: Die Welträthsel. Gemeinverständliche Studie über monistische Philosophie (Kröner, Stuttgart 1903).

Haeckel, E.: Die Lebenswunder (Kröner, Stuttgart 1906).

Haldane, J. B. S.: The Marxist philosophy and the sciences (Allen & Unwin, London 1938).

Haldane, J. S. B.: see Newman (1956).

Handler, P.: Biology and the future of man (Oxford University Press, New York 1970).

Hearn, L.: Gleamings in Buddha-Fields (Tauchnitz, Leipzig 1910).

Hearn, L.: Japan. An attempt at interpretation (Macmillan, New York 1924).

Heisenberg, W.: The physical principles of the quantum theory (Chicago University Press, Chicago 1930).

Heisenberg, W.: Physics and philosophy. The revolution in modern science (Harper, New York 1958).

Hering, E.: Das Gedächtnis als eine allgemeine Funktion der organisierten Materie. Vortr. Akad. Wien 1870 (Engelmann, Leipzig 1905).

Hesse, M. B.: Forces and fields. A study of action at a distance in the history of physics (Philosophical Library, New York 1962).

Hilbert, D.: Axiomatisches Denken. Math. Annln 78: 405–415 (1918).

Hilbert, D.; Bernays, P.: Grundlagen der Mathematik. 2 vols. (Springer, Berlin 1934, 1939).

Hintsches, E.: Kernphysik. Pufferzone zwischen Materie und Antimaterie. Max-Planck-Ges. Spiegel Nr. 5; pp. 1–2 (1977a).

Hintsches, E.: Genetische Manipulation. MPG führt Sicherheitsrichtlinien ein. Max-Planck-Ges. Spiegel Nr. 4, pp. 3–5 (1977b).

His, W.: Zur Geschichte des menschlichen Rückenmarks und der Nervenwurzeln. Abh. Kgl. Sächs. Ges. Wiss. 13: 477–514 (1886).

Hoagland, H.: The Weber-Fechner law and the all-or-none theory. J. genet. Psychol. 3: 351–373 (1930).

Hoagland, H.: Consciousness and the chemistry of time; in Abramson, Problems of consciousness, 1st Conf. Jos. Macy Jr. Found., 1950 (New York 1951).

Hobbes, T.: Leviathan (1651; Everyman's Library, Dent, London 1949).

Hoffmann, B.: The strange story of the quantum; 2nd ed. (Dover, New York 1959).

Horowitz, N. H.: The search for life on Mars. Scient. Am. 237/5: 52–61 (1977).

Hoyle, F.: Frontiers of astronomy (Harper, New York 1955).

Hoyle, F.: Astronomy and cosmology (Freeman, San Francisco 1975a).

Hoyle, F.: Highlights in astronomy (Freeman, San Francisco 1975b).

Hubble, E.: The realm of the nebulae (Yale University Press, New Haven 1936).

Hume, D.: A treatise of human nature. 2 vols. (1739–1740; Everyman's Library, Dent, London 1911).

Hume, D.: Philosophical essays concerning human understanding (1748). An inquiry concerning human understanding (1750; London, 1854, 1861).

Huxley, J.: The size of living things; in Man stands alone (Harper, New York 1941).

Jacobshagen, E.: Allgemeine vergleichende Formenlehre der Tiere (Klinkhardt, Leipzig 1925).

Jaensch, E. R.: Eidetic imagery (Paul, Trench, Trubner, London 1930).

Jaffé, G.: Drei Dialoge über Raum, Zeit und Kausalität (Springer, Berlin 1954).

James, W.: The principles of psychology. 2 vols. (Holt, Dover, New York 1890, 1950).

Jeans, Sir J.: Through space and time (Macmillan, New York 1931).

Jeans, Sir J.: Physics and philosophy (Cambridge University Press, Cambridge 1943).

Jung, R.: Physiologie und Pathophysiologie des Schlafes (Referat).
    Verh. 71. Kongr. dt. Ges. inn. Med., München (Bergmann, München 1965).

Kabir, P. K.: The CP puzzle. Strange decays of the neutral kaon (Academic Press, New York 1968).

Kant, I.: Prolegomena zu einer jeden künftigen Metaphysik, die als Wissenschaft wird auftreten können (Hartknoch, Riga 1783); (ed. Reclam, Leipzig, n.d.).

Kant, I.: Kritik der reinen Vernunft (Hartknoch, Riga 1781, 1787); (ed. Reclam, Leipzig, n.d.).

Kapp. E.: Grundlinien einer Philosophie der Technik (Westermann, Braunschweig 1877).

Karczmar, A. G.; Eccles, J. C.: Brain and human behavior. A symposium, Chicago 1969 (Springer, New York 1972).

Kempner, A. J.: Paradoxes and common senses (Van Nostrand, New York 1959).

Kenny, A. J. P.: Longuet-Higgins, H. C.; Lucas, J. R.; Waddington, C. H.: The nature of mind (Edinburgh University Press, Edinburgh 1972).

Kershner, R. B.; Wilcox, L. R.: The anatomy of mathematics (Ronald, New York 1950).

Kippenhahn, R.: Die Entwicklung der Sterne; in Scharf, Evolution, pp. 115–134 (Akademia Leopoldina, Halle 1975).

Kolata, G. B.: Catastrophe theory: the emperor has no clothes. Science 196: 287, 350–351 (1977a).

Kolata, G. B.: Bacterial genetics: action at a distance on DNA. Science 198: 41–42 (1977b).

Korschelt, E.: Lebensdauer, Altern und Tod (Fischer, Jena 1924).

Krause, F. E. A.: Ju-Tao-Fo. Die religiösen und philosophischen System Ostasiens (Reinhardt, München 1924).

Krause, F. E. A.: Geschichte Ostasiens. 2 vols. (Vandenhoek & Rupprecht, Göttingen 1925).

Kretschmer, E.: Medizinische Psychologie (Thieme, Leipzig 1922); 2nd ed. (1926); 14th ed. (Thieme, Stuttgart 1975).

Kuhlenbeck, H.: Das Positive in der Schopenhauerschen Philosophie, Inaug. Diss. Jena (1920).

Kuhlenbeck, H.: Vorlesungen über das Zentralnervensystem der Wirbeltiere (Fischer, Jena 1927).

Kuhlenbeck, H.: Die Grundbestandteile des Endhirns im Lichte der Bauplanlehre. Anat. Anz. 67: 1–50 (1929).

Kuhlenbeck, H.: Diskussionsbemerkung zu Hertwig, G.: Befruchtungs- und Vererbungsproblem im Lichte der vergleichend-quantitativen Kernforschung. Anat. Anz. 75: Erg. Bd., p. 71 (1932).

Kuhlenbeck, H.: The human diencephalon. A summary of development, structure, function and pathology (Karger, Basel 1954a).

Kuhlenbeck, H.: Some histologic changes in the rat's brain and their relationship to comparable changes in the human brain. Confinia neurol. 14: 329–342 (1954b).

Kuhlenbeck, H.: Die Formbestandteile der Regio praetectalis des Anamniergehirns und ihre Beziehungen zum Hirnbauplan. Okajima's Fol. anat. jap. (Nishi Festschrift) 28: 23–44 (1956).

Kuhlenbeck, H.: Brain and consciousness. Some Prolegomena to an approach of the problem (Karger, Basel 1957).

Kuhlenbeck, H.: Further remarks on brain and consciousness: the brain-paradox and the meanings of consciousness. Confinia neurol. 19: 462–485 (1959).

Kuhlenbeck, H.: Mind and matter. An appraisal of their significance for neurological theory (Karger, Basel 1961).

Kuhlenbeck, H.: The concept of consciousness in neurological epistemology; in Smythies, Brain and mind. Modern concepts of the nature of mind, pp. 137–161 (Routledge & Kegan Paul, London 1965a).

Kuhlenbeck, H.: Gehirn und Intelligenz. Confinia neurol. 25: 35–62 (1965b).

Kuhlenbeck, H.: Weitere Bemerkungen zur Maschinentheorie des Gehirns. Confinia neurol. 27: 295–328 (1966).

Kuhlenbeck, H.: Some comments on words, language, thought, and definition; in Buehne et al., Helen Adolf Festschrift, pp. 9–29 (Ungar, New York 1968).

Kuhlenbeck, H.: The central nervous system of vertebrates. A general survey of its comparative anatomy with an introduction to the pertinent fundamental biologic and logical concepts. Vol. 1 (1967a); 2 (1967b); 3/I (1970); 3/II (1973a); 4 (1975); 5/I (1977); 5/II (1978) (Karger, Basel 1967–1978).

Kuhlenbeck, H.: Some comments on psychophysics. Confinia neurol. *33:* 245–257 (1971).

Kuhlenbeck, H.: Schopenhauer's Satz 'Die Welt ist meine Vorstellung' und das Traumerlebnis. Schopenhauer Jahrbuch 53 (Hübscher Festschrift), pp. 376–392 (Kramer, Frankfurt 1972).

Kuhlenbeck, H.: Gehirn und Bewusstsein; transl. by J. Gerlach and U. Protzer. Erfahrung und Denken. Schriften zur Förderung der Beziehungen zwischen Philosophie und Naturwissenschaften, vol. 39 (Duncker & Humblot, Berlin 1973b).

Kuhlenbeck, H.; Voit, K.: Beobachtungen am Kernbild nach Hydrolyse und Nuklealfärbung. Weitere Beiträge zur Nuklealreaktion. Anat. Anz. *74:* 1–32 (1932).

Kuhlenbeck, L.: Im Hochland der Gedankenwelt. Grundzüge einer heroisch-ästhetischen Weltanschauung (Diederichs, Leipzig 1903).

Kuhlenbeck, L.: Giordano Bruno, Gesammelte Werke. Herausgegeben, verdeutscht und erläutert. 6 vols. (Diederichs, Leipzig 1904–1909); vol. 1: Das Aschermittwochsmahl (Diederichs, Leipzig 1904); vol. 3: Zwiegespräche vom unendlichen All und den Welten (Diederichs, Jena 1904).

Kuhlenbeck, L.: Giordano Bruno. Seine Lehre von Gott, von der Unsterblichkeit der Seele und von der Willensfreiheit. Die Religion der Klassiker, vol. 1 (Protestantischer Schriftenvertrieb, Berlin-Schöneberg 1913).

Kuiper, T. B. H.; Morris, M.: Searching for extraterrestrial civilizations. Science *196:* 661–662 (1977).

Küpfmüller, K.: Informationsverarbeitung durch den Menschen. Nachrichtentechn. Z. *12:* 68–74 (1958).

Lashley, K. S.: The behavioristic interpretation of consciousness. Psychol. Rev. *30:* 237–272, 329–353 (1923).

Laslett, P.: The physical basis of mind (Blackwell, Oxford 1950).

Lecomte du Noüy, P.: Biological time (Macmillan, New York 1937).

Lederman, L. M.: The Ypsilon particle. The heaviest fundamental particle yet discovered, it has led to the introduction of a fifth quark. Scient. Am *235/4:* 72–80 (1978).

Lee, T. D.: Weak interactions and nonconservation of parity. Science *127:* 569–573 (1958).

Lemaître, G.: Essai de cosmologie: l'hypothèse de l'atome primitif (Griffon, Neuchâtel 1946).

Levitan, M.: Textbook of human genetics; revised 2nd ed. Textbook by Levitan, M.; Montagu, A. (Oxford University Press, New York 1977).

Lilly, H. C.: The shape of intelligence. The evolution of the human brain (Scribner's, New York 1969).

Lilly, J. C.: Mental effects of reduction of ordinary levels of physical intact, healthy persons. Psychiat. Res. Rep. *5:* 1–28 (1956).

Lilly, J. C.: Man and dolphins (Doubleday, New York 1963).

Lilly, J. C.: Lilly on Dolphins. Humans and the sea (Anchor-Doubleday, Garden City 1975).

Lilly, J. C.; Miller, A. M.: Vocal exchanges between dolphins. Science *134:* 1873–1876 (1961).

Locke, J.: An essay concerning human understanding (1689). London 1854; Bell, London 1875).

Lodge, Sir O.: Pioneers of science (Macmillan, Dover, London, New York 1893, 1960).

Lorentz, H. A.; Einstein, A.; Minkowski, H.; Weyl, H.: The principle of relativity (Dover, New York n.d.).

Lorenz, K.: Analogy as a sommee of knowledge. Science *185:* 229–234 (1974).

Lorenz, K.: Evolution des Verhaltens; in Scharf, Evolution, pp. 271–290 (Akademia Leopoldina, Halle 1975).

Luther, M.: Tischreden oder Colloquia, so er in vielen Jahren mit gelehrten Leuten, fremden Gästen und seinen Tischgesellen geführt (Reclam, Leipzig n.d.).

MacColl, L. A.: Fundamental theory of servomechanism (Van Nostrand, New York 1945).

Mach, E.: Die ökonomische Natur der physikalischen Forschung. Populärwissenschaftliche Vorlesungen (Barth, Leipzig 1896).

Mach, E.: Die Analyse der Empfindungen und das Verhältnis des Physischen zum Psychischen; 9th ed (Fischer, Jena 1922).

MacKay, D. M.: Comparing the brain with machines. Am. Scient. *42:* 261–268 (1954).

Massey, H.: The new age in physics (Harper, New York 1960).

Maugh, T., II: The artificial gene: it's synthetized and it works in cells. Science *194:* 44 (1976).

Maugh, T., II: Phylogeny: Methanogens a third class of life? Science *198:* 812 (1977).

McCrea, W. H.: Die Entstehung der Planetensysteme, in Scharf, Evolution, pp. 135–144 (Akademia Leopoldina, Halle 1975).

McCulloch, W. S.; Pitts, W.: A logical calculus of the ideas immanent in nervous activity. Bull. math. biophys. *5:* 115–133 (1943).

McMillan, E. M.: Current problems in particle science. Science *152:* 1210–1215 (1966).

Metz, W. D.: Interstellar molecules were found in spite of the sages. Science *182:* 467–468 (1973).

Metz, W. D.: The new particle mystery: solid clues now lead to charm. Science *189:* 443–445 (1975).

Metz, W. D.: Violently active galaxies: the search for the energy machine. Science *201:* 700–702 (1978).

Miller, D. A.: Evolution of primate chromosomes. Man's closest relative may be the gorilla, not the chimpanzee. Science *198:* 1116–1124 (1977).

Minkowski, H.: Space and time (1908); reprinted in Lorentz et al., pp. 75–91 (Dover, New York n.d.).

Monod, J.: Le hasard et la necessité (Du Seuil, Paris 1970).

Montaigne, M. E. de: Essais (1595); Editio Leclerc (Garnier, Paris, n.d.).

Moore, G.E.: Philosophical studies (Routledge and Paul, London 1922).

Moritz, K. P.: Götterlehre der Griechen und Römer (1791); M. Obermeyer (ed). (Reclam, Leipzig n.d.).

Münsterberg, H.: Grundzüge der Psychologie (Barth, Leipzig 1900).

Ne'eman, Yuval: cit. Brancazio, P. 1975, p. 707.

Neumann, J. von: Mathematische Grundlagen der Quantenphysik (Springer, Berlin 1932).

Neumann, J. von: The general and logical theory of automata; in Jeffres, Cerebral mechanisms in behavior. Hixon Foundation, pp. 1–41 (Wiley, New York 1951).

Neumann, J. von: Probabilistic logics (California Institute of Technology, Pasadena 1952).

Neumann, J. von: The computer and the brain (Yale University Press, Yale 1958).

Neumayr, M.: Erdgeschichte. 2 vols.; 1st ed.; 3rd ed. by F. E. Suess (Bibliographisches Institut, Leipzig 1895, 1920).

Newman, J. B.: The world of mathematics. 4 vols. (Simon & Schuster, New York 1956).

Newton, I.: Philosophiae naturalis principia mathematica (1687); ed. Cotes (Tegg, London 1833); translated by A. Mott, revised and ed. by Cajori (University of California Press, Berkely 1934).

Nievergelt, J.; Farrar, J. C.: What machines can and cannot do. Am. Scient. *61 (May-June):* 309–315 (1973).

Ogden, C. K.; Richards, I. A.: The meaning of meaning. A study of the influence of language upon thought and the science of symbolism (Harcourt, Brace, New York 1923, 1946).

Olds, J.: Self-stimulation of the brain. Science *127:* 315–324 (1958).

Oort, J. H.: Galaxies and the universe. Properties of the universe are revealed by the rotation of galaxies and their distribution in space. Science *170:* 1363–1370 (1970).

Oort, J. H.: Evolution der Galaxien; in Scharf, Evolution, pp. 97–112 (Akademia Leopoldina, Halle 1975).

Oppenheimer, J.: in Willier, Weiss, Hamburger: Problems, concepts and their history (sect. I): Analysis of development (Saunders, Philadelphia 1955).

Ornstein, R. E.: The psychology of consciousness (Freeman, San Francisco 1972).

Ortega y Gasset, J.: La rebelión de las masas (Occidente, Madrid 1960).

Patton, R. L.: Introductory insect physiology (Saunders, Philadelphia 1963).

Pauling, L.: The nature of the chemical bond; 3rd ed. (Cornell University Press, Ithaca 1960).

Pavlov, I. P.: Conditioned reflexes. An investigation of the physiological activity of the cerebral cortex (Oxford University Press Dover, Oxford New York 1927, 1960).

Penfield, W.: The mystery of mind: a critical study of consciousness and the human brain (Princeton University Press, Princeton 1975).

Perry, J.: Spinning tips and gyroscopic motions (Dover, New York 1957).

Piéron, H.: Contribution à la psychologie du poulpe. L'aquisition d'habitudes. Bull. Inst. gén. psychol. *11:* 111–119 (1911).

Planck, M.: Positivismus und reale Aussenwelt (Akad. Verlagsges. Leipzig 1931).

Planck, M.: Die Kausalität in der Natur; in Wege zur physikalischen Erkenntnis, pp. 223–259 (Hirzel, Leipzig 1933).

Planck, M.: Scheinprobleme der Wissenschaft (Barth, Leipzig 1947, 1958).

Poincaré, H.: La valeur de la science (Flammarion, Paris 1909).

Poincaré, H.: The foundation of science; transl. by G.B. Halstead (Science Press, New York 1913a).

Poincaré, H.: Dernières pensées (Flammarion, Paris 1913b).

Poincaré, H.: La science et l'hypothèse, 1st ed. 1906 (Flammarion, Paris 1943).

Poincaré, H.: Mathematics and science. Last essays; transl. by J.W. Boldue (Dover, New York 1963).

Polyak, S.: in Klüver, The vertebrate visual system (Chicago University Press, Chicago 1957).

Popper, K.; Eccles, J. C.: The self and its brain (Springer, New York 1977).

Rank, D. M.; Townes, C. H.; Welch, W. J.: Interstellar molecules and dense clouds. Science *174:* 1083–1101 (1971).

Ranson, S. W.: The anatomy of the nervous system from the standpoint of development and function (Saunders, Philadelphia 1947).

Reichenbach, H.: Experience and prediction (Chicago University Press, Chicago 1938).

Remane, A.: Offene Probleme der Evolution; in Scharf, Evolution, pp. 165–170 (Akademia Leopoldina, Halle 1975).

Riese, W.: Hughlings Jackson's doctrine of consciousness. Some versions and elaborations. J. nerv. ment. Dis. *120:* 330–337 (1954).

Robinson, A. L.: Elementary particles: neutrino experiments suggest charm. Science *191:* 452 (1976).

Robinson, A. L.: Particle physics: new evidence from Germany for a fifth quark. Science *200:* 1033–1034 (1978).

Robinson, A. L.: What is unified in the unified field theories? Science *206:* 672–673 (1979).

Robson, D.: Isospin in nuclei. Science *179:* 133–139 (1973).

Rogers, M.: Biohazard (Knopf, New York 1977).

Rosenblueth, A.; Wiener, N.; Bigelow, J.: Behavior, purpose and teleology. Philosophy Sci. *10:* 18–24 (1943).

Rothman, M. A.: Things that go faster than light. Scient. Am. *203/1:* 142–152 (1960).

Rothmann, H.: Zusammenfassender Bericht über den Rothmann' schen großhirnlosen Hund nach klinischer und anatomischer Untersuchung. Z. ges. Neurol. Psychiat *87:* 247–313 (1923).

Russell, Bertrand: Mysticism and logic (Langmans Green, New York 1912).

Russell, B.: The analysis of mind (Allen & Unwin, London 1921).

Russell, B.: The problems of philosophy (London 1927).

Russell, B.: The history of western philosophy (Simon & Schuster, New York 1945).

Russell, B.: Human knowledge. Its scope and limits (Simon & Schuster, New York 1948).

Russell, B.: in Dennon: Dictionary of mind, matter and morals (Philosophical Library, New York 1952).

Russell, B.: The analysis of matter (Dover, New York 1954).

Russell, B.: in Rosten: A guide to the religions of America (Simon & Schuster, New York 1955).

Russell, B.: The ABC of relativity (Signet Science Library Book, New York 1962).

Sagan, C.; Drake, F.: The search for extraterrestrial intelligence; in Gingerich: Cosmology (Freeman, San Francisco 1977).

Sagan, C.; Sagan, L.S.; Drake, F.: A message from earth; in Brandt, Maran: The new astronomy and space science reader (Freeman, San Francisco 1977).

Sarkisov, S. A.: The structure and function of the brain (Indiana University Press, Bloomington 1966).

Scharf, H.-J.: Evolution (Akademia Leopoldina, Halle 1975).

Schilder, P.: Das Körperschema (Springer, Berlin 1923).

Schilder, P.: The image and the appearance of the human body; studies in constructive energies of psyche (Kegan, London 1935).

Schopenhauer, A.: Sämmtliche Werke (1813–1851). 6 vols. Handschriftlicher Nachlass. 4 vols. Ed. Grisebach (Reclam, Leipzig n.d.).

Schorr, R.: Simon Necomb's Astronomie für jedermann; 5th ed. (Fischer, Jena 1929).

Schrödinger, E.: Wave mechanics (Blackie, London 1928).

Schrödinger, E.: What is life? (Cambridge University Press, Cambridge 1946).

Schrödinger, E.: Science and humanism; physics in our time (Cambridge University Press, Cambridge 1951).

Schrödinger, E.: What is matter? Scient. Am. *189 (Sept.):* 52–57 (1953).

Schrödinger, E.: Science theory and man (Dover, New York 1957).

Schrödinger, E.: Mind and matter (Cambridge University Press, Cambridge 1958).

Schwartz, R. M.; Dayhoff, M. O.: Origins of protokaryotes, mitochondria, and chloroplasts. Science *119:* 395–403 (1978).

Schwinger, J.: A magnetic model of matter. Science *165:* 757–761 (1969).

Schwitters, R. F.: Fundamental particles with charm. Scient. Am. *237/4:* 56–70 (1977).

Semon, R.: Die Mneme als erhaltendes Prinzip im Wechsel des organischen Geschehens (Engelmann, Leipzig 1904).

Semon, R.: Die mnemischen Empfindungen in ihren Beziehungen zu den Originalempfindungen (Engelmann, Leipzig 1909).

Semon, R.: Bewußtseinsvorgang und Gehirnprozeß (Bergmann, Wiesbaden 1920).

Severtzoff, A. N.: Morphologische Gesetzmäßigkeiten der Evolution (Fischer, Jena 1911).

Shannon, C. E.: A symbolic analysis of relay and switching circuits. Trans. Am. Inst. elect. Eng. *57:* 713–723 (1938).

Sherrington, C. S.: The integrative action of the nervous system (Yale University Press, New Haven 1906; 2nd ed. 1947).

Sherrington, C. S. (1950); see Laslett, P. (1950).

Sherrington, C. S.: Man on his nature; 2nd ed. (Cambridge University Press, Cambridge 1951).

Singer, M. F.: The recombinant DNA debate. Science 196: 127 (1977).

Singh, J.: Great ideas of modern mathematics; their nature and use (Dover, New York 1959).

Singh, J.: Great ideas and theories of modern cosmology (Dover, New york 1961).

Singh, J.: Great ideas in information theory, language and cybernetics (Dover, New York 1966).

Skinner, B. F.: The behavior of organism: an experimental analysis (Appleton-Century-Crofts, New York 1938).

Skinner, B. F.: Contingencies and reinforcement: a theoretical analysis (Appleton-Century-Crofts, New York 1969).

Skinner, B. F.: Beyond freedom and dignity (Knopf, New York 1972).

Slater, E. T. O.: Consciousness; see Laslett, P. (1950).

Smyth, H. D.: Atomic energy for military purposes (Princeton University Press, Princeton 1945).

Smythies, J. R.: Brain and mind –modern concepts of the nature of mind (Routledge & Kegan Paul, London 1965).

Spengler, O.: Der Untergang des Abendlandes. 2 vols. (Beck, München 1919, 1927).

Sperry, R. W.: Neurology and the mind-brain problem. Am. Scient. 40: 291–312 (1952).

Spinoza, B.: Ethica ordine geometrica demonstrata (1677). Die Ethik des Spinoza im Urtexte (Leipzig 1875).

Stein, H.: Untersuchungen über den Zeitsinn bei Vögeln. Z. vergl. Physiol. 33: 387–403 (1951).

Steinbuch, K.: Automat und Mensch. Über menschliche und maschinelle Intelligenz (Springer, Berlin 1961).

Strümpell, A.: Ein Beitrag zur Theorie des Schlafes. Pflügers Arch. ges. Physiol. 15: 573–574 (1877).

Sussman, H. J.; Zahler, R. S.: Catastrophe theory: mathematics misused. Science 17: 20–23 (1977).

Tarski, A.: An introduction to logic and to the methodology of deductive sciences (Oxford University Press, New York 1946).

Thom, R.: 'Modern mathematics': an educational and philosophic error? Am. Scient. 59: 695–699 (1971).

Thomas, K.: Träume – selbst verstehen. Wie sie entstehen, was sie bedeuten, warum sie heilen; 3. Aufl. (Thieme, Stuttgart 1979).

Thompson, D'Arcy: On growth and form (Cambridge University press, Cambridge 1942).

Thorne, K. S.: The search for black holes; in Gingerich, Cosmology, pp. 63–74 (Freeman, San Francisco 1977).

Turing, A. M.: On computable numbers, with an application to the Entscheidungsproblem. Proc. Lond. math. Soc. Ser. 2, 42: 230–265 (1936); 43: 544–546 (1937).

Turing, A. M.: Computing machinery and intelligence (can a machine think?). Mind 59: 433–460 (1950).

Turner, B. E.: Interstellar molecules; in Brandt, Maran, The new astronomy and space science reader, pp. 221–236 (Freeman, San Francisco 1977).

Unsöld, A.: Evolution von Kosmos und Erde; in Scharf, Evolution pp. 91–95 (Akademia Leopoldina, Halle 1975).

Vaihinger, H.: Die Philosophie des Als Ob. System der theoretischen, praktischen und religiösen Fiktionen der Menschheit auf Grund eines idealistischen Positivismus (Reuther & Reichardt, Berlin 1911; 2. Aufl. 1913).

Vaucouleurs, G. de: The case for a hierarchical cosmology. Science *167:* 1203–1213 (1970).

Verworn, M.: Die Mechanik des Geisteslebens (Teubner, Leipzig 1919).

Vitruvius: De architectura. Latin text with English translation by F. Granger. 2 vols. The Loeb Classical Library (Heinemann, London 1934).

Voit, K.: Über das Verhalten der Bakterien in der Nuklealfärbung. Z. ges. exp. Med. *47:* 183–192 (1925).

Voit, K.: Über das Verhalten der Bakterien zur Nuklealfärbung. II. Mitteilung. Z. ges. exp. Med. *55:* 546–568 (1927).

Voltaire (Francois Marie Arouet): Memnon ou la sagesse humaine (1747); Micromégas, histoire philosophique (1752), pp. 17–22; 101–119; in Romans de Voltaire (Garnier, Paris n.d.).

Wade, N.: The ultimate experiment. Man-made evolution (Walker, New york 1977).

Wald, R.: Particle creation near black holes. Am. Scient. *65:* 585–589 (1977).

Watson, J. B.: Behaviorism (Kegan Paul, London 1925).

Watson, J. B.: Psychology from the standpoint of a behaviorist; 3rd ed. (Lippincott, Philadelphia 1929).

Watson, J. D.; Crick, F. H. C.: A structure for desoxyribose nucleic acid. Nature, Lond. *171:* 737–738 (1953).

Wegener, A.: Die Entstehung der Kontinente und Ozeane (Vieweg, Braunschweig 1915).

Weiskopf, V. F.: Quantum theory and the elementary particles. Science *149:* 1181–1189 (1965).

Weiss, P.: Principles of development (Holt, New York 1939).

Wells, H. G.: A short history of the world (Penguin Books, Hammondsworth, London 1947, 1949).

Whitehead, A. N.: The principles of human knowledge (1925); quoted after Craik (1952).

Whitehead, A. N.: Science and the modern world (Macmillan, New york 1925).

Whitehead, A. N.: Science and philosophy (Philosophical Library, New York 1948).

Whittaker, E.: Space and spirit (Regnery, Hinsdale 1948).

Wiener, N.: Cybernetics or control and communication in the animal and in the machine (Wiley, New York 1948).

Winterstein, H.: Kausalität und Vitalismus vom Standpunkt der Denkökonomie (Springer, Berlin 1928).

Winterstein, H.: Reizung und Erregung. Arch. Entw. Mech. Org. *116:* 7–19 (1929).

Wolff, G.: Leben und Erkennen. Vorarbeiten zu einer biologischen Philosophie (Reinhardt, München 1933).

Yang, C. N.: Law of parity conservation and other symmetry laws. Science *127:* 565–569 (1958).

Young, J. Z.: A model of the brain (Clarendon Press, Oxford 1964).

Young, J. Z.: The anatomy of the nervous system of *Octopus vulgaris* (Clarendon Press, Oxford 1971).

Ziehen, T.: Erkenntnistheorie auf psychophysiologischer und physikalischer Grundlage (Fischer, Jena 1913).

Ziehen, T.: Leitfaden der physiologischen Psychologie in 16 Vorlesungen (Fischer, Jena 1920).

Ziehen, T.: Grundlagen der Naturphilosophie (Quelle & Meyer, Leipzig 1922).

Ziehen, T.: Das Leib-Seele-Problem. Dt. med. Wschr. *50:* 1267–1269 (1924).

Subject Index